Medications

for
Attention Disorders
(ADHD/ADD)
and
Related Medical Problems

(Tourette's Syndrome, Sleep Apnea, Seizure Disorders)

A

Comprehensive

Handbook

by
Edna D. Copeland, Ph.D.
with
Stephen C. Copps, M.D.

Specialty Press, Inc.
Plantation, Florida
1995 Edition

Copeland, Edna D. with Copps, Stephen C.
   Medications for Attention Disorders and Related Medical Problems:
   A Comprehensive Handbook.
      p.

ISBN 1-886941-00-9 (Hardcover)
   1. Attention Deficit Disorders - Treatment
   2. Attention-Deficit/Hyperactivity Disorder - Treatment

Every effort has been exerted to provide accurate and authoritative
information and to insure that medication selection and dosage described
in this text are consistent with current recommendations and practice.
However, the book is not intended to diagnose or treat attention deficit
disorders or to render medical advice. Only a physician can medically
treat ADHD/ADD. In view of the constant flow of information relating
to drug therapy and drug reactions, both physicians and other readers
must constantly stay abreast of new developments. Package inserts on
each drug contain the most current changes in indications for usage and
dosage. They also contain added warnings and precautions. Neither is
this book intended to render legal or other professional advice. Rather,
its goal is to provide information. If expert assistance is needed, the
services of a professional should be obtained.

Specialty Press, Inc., first edition, 1995. 300 Northwest 70th Avenue,
Plantation, Florida 33317 (305) 792-8101

Manufactured in the United States of America

MEDICATIONS

FOR

ATTENTION DISORDERS

Dedication

This book is dedicated to my late husband, Frank Copeland, M.D., Psychiatrist and pioneer in Attention Disorders, with whom I worked for twenty years. His skilled clinician/scientist approach; his sensitivity, concern and respect for his patients; his unwavering optimism; and his ability to help people overcome adversity inspired me on a daily basis. He taught me much of what I know about the use of medications for attention disorders. He, in fact, taught me much of what I understand about life itself. I shall be eternally grateful for the opportunity to have known him, loved him, and practiced with him.

This book is also dedicated to my children, Frank and Anne, whose patience and encouragement have been unending, and to our patients and clients who allowed us to *practice* the arts of medicine and psychology with them as we persevered in our determination to deal effectively with this disorder.

Acknowledgements

The writing of a book is usually the accomplishment of a dedicated group of people. Such a collaborative effort was certainly true for *Medications for Attention Disorders*. I am especially indebted to the following: George Storm, M.D. for his contribution to the book and his editorial assistance; to Stephen Copps, M.D. for his medical expertise and consultation; to Vivian Bozeman for her enthusiastic support in overseeing the project; to Lanie Shaw and Cindy Lay for their preparation of the manuscript; to Ron Walker for his collegial support and commentary; to Beverley Bailey of Graphic Works, Inc. for her creative assistance, and to Laura Hall for her lay perspective. The assistance provided by these colleagues and associates, equally dedicated to recognizing and assisting those with attention disorders, is acknowledged with great appreciation.

Contributor

George Storm, M.D.
"ADHD and the Developmental Pediatrician"

Dr. Storm is especially qualified to share with other physicians and with families and educators his wealth of experience in both pediatric medicine and attention disorders. Since 1975, he has been a consultant to the "School Function Program" at Boston Children's Hospital. Dr. Storm was an instructor in Pediatrics at Harvard Medical School for eleven years. In addition to his pediatric training, he completed a fellowship in Child Psychiatry at Johns Hopkins Hospital. Among his community interests, he has served as a school board member, a school physician and on two Governor's Advisory Councils concerning children's issues. He maintains a busy private practice in Exeter, New Hampshire.

Wherever the art of medicine is loved, there is
also love of humanity.

—Hippocrates

Preface

Hippocrates' words, "Wherever the art of medicine is loved, there is also love of humanity," uniquely describe the efforts of all of those in medicine, psychology and education, who have feverishly worked on behalf of children and adolescents with hyperactivity and attention disorders for the past twenty years. One cannot sit with children and families day after day for years on end and watch the profoundly negative effects these disorders have on children's accomplishments, esteem, social relationships, and ultimate place in society without an intense urge to seek both causes and solutions. Neither can one witness, without an intense desire to intervene, the anguish parents experience as their best efforts fail or the frustrations of teachers who cannot educate their students.

In the 1990's the neurochemical basis of attention disorders is well-established. ADHD and ADD are unquestionably medical problems. This is perhaps the most basic concept with which each person affected by attention disorders must come to terms. It is my sincere belief that attention disorders may well be the neurological equivalent of visual problems: the difficulties can range from mild to severe; those affected number in the millions; and medical, behavioral, psychological and educational interventions can minimize the negative effects when the difficulties are identified early in the child's life. I also believe that early and appropriate intervention can easily relegate ADHD and ADD to the status of manageable problems in living.

When one fully understands attention disorders, the role of medication in their treatment is comprehensible and justifiable. Far from the assertions of those who do not understand, medication in the treatment of attention disorders neither drugs nor controls. Rather, it provides an individual with the freedom to function normally. Like the second-grader who can see the blackboard for the first time after donning glasses, the ADHD/ADD child or adolescent treated with medication can process information more normally, pay better attention to his teacher, control his impulsive responding, interact more sensitively and appropriately with his peers, come to terms with adult authorities, and develop the self-discipline, responsibility and skills to live a productive and fulfilling life.

The use of medication to treat attention disorders is an unknown for many. One's natural anxiety about drugs, especially their use in children and adolescents, causes understandable concern. This book attempts to address the concerns of the reader at both the cognitive and emotional levels, hopefully assisting those who struggle with the medication issue—whether children, adolescents, parents, educators or professionals—arrive at decisions which are both knowledgeable and comfortable.

Medication, however, is not an answer by itself, and using it as a primary solution is *not* recommended. For many people, nevertheless, it will become the cornerstone which enables other interventions to be effective. It is my hope that medication will someday not be needed. While this possibility exists, it is unlikely given our current state of knowledge. However, those who are willing to utilize all the other approaches recommended are most likely to maximize the potential benefits of the medication with the least amount needed. Eliminating stress, excessive indulgence, inappropriate educational practices, poor nutrition, and environmental toxins, and providing structure, organization, clearly-defined expectations and consequences, opportunities for achievement, and a sense of power, belonging and esteem will go far in eliminating the negative effects of this disorder. I both challenge and urge each educator, parent and professional to take all the necessary nonmedical actions available to manage attention disorders before, or concurrently, with the use of medication.

Until we have more successful genetic, physical, psychological, behavioral, educational or environmental interventions, most of us must come to terms with and accept the necessary role that medication will play in the overall treatment of the attention disorders of many children, adolescents and adults. Knowledgeable and responsible use of this therapeutic intervention has a well-established, important place in our armamentarium against the tyranny of these very treatable disorders. If this book assists the reader in arriving at a thoughtful and comfortable decision about medication, regardless of what it is, the goal of writing it will have been accomplished.

Edna D. Copeland, Ph.D.
January, 1991 • March, 1994

Contents

Preface

PART I. UNDERSTANDING ATTENTION DEFICIT DISORDERS

Chapter 1. What Are Attention Disorders?   **3**

History of Attention Disorders   5

Characteristics of Attention Disorders   9

Copeland Symptom Checklists for ADHD/ADD   10

Chapter 2. Neurophysiology of Attention Disorders   **17**

Structures and Functions of the Brain   18

What Is *Attention?*   39

Disorders of Attention versus Learning Disabilities   40

Summary   44

Chapter 3. Causes of ADHD/ADD   **45**
ADHD/ADD Syndrome Validity   46
Causes of Physiological ADHD/ADD   49
Other Causes of Attentional Problems   60
Summary   67

Chapter 4. ADHD and the Developmental Pediatrician   **69**
by George Storm, M.D.

The Developmentally Specialized Pediatrician   70
Family and School History   72
The Child's Appointment   74
The Interpretive Conference   77

PART II. MEDICATIONS: GENERAL PRINCIPLES

Chapter 5. The Role of Medication in Attention Disorders: **83**
Social and Emotional Issues
Accepting a Diagnosis of ADHD/ADD   85
Reluctance to Utilize Medication   86
Confusion and Anxiety about Stimulant Medication   88
A Personal Philosophy of Treatment   89
Rationale for Not Using Medication as a First Option   90

Chapter 6. Mechanisms and Goals of Medications   **95**
General Mechanism of Medications for ADHD/ADD   96
What Medications for ADHD/ADD Can Do   97
What Medications for ADHD/ADD Cannot Do   132

Chapter 7. Medication Usage: Practical Issues   **139**
Decision To Use Medication—Benefit:Risk Ratio   139
Deciding Which Medication Is Best   140
Administration of Medication   141
Issues in Medication Administration   147
Importance of Education and Counseling   151

PART III. MEDICATIONS

Chapter 8. Stimulant Medications   **161**
Definition of Terms   163
Ritalin (Methylphenidate HCL)[1]   163
Dexedrine (Dextroamphetamine Sulfate)   189
Desoxyn (Methamphetamine HCL)   196
Cylert (Pemoline)   197

Chapter 9. Antidepressants   **207**
Tofranil (Imipramine HCL)   208
Norpramin (Desipramine HCL)   219
Prozac (Fluoxetine HCL)   226
Monoamine Oxidase Inhibitors: Nardil (Phenelzine Sulfate))
   and Parnate (Tranylcypromine)   231

Chapter 10. Antihypertensives: Catapres (Clonidine HCL)   **237**

Chapter 11. Medications for Special Situations   **249**
Major Tranquilizers: Haldol (Haloperidol), Mellaril
   (Thioridazine HCL), Thorazine (Chlorpromazine),
   and Stellazine (Trifluoperazine)   249
Tegretol (Carbamazepine)   254
Lithium   255
Caffeine   260
Other Medications   261

PART IV. ASSOCIATED NEUROLOGICAL AND SLEEP DISORDERS

Chapter 12. Neurological Disorders   **269**
Simple Motor Tics   269
Tourette Syndrome   270
Seizure Disorders   276

Chapter 13. Sleep Disorders   **281**
Sleep: General Considerations   281
Sleep Apnea   284
Narcolepsy   287

[1]HCL = Hydrochloride

PART V. THE EDUCATOR'S IMPORTANT ROLE

Chapter 14. The Responsibility of the School under Federal Law   293

Chapter 15. The Teacher's Role in Monitoring Medications   305

Chapter 16. Medication Guidelines for Schools   317

Epilogue   329

Appendix   331
   1 Suggested Readings and Video Programs   333
   2 Review Articles on the Neurophysiology of ADHD/ADD   337
   3 List of Support Groups by State   339
   4 Symptom Checklists: Preschool and Elementary   341
   5 Sources of Tests Discussed in Chapter 4   347
   6 Selected Bibliography: Coping with the Grief
     of ADHD/ADD and LD   349
   7 Tourette Syndrome Associations and Suggested Readings
     in Tourette Syndrome   351
   8 Regional Offices of Civil Rights   353

Glossary   355

References   359

Subject Index   381

PART I

Understanding Attention Deficit Disorders

Likely as not, the child you can do the least with
will do the most to make you proud.

—Mignon McLaughlin

1

What Are
Attention Disorders?

She daydreams - she never knows what the assignment is.

He doesn't listen.

Her homework is so sloppy! But she can do it neatly when she tries.
She just isn't motivated.

Her room is a disaster. Even when she tries, she can't keep it straight.
She's just one of those disorganized people.

Driving with him scares me to death. He seems oblivious to the
traffic. He's almost had three wrecks and he's only been driving a
month.

He doesn't keep friends long. They bore him very quickly. He's
always looking for a new thrill.

I love him dearly, but he's driving me wild.

I can't count on him. He never keeps his word.

They told me she was so bright and had so much potential. What
happened? She's barely passing third grade!

These comments represent the feelings of helplessness and frustration of parents and teachers living with and educating children and adolescents with attention disorders. No matter how much adults care, there can be many frustrating moments.

Each of us looking back over years of teaching or parenting can recall saying things we wish we had not said and scenes we wish we could erase. Sharp words uttered in a moment of frustration, a tongue-in-cheek criticism that angered the child and ended further exchange; a child punished when already quite discouraged and having that punishment be the final straw for him; humiliation before others in a moment of confrontation; a stubborn unwillingness to admit a mistake, knowing in your heart that only such honesty will restore the child's faith and partially repair the damage you have inflicted ... these are the things which, I hope, do keep us awake at night, whether parent or teacher.

Despite the fact that we are human, we have neither the luxury nor the privilege of responding inappropriately and hurtfully to our young charges. They are defenseless in the face of our authority and, even when they fight back, they ultimately lose. We must begin a conscious, individual effort and a collective campaign to turn our homes and classrooms into sunny, happy learning centers and our roles as teachers, parents and professionals into that of facilitators and allies.

To do so, however, we must first understand the problem....

Attention deficit disorders, both ADHD and ADD,[1] are problems which usually begin in early childhood, usually by the age of four.

---

[1]ADHD is attention deficit-hyperactivity disorder; ADD is attention deficit disorder without hyperactivity. The terms *attention deficit disorders* and *attention disorders* will be utilized throughout this book to refer to both. However, it is important to recognize that the two entities represent different sets of problems and will probably be found to have somewhat different neurological and neurochemical causes. Nonetheless, at present, ADHD and ADD are utilized interchangeably most of the time.

However, they typically are not identified until the elementary school years or even later. For many, their attention disorders will continue into adolescence and adulthood and may well persist throughout their lives. Attention disorders can be difficult to recognize, for the symptoms masquerade as learning disabilities, emotional problems, bad behavior, poor parenting, overly stressful environments, demanding schools, laziness and lack of motivation, among others.

ADHD and ADD affect millions of children, adolescents and adults in every country in the world. They occur in people of every ability level and in every socioeconomic group. They are thought to occur much more frequently in males but may not, as girls with ADD are very underidentified. There are now international efforts to understand and treat attention disorders. England, calling these problems "conduct disorders," previously reported a much smaller percentage with ADHD/ADD than the U.S. When using similar diagnostic criteria, however, other countries, as reported by Drs. Shaywitz and Shaywitz (1988), have been found to have similar, and often even higher, percentages of ADHD/ADD children and adolescents than does the United States (3-8%): New Zealand - 13%; West Germany - 8%; Italy - 12%; Spain - 16%; Great Britain - 10%; and China - 11%.

HISTORY OF ATTENTION DISORDERS

Attention Disorders are not new problems. Rather, they have existed for hundreds of years. Only recently, however, have we begun to understand them and to know how to deal more effectively with them.

The complexity of these disorders has been staggering, for each child, adolescent or adult manifests the symptom complex in a unique and individual way. Our understanding has continued to evolve over the years as researchers have attempted to define the central problem in attention disorders.

One of the first mentions of this disorder is perhaps found in the writings of John Locke (1762), who wished for "A proper and effectual remedy for this wandering of the thoughts...." The date most frequently mentioned, however, is that of 1848, when *Fidgety Phil* appeared as a character in a story written for his children by Dr. Heinrich Hoffman, a German doctor. ADHD/ADD was next addressed in 1902 by Dr. George Still in *Lancet*, the premier medical magazine of its time. It is noteworthy that his descriptions are still quite appropriate today. However, he characterized these symptoms as "a defect in moral control". In the 1940's, an outbreak of encephalitis, which left many people with similar symptoms of hyperactivity, inattention and poor impulse control, suggested that attention disorders might be the result of organic problems. The notion that attention disorders are caused by brain damage has continued to persist. Other names by which ADHD and ADD have been known are *Minimal Brain Damage, Minimal Brain Dysfunction (MBD), Hyperkinetic Reaction of Childhood, Attention Deficit Disorder With and Without Hyperactivity, Attention-deficit Hyperactivity Disorder,* and *Undifferentiated Attention Deficit Disorder.*

The name has thus changed several times as research data and clinical experiences have accrued. In 1980, the American Psychiatric Association established the diagnosis of *Attention Deficit Disorder With and Without Hyperactivity*, and outlined inattention, impulsivity and activity-level problems as the major symptoms. This date is noteworthy, for it was the first time the term *attention* was used. Investigators had increasingly found that attentional problems, rather than hyperactivity, were the cardinal symptoms. In 1987, the name was changed to *Attention-deficit Hyperactivity Disorder, ADHD,* and *Undifferentiated Attention Deficit Disorder, UADD or ADD* (DSM-III-R).

In recent years (1987-1995), interest in attention disorders has exploded. As it has, both scientific and clinical understanding of the multifaceted dimensions of the ADHD/ADD continuum has increased. In 1994 the APA reconfigured the core symptoms to correspond with the most current research findings and professional opinions in the field.

The current diagnostic criteria for Attention-Deficit/Hyperactivity Disorder have been established by the 1994 *American Psychiatric Association Diagnostic and Statistical Manual of Mental Disorders (DSM-IV^(TM))*.[2] Although the term *ADD* has been dropped, it will continue to be used in this book to refer to attention deficit disorder without hyperactivity, i.e. *ADHD/Inattentive Type* because of its congruence with the actual symptoms manifested.

DIAGNOSTIC CRITERIA FOR
ATTENTION-DEFICIT/HYPERACTIVITY DISORDER

Either (1) or (2)

(1)   *six (or more) of the following symptoms of <u>inattention</u> have persisted for at least 6 months to a degree that is maladaptive and inconsistent with developmental level:*

INATTENTION
(a)   often fails to give close attention to details or makes careless mistakes in schoolwork, work, or other activities
(b)   often has difficulty sustaining attention in tasks or play activities
(c)   often does not seem to listen when spoken to directly
(d)   often does not follow through on instructions and fails to finish schoolwork, chores, or duties in the workplace (not due to oppositional behavior or failure to understand instructions)
(e)   often has difficulty organizing tasks and activities
(f)   often avoids, dislikes, or is reluctant to engage in tasks that require sustained mental effort (such as schoolwork or homework)
(g)   often loses things necessary for tasks or activities (e.g., toys, school assignments, pencils, books, or tools)
(h)   is often easily distracted by extraneous stimuli
(i)   is often forgetful in daily activities

(2)   *six (or more) of the following symptoms of <u>hyperactivity-impulsivity</u> have persisted for at least 6 months to a degree that is maladaptive and inconsistent with developmental level:*

HYPERACTIVITY
(a)   often fidgets with hands or feet or squirms in seat
(b)   often leaves seat in classroom or in other situations in which remaining seated is expected

---

[2]Reprinted with permission from the *Diagnostic and Statistical Manual of Mental Disorders, Fourth Edition.* Copyright 1994, American Psychiatric Association.

(c) often runs about or climbs excessively in situations in which it is inappropriate (in adolescents or adults, may be limited to subjective feelings of restlessness)

(d) often has difficulty playing or engaging in leisure activities quietly

(e) is often "on the go" or often acts as if "driven by a motor"

(f) often talks excessively

IMPULSIVITY

(g) often blurts out answers before questions have been completed

(h) often has difficulty awaiting turn

(i) often interrupts or intrudes on others (e.g., butts into conversations or games)

B. Some hyperactive-impulsive or inattentive symptoms that caused impairment were present before age 7 years.

C. Some impairment from the symptoms is present in two or more settings (e.g., at school [or work] and at home).

D. There must be clear evidence of clinically significant impairment in social, academic, or occupational functioning.

E. The symptoms do not occur exclusively during the course of, . . . or are accounted for, by another mental disorder . . .

Code based on type:

314.01 *Attention-Deficit/Hyperactivity Disorder, Combined Type:* if both Criteria A1 and A2 are met for the past 6 months

314.00 *Attention-Deficit/Hyperactivity Disorder, Predominantly Inattentive Type*: if Criterion A1 is met but Criterion A2 is not met for the past 6 months

314.01 *Attention-Deficit/Hyperactivity Disorder, Predominantly Hyperactive-Impulsive Type*: if Criterion A2 is met but Criterion A1 is not met for the past 6 months

Despite the many changes of name since 1902, the disorder itself has remained remarkably stable. The three most generally accepted components of attentional disorders continue to be (1) inattention/distractibility, (2) impulsivity, and (3) activity level or arousal problems, either overactive/overaroused or underactive/underaroused.

It is uniformly agreed among experts that these criteria are too broad and, when used by themselves, may overidentify or misidentify attention deficits in children, adolescents and adults. Educators are especially concerned that ADHD/ADD will be overidentified and place excessive and inappropriate burdens on the schools and encourage improper placements for students.

The Council on Child and Adolescent Health of the American Academy of Pediatrics has endorsed the following recommendations for diagnosing ADHD in children:

> To establish an accurate diagnosis, information must be obtained on factors such as: (1) the child's birth, developmental, family, medical, psychosocial, and scholastic history; (2) sensory screening; and (3) a physical, neurologic, and neuromaturational examination (Committee on Children with Disabilities - Committee on Drugs, 1987).

The evaluation process is discussed at length in Chapter 4.

CHARACTERISTICS OF ATTENTION DISORDERS

Each child, adolescent or adult with ADHD or ADD has a unique set of symptoms and characteristics. It is important to be aware of these, for each will need attention and intervention.

An exhaustive review of the literature on ADHD/ADD revealed that the majority of the symptoms occur in one of the following categories:

I	Inattention/Distractibility	VI	Immaturity
II	Impulsivity	VII	Poor School Achievement,
III	Activity Level or Arousal Problems:		Cognitive and Visual-
	Overactivity/Overarousal		Motor Problems
	Underactivity/Underarousal	VIII	Emotional Difficulties
IV	Noncompliance	IX	Poor Peer Relations
V	Attention-Getting Behavior	X	Family Interaction Problems

Subsequent to this review, the *Copeland Symptom Checklist for Attention Deficit Disorders (Children and Adolescents)* was developed to assess these ten areas of difficulty. A checklist for adults, the *Copeland Symptom Checklist for Adult Attention Deficit Disorders,* was later devised. These checklists, presented on the following pages, provide a guide—a guide only—for determining each person's unique constellation of difficulties, assessing strengths, targeting interventions and measuring progress. A diagnosis of ADHD should be made only by a professional thoroughly trained in attention disorders.

SPI

COPELAND SYMPTOM CHECKLIST FOR ATTENTION DEFICIT DISORDERS

Attention Deficit Hyperactivity Disorder (ADHD)
and Undifferentiated Attention Deficit Disorder (ADD)

This checklist was developed from the experience of many specialists in the field of Attention Deficit Disorders and Hyperactivity. It is designed to help you assess whether your child/student has ADHD or ADD, to what degree, and if so, in which area(s) difficulties are experienced. Please mark all statements. Thank you for your assistance in completing this information.

Name of Child _____ Date _____

Completed by _____

Directions: Place a checkmark (✓) by each item below, indicating the degree to which the behavior is characteristic of your child/student.

* denotes ADD with Hyperactivity (ADHD).
• denotes ADD without Hyperactivity (Undifferentiated ADD)

	Not at all	Just a little	Pretty much	Very much	Score	%
I. INATTENTION/DISTRACTIBILITY						
*• 1. A short attention span, especially for low-interest activities.						
*• 2. Difficulty completing tasks.						
• 3. Daydreaming.						
*• 4. Easily distracted.						
• 5. Nicknames such as: "spacey," or "dreamer."						
*• 6. Engages in much activity but accomplishes little.						
*• 7. Enthusiastic beginnings but poor endings.					= ___%
					21	
II. IMPULSIVITY						
* 1. Excitability.						
*• 2. Low frustration tolerance.						
*• 3. Acts before thinking.						
*• 4. Disorganization.						
*• 5. Poor planning ability.						
*• 6. Excessively shifts from one activity to another.						
* 7. Difficulty in group situations which require patience and taking turns.						
*• 8. Requires much supervision.						
*• 9. Constantly in trouble for deeds of omission as well as deeds of commission.						
*•10. Frequently interrupts conversations; talks out of turn.					= ___%
					30	
III. ACTIVITY LEVEL PROBLEMS						
A. Overactivity/Hyperactivity						
*• 1. Restlessness — either fidgetiness or being constantly on the go.						
* 2. Diminished need for sleep.						
* 3. Excessive talking.						
* 4. Excessive running, jumping and climbing.						
* 5. Motor restlessness during sleep. Kicks covers off — moves around constantly.						
* 6. Difficulty staying seated at meals, in class, etc. Often walks around classroom.					= ___%
					18	
B. Underactivity						
• 1. Lethargy.						
• 2. Daydreaming, spaciness.						
• 3. Failure to complete tasks.						
*• 4. Inattention.						
*• 5. Poor leadership ability.						
*• 6. Difficulty in learning and performing.					= ___%
					18	
IV. NON-COMPLIANCE						
*• 1. Frequently disobeys.						
*• 2. Argumentative.						
* 3. Disregards socially-accepted standards of behavior.						
• 4. "Forgets" unintentionally.						
5. Uses "forgetting" as an excuse (intentional).					= ___%
					15	

Published by **SPI** Southeastern Psychological Institute, P.O. Box 12389, Atlanta, Georgia 30355-2389

COPELAND SYMPTOM CHECKLIST FOR ATTENTION DEFICIT DISORDERS (Continued)

	Not at all	Just a little	Pretty much	Very much
V. ATTENTION-GETTING BEHAVIOR				
* 1. Frequently needs to be the center of attention.				
* 2. Constantly asks questions or interrupts.				
* 3. Irritates and annoys siblings, peers and adults.				
* 4. Behaves as the "class clown."				
* 5. Uses bad or rude language to attract attention.				
* 6. Engages in other negative behaviors to attract attention.				

= ____% 18

	Not at all	Just a little	Pretty much	Very much
VI. IMMATURITY				
*• 1. Behavior resembles that of a younger child. Responses are typical of children 6 months to 2-plus years younger.				
*• 2. Physical development is delayed.				
*• 3. Prefers younger children and relates better to them.				
*• 4. Emotional reactions are often immature.				

= ____% 12

	Not at all	Just a little	Pretty much	Very much
VII. POOR ACHIEVEMENT/COGNITIVE & VISUAL-MOTOR PROBLEMS				
*• 1. Underachieves relative to ability.				
*• 2. Loses books, assignments, etc.				
*• 3. Auditory memory and auditory processing problems.				
*• 4. Learning disabilities/learning problems.				
*• 5. Incomplete assignments.				
*• 6. Academic work completed too quickly.				
*• 7. Academic work completed too slowly.				
*• 8. "Messy" or "sloppy" written work; poor handwriting.				
*• 9. Poor memory for directions, instructions and rote learning.				

= ____% 27

	Not at all	Just a little	Pretty much	Very much
VIII. EMOTIONAL DIFFICULTIES				
*• 1. Frequent and unpredictable mood swings.				
*• 2. High levels of irritability.				
* 3. Underreactive to pain/insensitive to danger.				
* 4. Easily overstimulated. Hard to calm down once over-excited.				
*• 5. Low frustration tolerance.				
* 6. Temper tantrums, angry outbursts.				
• 7. Moodiness.				
*• 8. Low self-esteem.				

= ____% 24

	Not at all	Just a little	Pretty much	Very much
IX. POOR PEER RELATIONS				
* 1. Hits, bites, or kicks other children.				
* 2. Difficulty following the rules of games and social interactions.				
*• 3. Rejected or avoided by peers.				
• 4. Avoids group activities; a loner.				
* 5. Teases peers and siblings excessively.				
• 6. Bullies or bosses other children.				

= ____% 18

	Not at all	Just a little	Pretty much	Very much
X. FAMILY INTERACTION PROBLEMS				
1. Frequent family conflict.				
2. Activities and social gatherings are unpleasant.				
3. Parents argue over discipline since nothing works.				
4. Mother spends hours and hours on homework with ADD child leaving little time for others in family.				
5. Meals are frequently unpleasant.				
6. Arguments occur between parents and child over responsibilities and chores.				
7. Stress is continuous from child's social and academic problems.				
8. Parents, especially mother, feel: ☐ frustrated ☐ hopeless ☐ alone ☐ angry ☐ guilty ☐ afraid for child ☐ helpless ☐ disappointed ☐ sad and depressed				

= ____% 24

Copyright ©1987 by Edna D. Copeland, Ph.D.

7/90   Published by **SPI** Southeastern Psychological Institute, P.O. Box 12389, Atlanta, Georgia 30355-2389

sPI

COPELAND SYMPTOM CHECKLIST
FOR ADULT ATTENTION DEFICIT DISORDERS

Attention Deficit Hyperactivity Disorder (ADHD)
and Undifferentiated Attention Deficit Disorder (ADD)

This checklist was developed from the experience of many specialists in the field of Attention Disorders and Hyperactivity. It is designed to help determine whether you, or someone you are rating, has ADHD or ADD, to what degree, and if so, in which area(s) difficulties are experienced. Please mark all statements. Thank you for your assistance in completing this information.

Name _____ Date _____

Completed by _____

Directions: Place a checkmark (✓) by each item below, indicating the degree to which the behavior is characteristic of yourself or the adult you are rating.

	Not at all	Just a little	Pretty much	Very much	Score	%
I. INATTENTION/DISTRACTIBILITY, especially						
1. A short attention span, especially for low-interest activities.						
2. Difficulty completing tasks.						
3. Daydreaming.						
4. Easily distracted.						
5. Nicknames such as: "spacey," or "dreamer."						
6. Engages in much activity but accomplishes little.						
7. Enthusiastic beginnings but poor endings.					21	= ___%
II. IMPULSIVITY						
1. Excitability.						
2. Low frustration tolerance.						
3. Acts before thinking.						
4. Disorganization.						
5. Poor planning ability.						
6. Excessively shifts from one activity to another.						
7. Difficulty in group situations which require patience and taking turns.						
8. Interrupts frequently.					24	= ___%
III. ACTIVITY LEVEL PROBLEMS						
A. Overactivity/Hyperactivity						
1. Restlessness — either fidgetiness or being constantly on the go.						
2. Diminished need for sleep.						
3. Excessive talking.						
4. Difficulty listening.						
5. Motor restlessness during sleep. Kicks covers off — moves around constantly.						
6. Dislike of situations which require attention & being still—church, lectures, etc.					18	= ___%
B. Underactivity						
1. Lethargic.						
2. Daydreaming, spaciness.						
3. Failure to complete tasks.						
4. Inattention.						
5. Lacking in leadership.						
6. Difficulty in getting things done.					18	= ___%

Published by **sPI** Southeastern Psychological Institute, P.O. Box 12389, Atlanta, Georgia 30355-2389

COPELAND SYMPTOM CHECKLIST FOR ADULT ATTENTION DEFICIT DISORDERS (Continued)

	Not at all	Just a little	Pretty much	Very much
IV. NONCOMPLIANCE				
1. Does not cooperate. Determined to do things own way.				
2. Argumentative.				
3. Disregards socially-accepted behavioral expectations.				
4. "Forgets" unintentionally.				
5. "Forgets" as an excuse (intentionally).				

15 ___ = ___ %

	Not at all	Just a little	Pretty much	Very much
V. UNDERACHIEVEMENT/DISORGANIZATION/LEARNING PROBLEMS				
1. Underachievement in relation to ability.				
2. Frequent job changes.				
3. Loses things — keys, wallet, lists, belongings, etc.				
4. Auditory memory and auditory processing problems.				
5. Learning disabilities or learning problems.				
6. Poor handwriting.				
7. "Messy" or "sloppy" work.				
8. Work assignments are often not completed satisfactorily.				
9. Rushes through work.				
10. Works too slowly.				
11. Procrastinates. Bills, taxes, etc., put off until the last minute.				

33 ___ = ___ %

	Not at all	Just a little	Pretty much	Very much
VI. EMOTIONAL DIFFICULTIES				
1. Frequent and unpredictable mood swings.				
2. Irritability.				
3. Underreactive to pain/insensitive to danger.				
4. Easily overstimulated. Hard to stop once "revved up."				
5. Low frustration tolerance. Excessive emotional reaction to frustrating situations.				
6. Angry outbursts.				
7. Moodiness/lack of energy.				
8. Low self-esteem.				
9. Immaturity.				

27 ___ = ___ %

	Not at all	Just a little	Pretty much	Very much
VII. POOR PEER RELATIONS				
1. Difficulty following the rules of social interactions.				
2. Rejected or avoided by peers.				
3. Avoids group activities; a loner.				
4. "Bosses" other people. Wants to be the leader.				
5. Critical of others.				

15 ___ = ___ %

	Not at all	Just a little	Pretty much	Very much
VIII. IMPAIRED FAMILY RELATIONSHIPS				
1. Easily frustrated with spouse or children. Overreacts. May punish children too severely.				
2. Sees things from own point of view. Does not negotiate differences well.				
3. Underdeveloped sense of responsibility.				
4. Poor manager of money.				
5. Unreasonable; demanding.				
6. Spends excessive amount of time at work because of inefficiency, leaving little time for family.				

18 ___ = ___ %

7/90   Published by **SPI** Southeastern Psychological Institute, P.O. Box 12389, Atlanta, Georgia 30355-2389

sPi

SCORING THE COPELAND SYMPTOM CHECKLIST
FOR ATTENTION DEFICIT DISORDERS (ADHD/ADD)
(Child/Adolescent Checklist and Adult Checklist)

1. Scores for each category are as follows:

   Not at all = 0;   Just a little = 1;   Pretty much = 2;   Very much = 3

2. Each check receives a score from 0 - 3. Add the checks in each category. That score is placed over the total possible. Example:

	0	1	2	3		
* denotes ADD with Hyperactivity (ADHD). • denotes ADD without Hyperactivity (Undifferentiated ADD)	Not at all	Just a little	Pretty much	Very much	Score	%
I. INATTENTION/DISTRACTIBILITY						
*• 1. A short attention span, especially for low-interest activities.				✔		
*• 2. Difficulty completing tasks.			✔			
• 3. Daydreaming.		✔				
*• 4. Easily distracted.				✔		
• 5. Nicknames such as: "spacey," or "dreamer."		✔				
*• 6. Engages in much activity but accomplishes little.				✔		
*• 7. Enthusiastic beginnings but poor endings.				✔	16 / 21	76 %
II. IMPULSIVITY						
* 1. Excitability.				✔		
*• 2. Low frustration tolerance.				✔		
*• 3. Acts before thinking.				✔		
*• 4. Disorganization.			✔			
*• 5. Poor planning ability.			✔			
*• 6. Excessively shifts from one activity to another.				✔		
* 7. Difficulty in group situations which require patience and taking turns.				✔		
*• 8. Requires much supervision.				✔		
*• 9. Constantly in trouble for deeds of omission as well as deeds of commission.			✔			
*•10. Frequently interrupts conversations; talks out of turn.				✔	27 / 30	90 %

3. Compute the percentage for each category.

   Significance:*

   Scores between 35-49% suggest mild to moderate difficulties.

   Scores between 50-69% suggest moderate to severe difficulties.

   Scores above 70% suggest major interference.

   (*These scores represent clinical significance. The scale is currently being normed and statistical data should be available soon.)

   Children, adolescents and adults may have difficulties in only one area or in all ten. Those with undifferentiated ADD on the more daydreaming, inattentive, anxious end of the ADD continuum frequently manifest difficulties only in the "Inattention/Distractibility", "Underactivity", and the "Underachievement" categories, while those with overactive, impulsive ADHD will have difficulties in many more areas of their lives.

Published by sPi Southeastern Psychological Institute, P.O. Box 12389, Atlanta, Georgia 30355-2389

The characteristics which comprise these checklists are discussed at length in *Attention, Please! A Comprehensive Guide for Successfully Parenting Children and Adolescents with Attention Disorders and Hyperactivity (ADHD/ADD)* (Copeland & Love, 1991).

In this book, it is assumed that the reader has already obtained some information about attention disorders and their characteristics. Those who desire more information regarding a basic definition and overview of ADHD/ADD are referred to the Suggested Readings in Appendix 1.

*The brain is a physical structure of daunting
complexity, a veritable Chartres erected upon our
shoulders... a dazzling interplay of electrical
codes, neurochemical messages... electromagnetic
fields. Which of these is most important...?
One might as well ask, "Which is most important
to the Brandenburg Concerto: Bach, a Stradivarius
violin, or the concert violinist of your choice?"*

—Richard Restak, M.D., 1984

2
Neurophysiology
of Attention
Disorders

To understand more completely the concepts of attention efficiency and
attention disorders, one must have some understanding of the nature of
the brain itself. Its structures and functions hold the keys to attention,
disorders of attention, and the medications utilized to treat them.

The human brain, an unimposing three-pound mass of tissue in the
average person, is an amazingly complex and extraordinary universe
composed of an estimated ten billion nerve cells. The simplest brain cell
is more complex than an entire computer. Each cell is individual in
purpose and unique in function, yet each interweaves with hundreds of
others to form an exquisite network of over one quadrillion connections.
Within the brain's gray folds lies the power that allows man to think and
reason; to comprehend and understand; to feel and desire; to pay attention
and remember; and to create and achieve. It is this mass of electrical blips
and chemical drips that allows man to transfer thought into action and
dreams into reality.

It is this same brain which, when dysfunctional or damaged, can turn life into a nightmare—one filled with the uncontrolled, convulsive firing of neurons in an epileptic fit, or the schizophrenic terror of imagined horrors. It can produce rage and aggression, dull the senses, contort muscle movements into Parkinsonian spasms, or propel a person into a frenzy of hyperactivity and disorganization. The brain is both our greatest ally and our worst enemy. Understanding its structure, its functions, its complexity and its diversity is crucial in our attempts to insure its healthy functioning and thereby maintain control over our lives.

Our knowledge of the brain is currently in its infancy. We are, nevertheless, gradually unraveling some of its mysteries. The purpose of the following discussion is to provide an overview of the major structures and functions of the brain which have direct application for attention deficit disorders. Some may wish to skip this section, while others may find it critical in aiding their understanding of the role medication plays in treating this complex disorder. It is not necessary to understand how aspirin relieves pain, or antibiotics treat pneumonia, in order to receive their benefit. The knowledge that they do may be quite adequate. Likewise, many will accept that various medications assist those with ADHD and ADD without a desire to understand the neurologic mechanisms involved. Should you wish to omit this section, please continue with the discussion of "What Is *Attention*?" on page 39.

STRUCTURES AND FUNCTIONS OF THE BRAIN

The following structures of the brain and their contribution to both attention and disorders of attention will be discussed:
- The exterior casing of the brain (the outer membranes and skull).
- The cerebral hemispheres.
- The cerebral cortex.
- The four major lobes of each hemisphere.
- The cerebellum.

- Subcortical brain structures.
- The reticular activating system and the reticular formation.
- Other structures within the brain which affect attention, behavior and emotions, including the thalamus, hypothalamus, limbic system and basal ganglia.

Exterior of the Brain

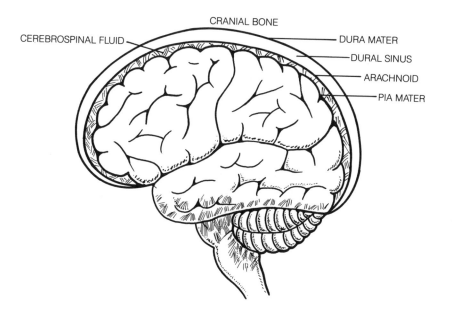

Beneath the bony structure of the skull are three membranes:

- The *dura mater* (hard mother)—a hard fibrous membrane beneath the skull.

- The *arachnoid* (cobweb)—the membrane that bridges the brain's many crevices and is located between the dural sinus and the pia mater.
- The *pia mater* (tender mother)—a firm, tight membrane which covers, like a glove, every nook and cranny of the brain's highly irregular surface.

Approximately six to eight ounces of cerebrospinal fluid flow between the pia mater and the arachnoid cushioning the brain from insult and filling every unoccupied space between the membranes and in the spinal cord. Despite this protection, injury can occur through *in utero* insults, birth trauma, and accidents, and cause attention disorders both with and without hyperactivity.

Cerebral Hemispheres

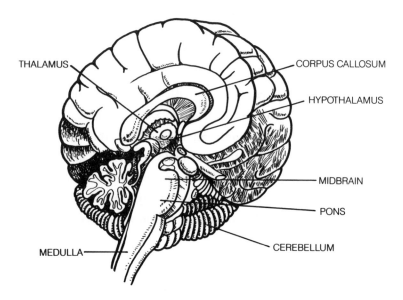

THALAMUS

CORPUS CALLOSUM

HYPOTHALAMUS

MIDBRAIN

PONS

CEREBELLUM

MEDULLA

The brain, for reasons not yet understood by neuroscientists, is divided into two cerebral hemispheres, the left and the right, which are connected by a bundle of tissue called the *corpus callosum*. The corpus callosum provides for communication between the hemispheres. While the cerebral hemispheres look and are in many ways alike, they are organized somewhat differently. Speech, hearing, language functions, logic, analytical thought and organization are, for most people, located in the left hemisphere, while spatial skills, wholistic learning, and the ability to visualize and see images are right-hemispheric functions. While everyone uses both sides of their brains, most people have a preference for one side over the other. This preference, or *brain dominance*, contributes to each person's unique personality, learning style and approach to many aspects of his life.

Brain preference or dominance occurs in the same proportions in both the ADHD/ADD and non-attention-disordered populations. Right-brain ADHD and ADD children, adolescents and adults often struggle more than those who are more left brain, however, because right-brain traits can compound the ADHD/ADD person's lack of organization, planning ahead, and sequential follow-through. The left-brain, high-energy ADHD person often accomplishes goals with enhanced speed and determination, while the right-brain ADHD/ADD person may have difficulty getting organized for the day. Since the American culture in general, and schools in particular, reward left-brain traits, those with more right-brain characteristics and ADD often are at a double disadvantage.

The brain is arranged contralaterally, that is, the right side of the brain controls the left side of the body and vice versa. This organization applies to handedness, footedness and most motor functions, as well as partially to vision. One side of the brain usually becomes more dominant by the age of five or six and controls both the flow of information received and the responses made.

Cerebral Cortex

The *cerebral cortex* is a layer of gray matter that covers the cerebral hemispheres. It is sometimes called the "bark" of the brain, for when the brain is cut into sections it looks like a tree trunk. Dark material called *gray matter* is on the outside, while light gray material, called *white matter*, composed of neurons covered by a sheath, connects various regions of the cortex to other brain centers.

The cerebral cortex is considered the *thinking* part of the brain and is responsible for the higher thought processes which separate man from all other species.

Lobes

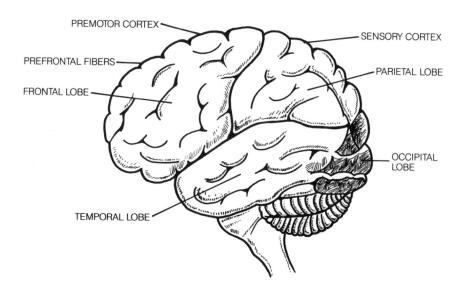

Each hemisphere of the brain is divided into four lobes by fissures, called *sulci* (singular: *sulcus*). They are the *frontal, parietal, occipital* and *temporal* lobes. Each has very specific functions in the overall organization of a person's life.

Frontal Lobes

The frontal lobes are perhaps the most important of the lobes. In each hemisphere they begin at the anterior of the brain and reach back to the central sulcus. The area between the central and precentral sulci helps control body movements and is called the *motor area*, while the remainder of the frontal lobes modulates various aspects of thinking, feeling, imagining and making decisions.

The frontal lobes are the primary areas for movement. Damage or dysfunction leads to impaired motor movements which may result in either hyperactivity or diminished movement and paralysis. Immediately forward of the frontal lobes is the *premotor cortex* where more complex motor movements are organized. Its role in the preparation of specific voluntary movement appears diminished in ADHD. Dysfunction in this region could be responsible for the motor restlessness of ADHD. The premotor cortex is also critical for suppressing motor responses to certain sensory stimuli. "Acting without thinking," or, more accurately, acting without appropriate inhibition, is seen frequently in the impulsive actions of ADHD children, adolescents and adults. Calling out in class, not waiting one's turn, interrupting, or hitting another person in a moment of frustration are examples of motor responses which should have been inhibited by the premotor cortex.

Involvement of the frontal lobes in hyperactivity has been proposed by several researchers (Mattes, 1980; Mesulam, 1986) and most recently in a landmark study by Dr. Alan Zametkin and his associates at the National Institute of Mental Health, published in *The New England Journal of Medicine* (1990). They found that hyperactive adults who have been hyperactive since childhood, and who also have hyperactive children, had decreased glucose metabolism rates in the prefrontal cortex and the premotor cortex, as well as a more global decreased rate of glucose metabolism in the brain.

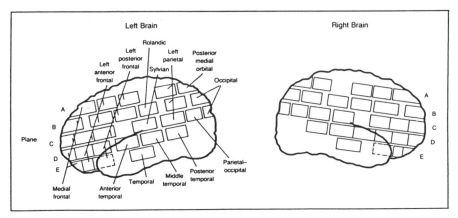

Figure 1. Schematic Representation of the Regions Sampled.

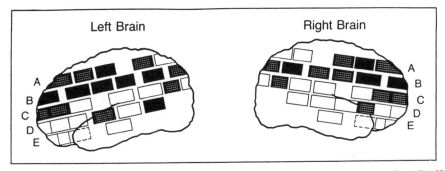

Figure 2. Regions of the Brain That Had Significantly Decreased Absolute Rates of Glucose Metabolism in Hyperactive Adults (N = 25) as Compared with Controls (N = 50).

No regions had significantly higher metabolism in patients than controls. The solid rectangles indicate that the P value for the difference between patients and controls was ≤0.01, the shaded rectangles that the P value was ≤0.05, and the open rectangles that the difference was not significant. The following subcortical regions of the right brain are not shown: right thalamus (P≤0.01), right caudate (P≤0.05), right hippocampus (P≤0.05), and cingulate (P≤0.01). All P values were obtained by two-tailed t-test. The middle medial cortical region in Plane A (not shown) had reduced metabolism (P<0.05).

Figure 1[1] is a schematic representation of the regions sampled.

Figure 2[1] shows the regions of the brain that had significantly decreased

[1]Reprinted by permission, *The New England Journal of Medicine*, November 15, 1990, Vol. 323: pp. 1363-1364.

absolute rates of glucose metabolism in hyperactive adults as compared with non-ADHD adults.

Dr. Hans Lou and his associates (1989) had earlier reported their findings that striatal regions in the frontal and central brain structures of hyperactive children were not receiving an adequate blood supply.

The prefrontal areas are also important biologic determiners of attention according to Dr. M. Marsel Mesulam, a Harvard University neurologist. Disorders or dysfunction in these regions, he stated, often result in inattention, distractibility and disinhibition (Mesulam, 1986).

Dr. Zametkin and his associates also found differences in the metabolic rate of other regions of the brain including the left parietal lobe, the left temporal lobe and bilateral rolandic structures, in addition to other subcortical structures, as can be seen in the figures on page 24.

The frontal lobes are part of the *frontal system*, which has important connections with other parts of the brain including the thalamus, hypothalamus, limbic system, and basal ganglia, among others. This system is an important coordinator of emotion, judgment, creativity and volition. It is sometimes referred to as the *seat of emotions.*

Early reports of those with accidental or surgical damage to the frontal system indicated that there were marked changes in the personalities of those affected. Phineas Gage, famous in the neurological literature, changed after frontal lobe injury from an intelligent, pleasant person to one who was impulsive, childlike, inappropriate in his actions, unable to follow through on tasks, and socially inept. Others with frontal lobe damage have changed from being shy and introverted individuals to assertive, boastful, careless, and mindlessly happy people.

It has long been observed that patients with frontal lobe injury frequently exhibit many of the same behaviors as those with severe ADHD. The role of the frontal lobes in some types of ADHD/ADD appears to have been firmly established at this time.

Parietal Lobes

The parietal lobes contain the primary sensory cortex and receive impulses from all the senses except vision and smell, which report directly to the cerebral cortex. The parietal lobes have been described as the *feeling* part of the brain, or the *somatosensory area*, since they receive information about various bodily sensations and are responsible for the experience of touch, pressure, pain and pleasure, among others. The hyperactive child's insensitivity to pain, or the often-noted inability to be satisfied (Levine & Melmed, 1982), might reflect a dysfunction in this region. One could also speculate that the decreased sensitivity to bowel and bladder pressures, often noted especially in ADHD, result from parietal-lobe dysfunctions. These are possibilities which are not, as of yet, explored, but ones which do have at least surface logic.

Temporal Lobes

While each lobe has its own critical functions, the temporal lobes are especially important because of their connections with our most primitive brain, the *medulla,* or the "reptile brain". The medulla is the part of the brain which developed first and continues to be more prominent in lower species. The connection between the temporal lobes and the medulla enables us to experience intense emotions such as fear, anger, lust, and even primitive jealousy.

The temporal lobes also receive auditory information and control auditory memory and language, as well as one's sense of time. The often-noted problems of short-term memory and language-processing problems in those with ADHD/ADD may have some of their origins in the under-stimulation of neurotransmitters in the temporal lobes. Dr. Zametkin's findings of decreased glucose metabolism in the left temporal lobe may possibly account for the much greater frequency of occurrence of short-term auditory-memory problems than of short-term visual-memory problems noted so often in those with attention disorders.

Occipital Lobes

Located behind the temporal lobes are the occipital lobes with their amazingly complex visual centers. The eyes have been called, by the Chinese, the "windows to the soul". The East values, too, what the eyes tell the brain: "The eyes believe what they see; the ears believe what other people tell them" (Chinese proverb). Complex visual transformations are produced in the brain by the signals conveyed from our eyes by way of the optic nerves. Although some do, most individuals with ADHD/ADD show little or no impairment of visual processing. By contrast, auditory processing problems are widespread in those with attention disorders.

Cerebellum

The *cerebellum,* termed "the diminutive brain," is located at the base of the cerebral hemispheres under the occipital and temporal lobes. It is sometimes considered part of the mid-brain and sometimes treated as a separate structure. It is a relatively large and intensely foliated structure that coordinates with all the motor regions of the cortex, as well as the basal ganglia, to coordinate and modulate movement.

Subcortical Brain Structures

Deep inside the brain are other structures critical to understanding attention disorders. Especially important are the thalamus, hypothalamus, limbic system and basal ganglia. The reticular activating system and the reticular formation serve critical functions in attention as well and will be discussed separately.

The cerebral hemispheres rest on the *thalamus*. The thalamus and hypothalamus are the most important structures in the midbrain. The thalamus, or *marriage bed*, joins many brain centers together and serves as a modulator of movement, sensation, emotions and behavior. All information except smell and sight must pass through the thalamus to the cerebral cortex, where the information is considered and analyzed and one's response is judiciously considered. The thalamus serves an important communication role between the limbic system and the basal ganglia as well.

The *hypothalamus* is located directly below the thalamus and regulates hormonal functions. Hunger, endocrine levels, water balance, sexual rhythms, and the autonomic nervous system are all controlled by the hypothalamus. It also controls many motivational states including anger, hunger, fatigue, arousal, tranquility and placidity. The behaviors that accompany emotional states are orchestrated by the hypothalamus as well. Damage to the hypothalamus, or the fiber tracks leading from it, can cause rage and aggressive attacks. Could the loss of control often observed in ADHD be a problem of hypothalamic function in some people? Could the excessive placidity of those with lethargic ADD also reflect hypothalamic dysfunctions? These are questions yet to be answered. Though small, less than four grams in the average adult, the hypothalamus regulates the body's most critical activities.

Many medications affect hypothalamic functions as can be seen from the side-effects of dry mouth and decreased appetite, among others. They have positive benefit on hypothalamic functions, enhancing emotional control and appropriate levels of arousal.

The *limbic system*, a rim of cortical structures tightly interconnected with the hypothalamus, has an important role in emotional states and attention. It forms a neural connection between the cerebral cortex and the hypothalamus, thus allowing for the interplay between thoughts and emotions. All of us easily recognize that one's thoughts affect one's feelings and, vice versa, that one's feelings can influence one's thoughts and behaviors. The components and connections of the limbic system are thought to contain most of the elements that define individual personality and patterns of behavior. It modulates emotions, memory and aspects of attention. It likewise influences a person's *cognition*, a neurological/educational term which refers to a person's thinking and reasoning.

The limbic system is not fully connected with the reticular system until adolescence. In ADHD/ADD children this connection occurs later than in their peers. The final completion of this complex inhibitory system usually results in greater impulse control, maturity and judgment (Healy, 1987).

The *basal ganglia* are nested deep inside the brain and are located near structures which are part of the limbic system. They are a group of nerve cell clusters, often called *nerve knots*, that serve important transmission and regulatory functions, primarily modulators of movement and integrators of sensory information. The basal ganglia help to coordinate physical movement by relaying information from the cerebral cortex to the brainstem and cerebellum. The basal ganglia are also activated when problems occur, serving a support role between various systems within the brain, assuring that they communicate effectively in times of distress.

The basal ganglia share with the limbic system a particular neurotransmitter, *dopamine*, that is considered important in the development of some psychiatric disorders, such as schizophrenia, and physical diseases such as Parkinson's disease and Huntington's chorea. Dopamine is thought to be implicated in ADHD/ADD as well.

Reticular Activating System

An understanding of the mechanisms of the reticular activating system and the reticular formation, among the first structures to be implicated in attention disorders, illustrates how neurochemical deficiencies and imbalances may affect all the attentional structures involved. It is stressed, however, that this explanation is simplistic and is used for illustrative purposes only.

The Role of the Reticular Activating System and the Reticular Formation in Attention, Concentration, Impulse Control and Behavior: A Model for Understanding the Processes of Attention

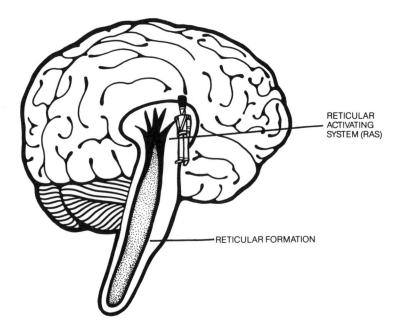

RETICULAR ACTIVATING SYSTEM (RAS)

RETICULAR FORMATION

A neurophysiologist, Dr. José Delgado, initiated much of the research on the brain using electrical stimulation, which in turn has provided much of the information on how the brain *attends*. Electrodes were implanted in the brain and the effects of stimulation on those areas were studied. It was shown that stimulation of the reticular formation produced a hyperalert animal. When the reticular formation was understimulated, sluggishness occurred and, if destroyed, a coma resulted.

The *reticular formation* consists of a group of densely packed nerve cells located in the central core of the brain stem. It runs from the top of the spinal cord into the middle of the brain (shaded area: illustration, p. 30). This small but crucial part of the brain contains nearly 70% of the brain's estimated 10 billion nerve cells.

A tiny, thimble-sized part of the reticular formation, called the *reticular activating system* (RAS), has a powerful role in determining our responses to the thousands of stimuli impinging on our brains every minute and thus a powerful role in directing consciousness. It serves as a kind of monitor (sometimes described as a "gatekeeper" to children), allowing selected stimuli to be relayed through the limbic system to the appropriate cortical areas. When a person has a deficient RAS, too many stimuli enter consciousness and result in poor attention, concentration and impulse control; distractibility; poor organization; low frustration tolerance; and many other symptoms associated with ADHD. An underaroused reticular formation, on the other hand, may not, in its sluggishness, transmit messages efficiently and effectively. Stimulant medications were initially thought to stimulate this arousal system so that it monitored, coordinated and organized incoming stimuli so they were transmitted properly to other centers in the brain, enabling them to perform their functions more efficiently. The role of the reticular system is not now considered central to ADHD/ADD symptoms but still appears to play a role. In both underaroused ADD and overaroused ADHD, stimulant medications appear to stimulate the reticular activating system and the reticular formation, along with other attention centers, thereby increasing, to a normal level, functions in both arousal and inhibition of the entire attention system.

Neurons: The Basic Structure of the Brain

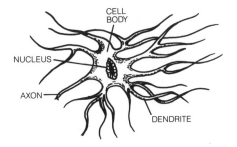

Each of the systems described consists of millions to billions of nerve cells. Nerve cells, called *neurons*, are the most basic units of the brain. Each is extraordinarily complex in function. Each consists of a cell body containing a *nucleus*; a long fiber called an *axon*; and an extensive number of branching fibers, or *dendrites*, that reach out to the other cells. The dendrites increase the surface of the neuron and enhance its receptivity to the influence of other cells. The more sophisticated the cell, the greater its number of dendrites. Also, the more advanced the species and the more efficient the brain, the greater the number of dendrites and neuronal connections. Cells in the cerebral cortex, the most advanced part of the brain, for example, may have 200,000 dendrites, while those in the medulla, the primitive brain, may have only 1,000 or so. In disorders such as Down's Syndrome, the dendrites are tiny, thinner, and fewer in number. The number and configuration of the dendrites is a rough approximation of the complexity of synaptic organization and, thus, the complexity of the brain itself.

The evolutionary process has resulted in an increased number of dendrites, thus increasing geometrically the number of possible neuronal connections. The more connections available, the more sophisticated the circuitry becomes. Thus, humans have more dendrites and neuronal connections than animals, and animals have more than insects. Experience and stimulation also increase the number of dendrites and thus the number of available neuronal connections. This is why early stimulation is critical to later ability and why those denied stimulation and exposure are not only duller intellectually and creatively, but emotionally as well. The death of infants from lack of contact with caregivers dramatically proves this point (Spitz, 1945). Spitz also found that children cared for in an institutional setting showed an average loss in developmental quotient from 124 to 72 within one year, while other researchers found that the I.Q.'s of thirteen mentally retarded children increased an average of 27.5 points over two years after they were removed from an overcrowded orphanage to living conditions where they became the center of attention (Skeels & Dye, 1938-1939).

Appropriate levels of early stimulation of infants and young children do, in fact, increase their potential in all areas. Rats raised with little or no stimulation showed adverse effects ranging from decreased problem-solving ability, to fear of exploration, to a reduction in the size of their brains (DeNelsky & Denenberg, 1967; Hebb, 1947; Rosenzweig, 1966). A striking finding of a study by Schwartz (1964) was that brain-injured rats raised in sensory-rich environments performed better than normal rats raised in sensory-poor environments. If ADHD/ADD were recognized in infancy, one can conjecture that it might be possible to intervene early with the appropriate stimulation, thereby increasing the number of dendrites and the neuronal connections available. While certainly an untested hypothesis, it is a possibility worth exploring. *Excessive* early stimulation does not, however, appear to be helpful, and can, in fact, be counter-productive.

I cannot resist stressing at this point how important habit and training are. Each new experience charts a unique neuronal course. After several repetitions, however, the activity becomes automatic, with the appropriate neurons firing easily and with little expenditure of energy or planning. It is like a path in the woods. Each time it is walked, the deeper and more permanent it becomes. Soon one can traverse the path with no thought at all. Unlike nature paths, neuronal pathways can remain for a lifetime. Driving a car is an example. One of the most complicated activities in which humans engage on a daily basis becomes a set of automatic responses because of the neuronal connections established.

With this knowledge, it makes sense to look at all those behaviors we desire in our children. Parents who are willing to insist that their children get up by alarms, put the top back on the toothpaste, put their dishes away, say "please" and "thank you," and organize their papers in special ways in notebooks can be assured that within a few months their children's brains take control and these very desirable traits become habitual neuronal patterns. It is important to remember that, at the neuronal level, good habits are as easy to establish as bad ones. It is as easy to put dirty clothes in a hamper as to throw them in a chair. While your children may resist such training, they will be grateful for their good neuronal pathways as adults. Even more grateful will be their spouses and employers!

ADHD/ADD children and adolescents seem to require more repetitions than average to establish these neuronal patterns. However, they do establish them if parents persist. You are encouraged to understand the way your child's brain functions and is organized to assist him in the greatest way possible. "I shouldn't have to tell you more than once!" may well become "I may have to tell you twenty times and follow through each time with consequences, but I *will* persist and you *can* learn." It is critical that positive reinforcement of the correct behavior be given immediately upon compliance to assist the learning process. This attitude, positive but persistent, is essential for all who live and work with ADHD/ADD children and adolescents.

Nerve Transmission

When a stimulus impinges upon the brain at a level strong enough to reach excitatory potential, the neuron "fires" and a nerve impulse is conveyed from the nucleus of the nerve body out the length of the axon to varying numbers of dendrites of other cells. To pass to another cell, the nerve signal must cross a tiny gap called a *synaptic cleft* at the *synapse*.

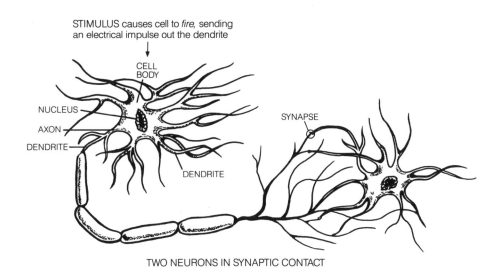

TWO NEURONS IN SYNAPTIC CONTACT

The power of determining one's own behavior is not the power of one entity (the mind) over another (the body), but the influence the brain has on itself. In other words, we are our brain.

—**Eric Hearth**
Researcher

Action at the Synaptic Cleft

At the synapse, the *electrical* signal releases a chemical called a *neurotransmitter* which is stored in vesicles, or packets, on the *presynaptic neuron*, i.e., the nerve cell before the synapse. Once the neurotransmitter has been released and is absorbed by an appropriate receptor on the *postsynaptic neuron*, i.e., the nerve cell after the synapse, the message continues its electrical transmission to the next synapse.

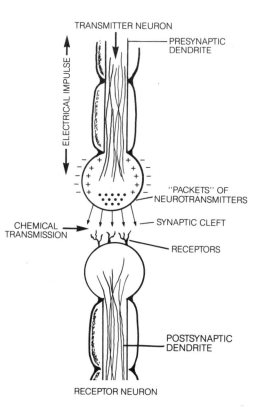

It is the neurotransmitters which enable the electrical impulse to be transmitted from one dendrite to another.   Without these neurotransmitters, the relay of impulses in the brain would be impossible.

Neurotransmitters: Chemical Messengers

There are many different neurotransmitters including norepinephrine, dopamine, choline, and serotonin, among others. Each neurotransmitter seeks a specific receptor on the postsynaptic neuron and cannot be absorbed by a receptor for another transmitter. For example, norepinephrine can only be absorbed by a norepinephrine receptor. Likewise, dopamine seeks out its own specific receptor.

Many disorders are known to be the result of specific neurotransmitter deficiencies. The level of dopamine, for example, is deficient in Parkinson's disease, while choline has been implicated in Alzheimer's disease. Some disorders result from an excess of a neurotransmitter, others from a deficiency, while still others may result from the neurotransmitters being out of balance.

The neurotransmitters most frequently implicated by the research in ADHD/ADD are norepinephrine and dopamine. Serotonin appears to be the significant neurotransmitter in Tourette Syndrome, obsessive-compulsive disorders and the overfocused behavior sometimes mistaken for underaroused ADD. The neurotransmitters will, in all likelihood, provide the keys to understanding many of man's most perplexing physical, behavioral, emotional and attentional disorders.

Neurotransmission is a complex process and involves both excitatory and inhibitory neurons. Inhibition is equally, if not more, important than excitation. In fact, the more sophisticated the organism, the more inhibitory neurons it has. Each physiological response is a complex interplay between all those inhibitory and excitatory neurons being stimulated and transmitting impulses at any given time.

Each neurotransmitter has a special function and each affects particular nerve cells in particular parts of the brain. ADHD and ADD have, for several years, been considered neurotransmitter disorders. Some medications used to treat attention disorders increase the availability of neurotransmitters on the presynaptic neurons (Ritalin and Dexedrine, for example), while others prevent the re-uptake of them on the presynaptic neurons, leaving more available at the synaptic cleft (Norpramin and Tofranil, for example).   The exact mechanisms of the medications traditionally used for ADHD and ADD will be addressed as each is reviewed in Section III.

Brain functioning is obviously a very complicated process with many potential sources of breakdown. Its complexity renders a search for easy solutions a futile endeavor. A comprehensive understanding of attention disorders is years away. A rudimentary knowledge of the brain does, at least, give us a roadmap. It helps us understand the effect of various interventions, both medical and nonmedical, and have greater confidence in the benefits of these treatments. Until the day that full knowledge of the brain is possible, we must rely upon clinical experience and observable effects for treatment protocols. We can then use that knowledge to develop hypotheses which will assist us in further researching the neurophysiology of this elusive disorder.

An understanding of neurological development is important, for it is more often delayed than not in those with ADHD/ADD and partially accounts for the immaturity of judgment and behavior noted so frequently in those with attention disorders. This delayed neurologic development should be a key consideration in all major academic and social decisions for the ADHD/ADD child or adolescent. The impact on school placement and academic performance are discussed at length in *Attention Without Tension: The Teacher's Handbook on Attention Disorders* (Copeland & Love, 1990).

WHAT IS *ATTENTION*?

Each moment the brain is constantly bombarded by thousands of stimuli, both externally from the environment and internally from the body and mind. It can process only a limited amount of this myriad of information impinging on it at any given moment. To make some sense of it, the brain must have a way to narrow the scope and focus of the information available. While no one knows exactly how this occurs, scientists do know that it is a highly directed process and one which follows certain rules. When attending to one activity, the brain ignores other sights, sounds and activities in the environment. This is beautifully illustrated by the child playing Nintendo who is oblivious to everything else around him. When the focus of interest and attention shifts, i.e., when he becomes hungry, totally different sensory data are acknowledged by the brain. When brain injury or neurochemical imbalances occur, the normal processes of attention break down.

As our previous discussion of the brain suggests, attention is also a distributed process that involves extensive areas of the brain, with each area making its own special contribution. Unfortunately there is not one *attention center* which might simplify both the process and our understanding of it. Rather, there is a complex network of neuronal connections throughout many structures of the brain, which function as a whole when attending, relating, organizing, assimilating and responding to stimuli. The term *attention* is a generic term, devised by professionals and researchers, to designate these many different processes.

Attention is clearly not one ability but many different skills. There are, likewise, different kinds of attention, including focused attention, selective attention, divided attention, sustained attention, and vigilance, among others. These different kinds of attention are unique; they also overlap in significant ways. Continued investigation and research are needed to assess the role of each in attentional problems and the contribution of each one to a particular individual's difficulties.

Attention, then, is a generic term used to indicate all those processes involved in a person's ability to discriminate adequately and to selectively respond to the myriad of information impinging on the brain at any given moment in time.

DISORDERS OF ATTENTION VERSUS LEARNING DISABILITIES

The relationship between learning disabilities, of which language disorders and reading disorders comprise a major portion, and attention deficit disorders is of increasing interest to researchers, educators and clinicians alike. ADHD and LD can occur independently or the two may co-occur. August and Garfinkel (1989) have coined the names "Behavioral ADD" for those who have ADHD/ADD without learning disabilities. They found that 80% of the group they studied met the criteria for ADHD but not for reading disability (Reading Disorder). By contrast, 20% of those diagnosed with ADHD also had a reading disorder. This group, with a co-occurrence of ADHD and RD, were called "Cognitive ADD."

Shaywitz (1986) had earlier found that 11% of ADHD-school-age children were also classified as learning disabled, while 33% of students classified as LD by the schools also had attention disorders. Holborow and Berry (1986) found that 41% of the LD school population they studied showed significant symptoms of ADHD, while Harter and his associates (1988) found that 16 of 27 (59%) of those they surveyed with a primary diagnosis of reading disorder also met ADHD diagnostic criteria.

The co-occurrence of ADHD/ADD and learning disabilities is an important finding and one which has significant treatment and educational implications. Public Law 94-142 provides for special education services for those who meet a statistical criterion of eligibility as learning disabled. The majority of ADHD/ADD students obviously will not meet these criteria, except the 11% to 30% who are also learning disabled. Those with ADHD or ADD without LD are increasingly demanding services under the provisions of Section 504 of P.L. 93-112.

The co-occurrence of language disorders and ADHD/ADD in preschoolers is so great as to suggest some causal connection. Baker and Cantwell (1987) found that 42% of the preschoolers they studied with diagnosed language disorders met the DSM-III-R criteria for ADHD/ADD. Love and Thompson (1988) did the converse of Cantwell. They studied the preschoolers referred to a psychiatric outpatient clinic and found that 48% had a dual diagnosis of language disorder and ADHD. The actual numbers are quite revealing: 56 of the 75 (75%) with language disorders also had an ADHD diagnosis, and 56 of the 85 (66%) with an ADHD diagnosis also had an independently diagnosed language disorder. Such co-occurrence is too significant to be ignored. It not only suggests that attention disorders and language disorders co-occur, but suggests that the difficulties compound each other to such a degree that the children are referred early in their lives to psychiatric outpatient facilities. Only children with major problems are referred at this age to this kind of treatment center.

In clinical practice similar findings have emerged. We have begun treating preschoolers as young as 3 1/2 and 4 who have dual diagnoses of language disorders and attention disorders with stimulant medication. Significant impact on their language development has occurred as a result of the medication, many times prior to the benefits of language therapy. Clinical observations suggest that ADHD preschoolers with language disorders who are treated with medication make significantly more progress in language development than those not medically treated.

While stimulants are not utilized routinely in most practices for behavioral assistance with preschoolers, the positive effect on language development will perhaps require a rethinking of our position on the use of medication in young children, especially if our goal is to prevent, as much as possible, future reading disorders and language disabilities. In my opinion, the latter two can often be far more devastating than an attention disorder.

Brain differences and similarities between those with language disorders, reading disorders, learning disabilities and attention deficit disorders are already the subject of investigation. Gross-Glenn et al.

(1986), in their study of dyslexics, showed decreased glucose metabolism in left hemispheric areas associated with language while engaged in a reading task. Zametkin's study, previously cited, showed decreased glucose metabolism in frontal areas associated with attention and impulse control while subjects performed an auditory attention task (auditory CPT). Harter et al. (1988) found a population-specific pattern of ERP (evoked response potential on EEG) when reading disabled students were excluded from the ADHD population and vice-versa.

In a study of major significance, Hynd et al. (1990) studied the planum temporale region of the brain previously found significant in dyslexic populations. They obtained ROI (region of interest) measurements on MRI scans for the width and area of the left and right anterior and posterior regions, length of left and right insular regions, and for the total brain area. ADD/H, severely dyslexic and normal subjects were studied. Their findings were as follows:

1)   Seventy percent of the normal and ADD/H populations had the expected left greater than right (L>R) pattern of brain asymmetry. Only 10% of the dyslexic children had L>R; 90% had R>L asymmetry. This pattern appears unique to dyslexics and may be related to deviations in normal patterns of cortical development during the fifth to seventh month of fetal gestation.

2)   Dyslexics had a bilaterally smaller insular region and a significantly smaller left planum temporale than did normals or ADD/H subjects.

3)   Both the dyslexic and ADD/H children had significantly smaller right anterior-width measurements of the insular region.

In summary, ADHD and normal children manifested similar brain morphologic findings in every area except the width of the anterior planum region. This would suggest that, while ADHD children are more like normals, they do share at least one characteristic in common with reading disabled students.

Medications such as the stimulants or tricyclic antidepressants improve the attention system. It is currently believed that they do not improve the functioning of the cortical neurons and the neurotransmitters in those regions involved in specific learning tasks such as phonetic decoding, word naming, reading comprehension and math conceptualization, among others. When a child or adolescent's academic and learning difficulties have their root cause in attentional problems, medicating for the ADHD or ADD can be quite helpful. By contrast, medications for attention disorders rarely improve true learning disabilities. For example, the attention system involves cortical neurons and specific neurotransmitters which regulate the child's ability to concentrate when reading. Other cerebral cortical centers and neurotransmitters determine his ability to read and to comprehend what he reads. Improving a child's attention, concentration, and impulse control can improve his ability to settle down to the reading task and his ability to focus. This ability to concentrate and accomplish tasks usually improves reading skill. While this is a secondary effect, it is one which can be quite dramatic. It is especially astounding when the child's academic deficiencies are primarily attentional in nature. Many parents have been pleasantly surprised by their ADHD/ADD child's newfound ability to read a book for pleasure after treatment of the attention disorder. On the other hand, no amount of medication will enable the truly dyslexic child to read as most other children do.

It is often confusing to the novice, and to professionals as well, which effect may be primary and which secondary. Effective intervention, however, necessitates separating, as much as possible, the neurologic etiology of learning disabilities from the neurologic regulatory problems in attentional disorders and determining the contribution of each to a child's academic difficulties so that both can be treated simultaneously as needed. Treating ADHD/ADD will not cure language disorders, dyslexia, true auditory discrimination problems, or math disorders, for example. Likewise, tutoring and remediation will not effectively diminish attention disorders. The importance of recognizing brain differences very early in a child's life cannot be overstated. By doing so his neurologic processing can perhaps be maximized, at this pliable and compensatory age, with both medication and appropriate stimulation such as language therapy or visual-motor assistance, for example. By doing so we may be able to enhance the development of those areas affected. Awareness of both the complexity and the overlap of LD and ADHD/ADD behooves us to seek intervention at the earliest possible age.

SUMMARY

It is hoped that this brief description of the structures, functions and organization of the brain have helped the reader understand the neurologic mechanisms involved in ADHD/ADD and the role medicine can play in altering the abnormalities of neurotransmitter production and transmission involved. Those who desire a more comprehensive understanding of the neurophysiology of attention disorders are referred to Appendix 2 for a listing of excellent review articles by leaders in the field.

*No forms of raising can produce ADD
[ADHD] problems in a child not
temperamentally predisposed to them.*

—Paul Wender, M.D., 1987

3
Causes of
ADHD/ADD

After one has a good understanding of the problems characteristic of ADHD/ADD and their neurophysiology, "What causes attention disorders?" is usually the next question. Attention disorders are especially perplexing since they manifest in biological, psychological, educational and social ways.

Nature or nurture ... genetics or environment? Which is the *true* source of a person's being? This debate has been waged for decades by scientists attempting to understand the forces which determine man's behavior. Is it his biological heritage which determines his destiny? Or is it the environment in which fate places him? Is it his home? ... his school? ... or his neighborhood which causes him to have difficulty? Or is it a combination of all of these?

Responsibility for ADHD/ADD has swung with the pendulum between biological and environmental explanations. In the last decade, however, increasing evidence mounts that, like many other disorders previously considered *behavioral, emotional*, or *environmentally induced*, many attention deficit disorders are part of our genetic inheritance—a factor of our biological constitutions at birth. Genes and physiology, at this juncture in history, are believed to play a greater role than environmental factors. Psychosocial and educational factors must not be underestimated, however, for they significantly determine how one's genetic script and one's physiologic nature will be acted out upon the stage of life. In our experience, and that of others, a person's adjustment is ultimately determined by the interplay of all of those biological, psychological, educational and social factors which simultaneously prevailed in his developmental years and those operating at any given moment in the present.

ADHD/ADD SYNDROME VALIDITY

Before addressing causes, however, it is important to address an issue that periodically arises about ADHD/ADD, i.e., "Is there such an entity and can we accurately distinguish it from other behavioral syndromes?" This issue has produced confusion among those responsible for assisting children and adolescents with attention disorders, especially school personnel, and has resulted in delays in addressing those students' academic, social and emotional needs in the school setting.

In 1970, *The Myth of the Hyperactive Child* was written in response to increased use of stimulant medication in California (Schrag & Divoky, 1970). Fear and uncertainty prevailed in the minds of many as a result of the authors' negative portrayal of hyperactive children and the use of medication to treat them. Despite a Congressional investigation which supported the concept and the medical management of hyperactivity in children (U.S. Office of Child Development, 1971), this book is believed to have delayed the investigation and treatment of attention disorders for many years.

In the mid- to late 1980's, the Church of Scientology supported litigation in several states whereby parents filed lawsuits against school boards, physicians, the American Psychiatric Association and teachers, among others. This group sensationalized ADHD/ADD, especially the use of medications such as Ritalin in the treatment of it (CCHR, 1987). Widespread media attention was subsequently given to attention disorders, particularly to the use of stimulant medication. Most of the publicity was quite negative (*New York Times*, May 5, 1987; *Atlanta Constitution*, April 13, June 8, November 10, November 29, 1987).

These complaints led initially to a task-force study in Georgia where the first major lawsuit was filed (Georgia DOE, 1987) and then to an investigation by Congress. The Secretary of Health and Human Services convened an Interagency Committee of the National Institutes of Health to report to Congress on Learning Disabilities. The Committee concluded that "Pharmacotherapy for ADD originated 50 years ago, and at the present time the ameliorative effects of medications in ADD are well established." It also recommended a greater research focus on defining characteristics of the whole spectrum of ADD patients, noting that currently "... the number of affected children may be seriously under-estimated" (Interagency Committee, 1987). CIBA Pharmaceutical Company, the manufacturer of Ritalin, was investigated that same spring of 1988 by the FDA and given a letter of complete compliance and safety (U.S. Department of Health and Human Services, 1988).

Despite continued investigation by some of the best researchers in the field of medicine and affirmative documentation by unbiased agencies, including Congress itself, some continue to question whether "hyperactivity ... is really a disorder at all" (Salholz, 1987; Vatz & Weinberg, 1988; Toufexis, 1989; & Kealy, 1990). Alfie Kohn, in an article written for the *Atlantic Monthly* (November, 1989) and reprinted in part in *Education Week* (November 22, 1989), questioned the existence of the disorder itself. Because he is well-respected as a writer, his article created confusion and skepticism and has helped delay understanding of this disorder. His criticisms appear more accurately directed at diagnostic and treatment methodologies than to the physiologic nature of these problems. Only a knowledgeable reader, however, would understand this distinction. Many, most in fact, did not.

The findings of the investigation by Dr. Zametkin, mentioned earlier, which demonstrated reduced glucose metabolism in various areas of the brain associated with the regulation of attention and motor activity, as well as the findings of others, represent a major advance in establishing the neurophysiologic nature of attention deficit disorders (Zametkin et al., 1990; Lou et al., 1989; Harter et al., 1988; Hynd et al., 1990). Much work remains to understand, more completely, the nature of these diverse and complex disorders, but a clear breakthrough in establishing the neurologic validity of attention disorders has certainly occurred. Those who would argue that ADHD or ADD is a "yuppie disease," "a parent's excuse" or "the latest vogue" will have difficulty supporting such a view. From this time on, no one can write, "No generally accepted evidence of an organic, or biological, cause of hyperactivity has been found" (Kohn, 1989).

It is important that parents, educators and professionals be assured of, and comfortable with, the validity of the concept of attention deficit disorders, for they will, in all likelihood, be exposed to controversy surrounding ADHD/ADD. One of the most important jobs of professionals and teachers will be that of first educating themselves and then educating parents to help them overcome their misinformation and anxiety about attention disorders and the treatments for them. Parents must become well informed if they are to be of assistance to their children. Each reader, whether parent, teacher, physician, or health professional, is encouraged to investigate all points of view. Only when fully informed can one be satisfied that one's knowledge and actions are consistent with the truth, as best it can be known at any given moment, and ultimately at peace with one's goals and treatments for the ADHD/ADD child, adolescent or adult.

CAUSES OF PHYSIOLOGICAL
ADHD/ADD

ADHD/ADD are complicated problems and, like other complex physiological problems, they have multiple causes. A close analogy is that of vision. One might experience visual problems, i.e., the inability to see correctly, as the result of a wide variety of factors such as disease (glaucoma), structural abnormalities (near-sightedness), injury, genetic defect, or even emotional disturbances. As in the area of visual problems, there is no single cause of attention disorders, nor is there any single solution. However, ADHD/ADD are, at this time, considered by most researchers and practitioners to be physiological problems. Accurately diagnosed attention disorders are not considered behavioral, emotional, learning, or environmental problems, although such problems may occur concurrently with attention disorders. Recent scientific investigations show quite conclusively that there are physiologic differences from the norm, primarily in the neurochemistry of the brain. Structural differences may also exist in some people with attention disorders, especially those who have experienced even minimal brain damage from accidents, infections or epilepsy, for example. New techniques for studying the brain offer great hope for further understanding in the future. Computerized brain scans (BEAMS), blood flow studies, positron emission tomography (PET) and magnetic resonance imaging (MRI) will contribute significantly to our growing body of knowledge about ADHD/ADD.

Causes of attention problems are grouped into four major categories. These include:

1) Constitutional or innate biological factors. These relate particularly to heredity, temperament and genetic makeup.
2) Organic factors. Organic factors include all physiologic insults and damage to the central nervous system and/or brain.

3) Attention disorders secondary to other medical problems.

4) Environmental toxins, including lead, formaldehyde, mercury and chemical pesticides.

Diet, nutrition, allergies and food intolerances appear to play a role in the attentional problems of a few. Likewise, some educational practices, as well as social, cultural and stress factors, contribute to attentional problems in many children and adolescents and can exacerbate markedly the symptoms of true ADHD and ADD.

Heredity

Heredity, at this time, is the most common identifiable cause of ADHD/ADD symptoms. Those of us working in the field have, throughout the years, noticed that many of the children and adolescents with attention disorders with whom we have worked have ADHD or ADD parents. Parents of ADHD and ADD children and adolescents quickly identify the symptoms in themselves as adults or in their early years, especially while in school.

The role of heredity in ADHD/ADD is an area of significant investigation at this time. Most of the investigations have compared hyperactive (ADHD) children with non-ADHD peers. Willerman (1973) studied 93 sets of twins and found that identical twins are much more likely than fraternal twins to both have attention disorders. Identical twins have the same genetic make-up, whereas, in fraternal twins, only one of the twins may have the faulty gene. Twin studies are among the most frequently used to study genetic determination of characteristics.

Researchers have found that there are four times as many hyperactive parents of hyperactive children as there are hyperactive parents of non-ADHD children (Morrison & Stewart, 1971; Cantwell, 1972). These same researchers also found that ADD is more common in fathers and uncles of ADD children than in the relatives of non-

ADHD/ADD children. The genetic contribution to this disorder has become increasingly apparent and is being investigated intensively as we attempt to understand attention disorders and to intervene effectively in them.

In working with the parents of children with attention disorders, we have found them eager to describe their own difficulties if they find someone willing to listen. It is, therefore, crucial that assistance in the form of support groups or educational groups be available, as well as medical and psychotherapeutic interventions for parents. Long histories of underachievement, negative feedback, and an ongoing sense of failure often result in problems with depression, marginal adjustment and other symptoms of emotional, social and economic distress. ADD parents have much more difficulty than non-ADD parents in meeting their children's needs for organization, structure, routine, limit-setting and rational discipline. Those who truly wish to help children must assist their parents simultaneously. A major recommendation of a task force reporting to the Governor and General Assembly of Virginia on "The Effects of the Use of Methylphenidate" (1991) was:

> The task force recommends that parents and families of ADHD children participate actively in the professional management of these children. Membership in organizations of ADHD parents and families is encouraged as a means for understanding the disorder, its treatment, and the vital role played by the family in the homes of ADHD children.

In addition to seeking assistance through support groups, parents are encouraged to seek help through medical and psychotherapeutic intervention when needed. A listing of support groups is given in Appendix 3.

Organic Factors

Since the 1940's, when an outbreak of encephalitis revealed a marked similarity of symptoms of brain-damaged children to those of hyperactive children, investigators have continued to look for organic causes of attention disorders. While organic factors lost much credence in the years from 1960 to 1980, they have recently regained some scientific support. Many early studies suggested that brain damage or minimal brain injury as a result of factors related to difficult pregnancies or deliveries might be the cause of ADHD and ADD. Unusually short or long labors, post-maturity, very young mothers, mothers who smoked, fetal distress both before and during delivery, toxemia and eclampsia have all been suggested as causative factors and may, in fact, contribute to these symptom complexes (Hartsough & Lambert, 1985; Denson, et al., 1975).

Other studies cast doubt on the importance of these factors. One of the largest studies of pregnancies, the Collaborative Perinatal Project of the National Institute of Neurological and Communicative Disorders and Strokes (Nelson & Ellenberg, 1979), was a multicenter, collaborative project that studied all aspects of pregnancy, labor and delivery. On long-term follow-up of the 550,000 children originally evaluated at birth, they found no correlation between Apgar scores and attention disorder symptoms. Both they and those who have found differences between normal and ADD groups in incidence of pre- and post-natal complications concluded that these variables had only minor significance.

Of growing concern in the field, however, is the number of babies being born whose parents used and/or abused drugs such as cocaine, crack and heroin either before pregnancy, affecting the sperm or egg, or during pregnancy, harming the developing fetus. There are also increasing numbers of *Fetal Alcohol Syndrome (FAS) babies*. Problems of ADHD/ADD and learning disabilities (LD) are especially acute in states where drug and alcohol abuse is widespread. In addition, premature infants as tiny as two and one-half pounds are routinely being saved with our advances in medical technology. These children are at much greater risk for learning disabilities, attention disorders and hyperactivity. The educational system must brace itself for a significant increase in the need for special education services for organically-caused attention disorders and learning disabilities over the next decades.

Dr. Hans Lou and his associates (1989), using emission-computed tomography blood-flow studies, found a consistent pattern of decreased blood flow in the basal ganglia and in the border zones between the major arterial distributions within the brain. They suggested that these differences were caused by hypoxic ischemic brain injury. While their conclusions are still tentative and require further investigation, their findings do support the existence of physiological differences between normal and ADD children's blood-flow patterns. Parenthetically, they showed that Ritalin (methylphenidate) increased the profusion of blood to these areas, thereby decreasing the symptoms of attention deficits.

As our understanding of the brain increases and improved measurements of structural and neurochemical differences are available, these early insults may, indeed, prove predictive. The crucial difference for long-term handicap may rest, not in whether there is early minimal injury, but in how well the infant and young child's environment enables him to overcome these early effects. A follow-up study of a group of Hawaiian Island infants, by Emmy Werner (1989), showed that the long-term effects of risk factors could be overcome if the environment provided adequate protective factors and good sources of support. The family and its social and emotional resources were crucial to good long-term prognosis. The importance of early identification and the ability of a positive environment to overcome early insult were, likewise, revealed in the study reported previously by Schwartz (1964). His findings revealed that sensory-rich environments significantly aided performance in brain-injured rats. They, in fact, performed better than normal rats raised in sensory-poor environments. The implications for early identification and intervention are profound. For the interested parent, teacher or professional, a preschool symptom checklist for attentional, learning and behavioral disorders is included in Appendix 4.

In summary, it appears that organic factors do contribute to attention disorders in some children. However, while a significant finding, organically-caused attention disorders are not believed to contribute substantially to the ADHD/ADD population at this time. In ten years, however, they may represent a very significant percentage of those affected.

Attention Disorders Secondary to Other Medical Problems

Most investigators state very strongly that the diagnosis of attention disorders is not appropriate to characterize behaviors seen in children with other medical problems. I certainly concur with their judgments and believe that part of the purpose of the medical evaluation is to rule out any possible contribution of such medical problems as hypo- or hyperthyroidism, pituitary problems, narcolepsy, hypoglycemia and seizure disorders, among others, to the symptom-complex presentation. Likewise, bipolar disorder, depression and other disorders considered *emotional* may mimic ADHD or ADD and should be ruled out.

The necessity of a complete medical evaluation was dramatically illustrated to me by a first grader referred to us by her teacher who suspected an attention disorder in her young student. The symptoms were classic.

Sarah presented for the evaluation as a very tall, thin, beautiful first grader whose slightly bulging, large blue eyes were her most prominent feature. She was restless and fidgety, very tense, and had great difficulty attending. After thirty minutes, the evaluation was discontinued. Sarah's eyes were too reminiscent of patients with whom I had worked when teaching in medical school.

I expressed my concerns to Sarah's mother, who then described events which had not seemed relevant earlier and that she had omitted in the initial interview: Sarah had grown over two inches in three months, she had become very thin, and she was irritable and tense. Sarah was referred to her pediatrician who hospitalized her immediately for acute hyperthyroidism. Treating her for attention deficit disorder, especially with stimulant medication, could well have been a disaster.

While most medical disorders are not considered to cause ADHD/ADD, there are noteworthy medical problems which co-occur with ADHD/ADD a great percentage of the time and may have common origins. One is Tourette Syndrome, which is discussed in detail in Chapter 12; another is otitis media, or ear infections. Those of us working in the fields of attention disorders and learning disabilities are struck with the number of children who present with histories of chronic ear infections. Recent research in this area has confirmed clinical suspicions. One investigation found that in a group of children experiencing school failure, 69% of the hyperactive children had a history of ten or more ear infections, while only 20% of the nonhyperactives had more than ten (Hagerman & Falkenstein, 1987). This finding is too significant to ignore. This same investigation found that 94% of the hyperactive children studied had had more than three ear infections, while only 50% of the non-hyperactive children who were experiencing significant school difficulty had had more than three. We are increasingly aware of the relationship between language disorders, reading disorders and attention disorders (Masland & Masland, 1988; Gray & Kavanaugh, 1985). The implication of allergies and ear infections, as well, in this constellation of difficulties is certainly one we need to pursue.

Another possible source of ADHD/ADD problems secondary to medical problems is seizure disorders and the medications involved. Research has demonstrated that children with epilepsy have more inattention, impulsivity and other characteristics of ADHD/ADD (Holdsworth & Whitmore, 1974). Those treated with phenobarbital and other anticonvulsant drugs tend to have an exacerbation of their attention deficit symptoms (AAP, Committee on Drugs, 1985). According to Drs. Trimble and Thompson (1982), sedative anticonvulsants, such as phenobarbital and clonazepam, as well as phenytoin, can decrease the child's ability to concentrate and learn. "Adverse behavioral responses to anticonvulsants such as the syndrome of hyperactivity, aggressiveness and irritability secondary to phenobarbital" occur in others (Silverstein et al., 1982). Anticonvulsants are thought to depress the reticular and other attention centers, thus making the attention system even more sluggish and inefficient.

In recent years, many of those with seizure disorders have been placed on Tegretol (carbamazepine). They are showing significant improvement in their attention deficit symptoms as well as their seizures. Other children, adolescents and adults are now being diagnosed as having *complex partial seizures* that are causing symptoms which mimic ADHD or ADD. They obviously improve much more readily when treated with Tegretol than with stimulant medications. Those with ADHD/ADD and *grand mal seizures* may require phenobarbital or Dilantin in combination with stimulant medications. Seizure disorders will be addressed in greater detail in Chapter 12.

Another medical area of concern is that of allergies. Clinical judgment and some research suggest an association between asthma, allergies and attention deficit disorders (Marshall, 1989). Others have not found a higher incidence of allergies and asthma among those with ADHD and ADD, although every parent and teacher knows that a child in the throes of allergies is less attentive, more lethargic and less productive. It is important to be aware of this relationship and also of the medications children take for control of allergy symptoms. Clinical evidence suggests that some of the medications taken for asthma and allergy may cause or exacerbate attentional difficulties and thus mimic ADD. Antihistamines taken with stimulants are believed to decrease slightly the effectiveness of the stimulant medications. If a child needs both, care is needed in the administration of each to maximize their benefits.

Environmental Toxins

Environmental toxins including lead, formaldehyde and chemical pesticides, among others, can cause ADHD and ADD symptoms. Research shows that elevated lead levels produce symptoms of inattention, impulsivity, over-arousal and others associated with attention disorders (Needleman et al., 1979; David et al., 1972). Lead is a toxic substance. Over the years the acceptable lead level established by the Communicable Disease Center (CDC) has been consistently decreased. A report by the CDC stated that "new research shows that low levels of lead contribute to childhood learning disabilities and high school dropout rates" (Seabrook, 1990). The U.S. Centers for Disease Control were expected to urge new public health measures, the first since 1985, to reduce the health effects of lead. "Numerous studies leave no doubt that low levels of lead have profound effects on children" (Kate Mahoffey, Lead Expert, EPA). Dr. Herbert Needleman, a University of Pittsburgh pediatrician, suggested that "brain damage from lead may also play a major role in the school's drop-out rate" (Seabrook, 1990).

Lead lurks, according to the findings of the Agency for Toxic Substances and Diseases, in the following:

- Plumbing: Lead pipes and pipes soldered with lead may contaminate water for 10.4 million children.
- Cans: About 1 million children may be exposed to lead from the few cans that are still sealed with lead, which can leach into food.
- Auto emissions: About 5 million children live where they may inhale lead from the burning of leaded gasoline.

- **Dust and soil:** Lead deposits from paint or gasoline endanger 5.9 to 11 million children.
- **Paint:** Old paint, especially in deteriorating housing, endangers about 12 million children. (Agency for Toxic Substances and Disease Registry)

While no one is certain of the precise effects of low lead levels in the brain, we can surmise from these investigations and reports that low lead levels may well produce low levels of attention deficit symptoms. In addition to the sources cited, it is noteworthy that children's text and library books continue to be printed with lead-based ink, as is wrapping paper.

Parents of children with attention disorders would do well to examine all potential sources of symptoms. Elevated lead levels can be accurately determined by appropriate laboratory tests, primarily those measuring the lead content in urine samples collected over 24-48 hours. Blood tests are not generally helpful in assessing chronic, low-level exposure to lead.

Chemical pesticides are also clearly a problem in many children. They can cause not only ADHD/ADD symptoms, but can produce life-threatening asthma and allergic reactions as well.

Formaldehyde is also becoming implicated in attention. This toxin has crucial implications for all who use duplicating machines, both schools and offices. Many copying machines produce methanol fumes which are converted by the body into formaldehyde. According to the U.S. Environmental Protection Agency, repeated exposure to formaldehyde can cause sensitization in an estimated "fewer than 20% but perhaps more than 10% of the general population ... who may respond to extremely low levels of formaldehyde" (Carey, EPA Technical Report, 1983).

Some schools have already had to take corrective measures to remedy the condition (Maloney, 1982), especially to increase ventilation. Those schools which may still use ditto machines are especially at risk for problems. The purple ink of dittos is made with formaldehyde. Students who are sniffing their ditto sheets may be particularly vulnerable. Levels of methanol can be measured by a device from the National Institute of Safety and Health (NIOSH).

Most schools that are aware of the dangers are eliminating this potential source of aggravation. Parents of formaldehyde-sensitive children should also become wary of the many other sources of formaldehyde exposure, including fabric, clothing, carpet, paint, wallboard, and pressed wood in furniture, among others. One child with whom we worked became almost stuporous after his room was redecorated. The new paint, carpet and furniture were saturated with formaldehyde, to which he was quite sensitive. One wonders if children from low socioeconomic backgrounds are not particularly exposed since less expensive building materials (paneling, for example) contain significant amounts of formaldehyde.

Household pesticides are also a problem for many. The EPA, in a major study released in 1990, found these chemicals "dozens of times higher than outdoor concentrations" (Weisskopf, 1990). The neurologically and physiologically damaging effects of lead and chemicals are much greater in children because their bodies are still in the formative stages of development. Adults, too, can have major adverse consequences from low levels of exposure to these toxins.

The potential sources of environmental contribution to attention disorders is an area we must begin to address as a professional and scientific community. The risk posed by these toxins should also be assessed by every parent of an ADHD/ADD child or adolescent. Medications for attention disorders can mask critical underlying causative factors. Suspected environmental sources of difficulty should be ruled out before beginning a medication regimen to alleviate the symptoms.

"The important thing is not to stop questioning. Curiosity has its own reason for existing. One cannot help but be in awe when he contemplates the mysteries of eternity, of life, of the marvelous structure of reality. It is enough if one tries merely to comprehend a little of this mystery every day. Never lose a holy curiosity."

—Albert Einstein

OTHER CAUSES OF ATTENTIONAL PROBLEMS

Diet, Nutrition, Allergies, and Food Intolerances

There has never been an area of behavioral research more controversial than this one. Drs. Ben Feingold (1975) and Lendon Smith (1976) began making assertions about sugar, food additives and salicylates some 15 years ago. I remember vividly trying these diets with patients from 1975 to 1980 and, like others, becoming very discouraged at the few who responded significantly to the very rigorous diets imposed. However, these men were pioneers and, while their notions were simplistic, they may have been on the right track. In our own practice, we have found that many children do have allergies, and there is a history of food intolerance in others, dairy products being the most common by far. While the medical community has rightfully been suspicious of theories not rigorously proven in scientific investigations, recent work suggests that there may, perhaps, be a link between food intolerances and ADHD/ADD symptoms.

Dr. Keith Conners, one of the foremost pioneers in attention deficit disorders, is now devoting much of his research to food-related problems. Early studies conducted did not support evidence of a dietary link to attention disorders (Conners, 1980). However, recent investigations that have eliminated multiple food offenders, instead of single foods, suggest that such diets may be effective in treating some children and adolescents with attention disorders (Egger, et al., 1985; Kaplan, et al., 1989). A definitive answer on the role of diet and food intolerances will require much more rigorous research. Conners (1990) has also found a link between when certain foods are eaten and the effect on behavior. For example, sugar and carbohydrates eaten alone for breakfast cause problems. However, they are tolerated if eaten with protein. As he jokingly says, "You can have doughnuts for breakfast if you eat tuna fish as well."

It can be helpful to screen for allergies and food intolerances. Both are usually apparent from clinical observations, developmental history and the family's medical background. Those who may have allergies are encouraged to have an allergy workup by an allergist, while those with possible food intolerances are encouraged to consider an elimination and challenge diet for approximately ten days to two weeks, if the family is willing and able to do so. If there is adequate indication, it can be worthwhile to investigate this area of difficulty because it is one over which both parents and children have control. Many parents are more comfortable using medication when they feel they have exhausted all other avenues of intervention. On the other hand, delaying the use of medicine unnecessarily for weeks or months can be detrimental. Giving the family unrealistic hope of a "cure" or causing undue stress and expense for the family are, likewise, not recommended.

Educational Factors

Attentional difficulties are inadvertently being created by some of our current educational practices and emphases. It is critical that these educational issues be addressed separately and problems originating from them not be confused with or allowed to cloud a clear approach to ADHD/ADD. Some of these problematic educational practices include:

a)   The current curricula of many schools are too advanced for the level of neurologic development of most kindergarten through third and fourth grade students. These children, taught with methods neurologically *over their heads*, cannot cope with the excessive demands for sustained attention and the emphasis on left-brain learning strategies.

b)   Many children, from kindergarten through college, are overplaced in school. Developmentally and neurologically immature children have shorter attention spans than neurologically mature students and cannot compete successfully with their same-age peers.

c)   Much of our information on *how* people learn is being ignored. Teachers are inadvertently only exacerbating problems of attention with inappropriate teaching methods.

d)   There is a noticeable decrease in opportunities for physical exercise during the school day and, thus, children are not getting desperately needed energy-releasing, tension-modulating, physical-activity breaks which reduce restlessness and enhance attention.

These educational factors, and others, are addressed in depth in *Attention Without Tension: The Teacher's Handbook on Attention Disorders* (Copeland & Love, 1990).

While I could cite other problems, a treatise on the problems with our current curricula and our methods of teaching is not our purpose here. However, it is important to recognize other causes of inattentive and distractible behavior in our classrooms. Only by acknowledging these difficulties can parents and teachers help restructure and redirect our educational system to eliminate the problems.

CULTURAL, SOCIAL AND EMOTIONAL FACTORS

While attention deficit disorders are physiologic in origin, there are many cultural, social and emotional factors which are creating symptoms of attention disorders in some, and exacerbating significantly the ADHD/ADD symptoms of others.

Decline of Discipline, Responsibility, and the American Work Ethic

Few things help an individual more than to place responsibility on him, and to let him know you trust him.
—Booker T. Washington

From the early years of America's development through World War II, emphasis on the work ethic and individual accomplishment through one's own efforts were the prevailing values. Perseverance, hard work, determination and an unwillingness to accept defeat were characteristic of both the individual and the culture at large.

With the advent of technology and the unprecedented wealth which was amassed following World War II, people's pursuits gradually shifted to enjoyment, leisure and personal fulfillment. Children, historically desired partially because they contributed to the work force, were no longer needed to meet labor needs, but were now wanted to meet adults' emotional needs. Parents' goals for their children also changed. Traditional attitudes and values, summed up in the parental declaration, "You are part of the family and *must* help," were abandoned, as our goals focused on pleasing the child ... making him happy. If he were happy, we as parents thought we would be fulfilled. As our child-oriented society evolved, permissive and democratic child-rearing practices replaced the autocratic principles which previously guided parents.

Our society has been in the throes of self- and child- indulgence since the 1950's. The effect of this philosophy has had far-reaching consequences, culminating in the '80's in unprecedented materialism and self-interest. Narcissism and materialism are insidious. Christopher Dickey perhaps said it best: "To rich and poor alike the pervasive consumerism of the last twenty years has left a hollow sense of purposelessness" (*Newsweek*, 1991).

Other effects of our shift in values have not been as obvious but have had equally negative repercussions for our youth. Many children, adolescents and young adults today lack the self-discipline which is learned from enforced structure, responsibility and consequences. This is evidenced by the twenty-two million adult children over the age of eighteen who are either unable or unwilling to support themselves and have returned home to live with their parents (Okimoto & Stegall, 1987). Many also lack the internalized structure and organization which come from years of following Mom and Dad's rules and schedule. Many verbalize feeling lost and have little sense of purpose or direction.

While indulgence and the lack of self-discipline and strength to overcome adversity have not caused physiologic ADHD or ADD, it can be reasonably asserted that they have resulted in very similar symptoms. For those with attention disorders, the societal undermining of structured demands, firm expectations and unwavering consequences for compliance or noncompliance, has made the road they travel infinitely more difficult. Many ADHD/ADD children raised in the 1920's, '30's and '40's succeeded because there was, perhaps, no choice.

Instability in Children's Lives

Never before in the history of our country have our children been asked to cope with so many changes. Before they are two months old and have bonded with their mothers, many are whisked off to daycare where they may be expected to relate to ten to thirty people in an eight-hour period. By the time they are in school, they may go to daycare, then to school, back to daycare and perhaps home ... or off to another location. Some even wonder *who* will pick them up ... or *if* they will.

Added to this instability of daily location is the increasing fragmentation of the family itself. Frequent moves by the family, disorganized environments, endless fast-food meals, exhausted and frequently absent parents ... all render organization and predictability for the child mindless euphemisms. Divorce, single-parent homes, step-families, sleeping in a different home three or four times a month ... the adjustments we expect children to make happily and successfully are endless.

If the instability of the home environment were not adequate to create fragile personalities, schools are unwittingly doing their fair share. Many schools have given up the stability of the traditional class, with only one teacher and only twenty-five children with whom one must learn to cope. Instead, children as young as five and six may change classes or teachers three or four times a day. Those who have any problems with organization easily feel overwhelmed and helpless. Attention-disordered children do not have a prayer. In addition, a child or teen may attend a school of several hundred to two thousand students. It can be very hard to feel special and unique when surrounded by hundreds of others like yourself, each vying for a moment of notice, a chance to succeed. Only a superstar can make a team for which there are dozens of hopeful candidates. Even the slightest attention disorder will be magnified under these conditions.

Not only are home and school unstable, but the world is as well. Nightly TV viewing of national and international events either dulls the senses to stupefaction or creates so much anxiety one can hardly function, yet we expect our youth to carry on as though the world were a sensible place.

Stress

Stress is a well-documented source of inattention, disorganization, frustration, inability to concentrate, anger and the many other symptoms so characteristic of ADHD and ADD. Stress often causes attentional symptoms in those who do not have ADD, and greatly exacerbates the problems of those who do.

While some of our children suffer stress from neglect, others experience stress as a function of enormous pressure to succeed. America has recently begun to question its "Supermom"-"Superdad"-"Superkid" mentality, but most concur that in the competitive international arena into which the whole world is thrust, only those with an edge are likely to be successful. Those who can, push their children hard to insure later success. Those who cannot, try to survive and pray their children can do the same.

Against this backdrop of cultural, social and emotional stresses, each family does its best to raise its children. Those whose children have attention disorders are especially vulnerable to the vicissitudes of their worlds. These children will require a concerted effort on the part of parents, teachers and professionals to guide them through.

Despite the problems, and they are legion, America has a resiliency which has always surfaced in times of greatest need. Our return to many of the principles which made our country great is promising. These are, in fact, the principles advocated for our attention-disordered children. Perhaps in treating those with ADHD/ADD we will, in some small way, help shift the national focus to a return to structure, organization, discipline, predictability, individualization, responsibility, esteem, respect, and concern for others. If so, in helping our children with attention disorders, we will have helped our world. It is a worthy goal to which to aspire.

SUMMARY

There are many potential causes of attention disorders and many factors which may contribute to attentional problems in children, adolescents and adults. The exact causes and mechanisms of these disorders are still unknown and may continue to be something of a mystery for many years. To further complicate the picture, ADHD and ADD manifest very differently and may well represent different neurochemical pictures. Neither is believed to have a single cause, but both probably, in the words of Dr. Gabrielle Weiss (1990), "represent a final common pathway of various interacting biologic and psychosocial variables." To decipher successfully the mysteries of our brain's functioning and malfunctioning, we must acknowledge complexity rather than seek simplicity. We must be willing to expend the painstaking energy it will require to understand the many facets of these disorders. Only when we do will we be able to make our interventions as specific to each problem as are the neurotransmitters and neuroreceptors themselves. When our work is complete, we can expect to have not only ADHD and ADD, but, rather, many varieties of attention disorders, each representing a more specific understanding of both the brain structures affected and the neurotransmitters involved.

As educators seek to abolish labels, physicians and scientists will, of necessity, create more as specific manifestations are identified and require a name. Labels, which are merely a form of medical shorthand, do not do harm to children. Misuse of those labels, on the other hand, to classify but not assist can be a source of great harm. In our frustration at being unable to find easy solutions to this complex set of problems, we are in danger of throwing "the baby out with the bath water." All who live and work with ADHD/ADD children, adolescents and adults must finally acknowledge and address both the uniqueness and the complexity of this disorder in each person if true assistance is to be provided. We have accomplished this goal in many of the disorders affecting the body. We must now aggressively address the last and perhaps most challenging frontier of all—the brain itself. An awesome challenge, a tremendous responsibility, and an exciting adventure await.

A challenging role lies ahead for the developmental pediatrician as "demystifier," informed advocate, a community resource for assessment of scientific information, monitor of progress, and link with school as well as family ally.

—George Storm, M.D., 1990

4

ADHD and the Developmental Pediatrician*

By George Storm, M.D.

Many parents are sufficiently struck by the numbers of children with infection, injury, and regular appointments in the pediatrician's waiting room to feel embarrassed about "bothering the doctor" with issues pertaining to behavior, attention efficiency, or learning. In fact, a parent's hidden agenda about developmental issues often has the potential for a more profound impact on future overall adjustment than the acute difficulties which require care but often crowd out the chance for more reflective discussions. Virtually every physician has had the experience of hearing a parent casually reveal very significant concerns, as if an afterthought, while zipping up their child's snowsuit, one foot out the door: "Oh by the way, the school says he can't follow directions,

---

*This chapter was originally written for and published in CHADDER, Fall/Winter, 1990. It is included in this book with the permission of Dr. Storm and CH.A.D.D.

is a handful, upsets everyone, and should repeat . . . do you think it's maturity or because his father's that way?" An article appeared in a pediatric journal several years ago entitled "Got A Minute?" The researchers observed the transactions in a regular office visit and determined, with regret, that developmental issues were pushed into a tiny fraction of total contact time between parent and doctor and, as expected, into much less time when appointments involved acute care. Allowed to continue, this situation promotes frustrating outcomes, for no human relationship is improved by speeding up the time needed for sharing and assimilation. The pressure on the M.D. to "come to closure" prematurely may lead to a pat answer, mindless enthusiasm, or false hope in the mistaken belief that the matter is solved. Still mystified by their child's behavior, the parent may then leave convinced the question was foolish in the first place, wondering about his or her competence since "probably no one else" had these worries!

THE DEVELOPMENTALLY SPECIALIZED PEDIATRICIAN

Fortunately, times are changing. Many pediatricians are increasing their training and practice commitment in developmental pediatrics. Parents are less hesitant to call their concerns to the physician's attention. This approach is certainly to be recommended and means requesting from the physician a "special" (longer) appointment to discuss developmental concerns (preferably when both parents can be present), writing a short note to the physician before a scheduled appointment headlining the areas of concern, or calling the office and telling the secretary that, because of a "personal matter," a call is needed from the physician to the parent. When the call is returned, it is easier to determine if the physician may have special training and is willing to make special time. These parent actions are perhaps analogous to the referee's gesture on the playing field signalling: "time out!"

At this juncture a parent may be very favorably surprised. The physician may have a special interest in developmental/behavior disorders, save special periods when interruptions are less likely to meet with parents, or may have cultivated helpful and experienced resources. Or, if one then feels the physician is knowledgeable in a number of areas but not behavior and development, or not interested or unable, then the quest for a second opinion should proceed. Can the physician recommend someone to review the concern? Can their local or teaching hospital provide resources? Can support group members share their experiences regarding helpful resources? The goal is to find a pediatrician with additional training, a child psychiatrist, or a child neurologist willing to systematically review issues pertaining to attention efficiency, self-control, compliance, and distractibility. Thus, a process of demystification begins. If it is determined that ADHD exists and, after a careful diagnostic formulation is constructed, it is also decided that medication may be an important aspect of multi-modal treatment, the M.D. is the responsible professional prescribing and monitoring medication with appropriate links to school. The same physician, if indicated, should be able to interact in a transdisciplinary fashion with other specialists involved in treatment possibly including: a psychological or neuropsychological consultant, speech/language consultant, and/or psychoeducational consultant. In such a team approach, the physician may serve as an orchestrator of selected services. (Not all services are needed for every child.) In this format the developmentally specialized physician is not superior to the other professionals but rather an informed generalist with a contribution to make in diagnostic overview and management.

In addition to time allotment, the developmentally specialized pediatrician will likely have recognized other practice differences in contrast to "regular" pediatrics. For example, the ADHD child usually will have a potent effect on the entire family system—i.e., siblings, parents, and perhaps other relatives. Also the ambiguity and stress associated with ADHD is chronic, involving management rather than cure, versus the pattern of care required in self-limited diseases. Also the "advice imposed" upon parents is quite different in the context of acute medical care than the "purposes mutually arrived at" which generally characterize the successful parent/child/ physician relationship in more chronic developmental disorders. Finally, the physician should be mindful that early recognition (early diagnosis), which is to be encouraged to promote prevention, should be formulated with care lest premature labeling or unnecessary stereotyping occur.

FAMILY AND SCHOOL HISTORY

Parents starting the evaluation process have often already experienced accusatory judgments about their child, feel intimidation, guilt, confusion, and even may be at odds with each other about the interpretation of the behavior. It should surprise no one that confusion and frustration lead to blaming one another. This does not promote consistent or effective parenting. The evaluation process begins with data collection about the child's early development as well as the family's interpretation of past experiences.

To make this process more focused, many physicians find that parent's developmental questionnaires, completed before the first appointment, serve to put current observations into perspective, creating a tapestry of family, medical and developmental history, including peer and academic problems. The family history emphasizes developmental learning, psychological and coping patterns. Often the collaboration on a questionnaire by both mother and father strengthens the teamwork and brings up events that one or the other parent may have forgotten.

A complete physical evaluation should have been performed within the past year including vision and hearing. While it is unusual for children with ADHD to have significant physical abnormalities, it is important to rule out physical disorder, exposure to lead, anemia, low grade infections, etc. In special circumstances, chromosome, thyroid, blood sugar, and brain wave (EEG) tests may be indicated— but not routinely.

With this background information available, every effort is made to include both parents in the initial parent interview. Even in instances of divorce or separation when parents may have strong residual anger, failed expectations, and mistrust between them, a child-centered review of relevant information with both parents can be constructive. This process offers an opportunity to define the symptom pattern, significant variables, assess what has been done thus far, explore apparent theories of causation, and become acquainted with parent fears of the future should the problem remain unchanged. While some physicians would prefer to interview parents and child together, there is an equally strong argument to support the freedom an adult session permits to discuss complaints, differing perceptions, and fears. Since a child's clinical presentations may appear to satisfy many of the criteria for ADHD, but be caused by anxiety, depression or inappropriate expectations, it is particularly important in this adult setting to assess family mutual respect and functioning. In a world characterized by an alarming rate of marital disruption, an awareness that residual turmoil and loyalty conflicts can aggravate attention disorders is important.

ADHD children may have a history of significant neurologic precursors during pregnancy (i.e., toxemia, prematurity, alcohol exposure, etc.) and/or temperamental dysfunction in early childhood with difficulties accepting nurturance and adapting to newborn routines. Chronic patterns of restlessness, attention difficulties and impulsivity across different settings are reported with an onset often before 4 years and almost always before 7 years. The assessment of historic data also looks carefully for patterns of significant school achievement problems.

School information is also very important to obtain by contact with teachers, principals, or school nurse after release of information is granted by parents. At times, physicians may wish to use a school inventory which taps aspects of a child's adjustment in the class, learning patterns, academic competence and attention efficiency when compared to peers. Any intelligence assessments, language evaluations or L.D. testing performed by the school are important to incorporate in the clinical profile.

In short, how does the child cope at home, with peers, with authority, with rules, with school?

THE CHILD'S APPOINTMENT

The child's appointment provides the physician with an opportunity to meet one-to-one, establish rapport, conduct a brief, psychologically sensitive interview and perform a neurodevelopmental exam. Several excellent formats for this exam have been standardized and developed under the supervision of Melvin D. Levine, M.D. (see *Peeramid*, Appendix 5). Since it is well known that physicians' appointments of 10 or 15 minutes are notoriously unreliable to determine the presence of ADHD because of a child's ability to remain "tuned in" in short, novel situations, it is very helpful to have a standardized "package" of developmental tasks. These provide a systematic overview and functional profile of motor, language, perceptual abilities as well as an opportunity to observe selective attention. Strengths and weaknesses can be defined and assigned priorities in order to coordinate any future relevant diagnostic or management referrals. It is important to emphasize that this evaluation does not produce a total score, such as an IQ, but does provide an overall approach to learning style. This examination is also different than the traditional neurological exam which searches for specific lesions or diseases of the nervous system. The findings of the neurodevelopmental (N-D) exam are likely to have therapeutic implications, especially if combined with related observations of the team.

It is important that highlighted deficit areas be documented by an expert in the field of the suspected disability (i.e., language, psychological, educational issues). The component parts of the N-D exam may consist of the following:

A. *Minor Neurologic Indicators:*   Tasks which may suggest problems with "fine tuning" of the central nervous system often associated with the need for help in study skills or related aspects of processing and output.

B. *Fine-Motor Function:* A series of tasks relating to the increasingly important demands for written output in later school years. Even beyond writing, fine-motor skills have importance in tasks relevant to life skills such as keyboarding, repairing, constructing, crafts, etc. Eye/hand coordination, motor speed, planning, the capacity to feel non-visual feedback from fingers, sequencing and the ability to perform efficiently are assessed.

C. *Language Screening:* Especially important for the ADHD child since language processing disorders often accompany attention deficits. A child may have problems deriving meaning in a listening environment, find listening unrewarding and is then more vulnerable to distractibility. Also, language competence directly relates to school performance. It is now clear that children with language difficulties may have serious problems with reading, written language, new concepts, or the processing of directions with increasingly complex demands in upper grades. Even social success and self-esteem are dependent upon the language subtleties of personal interaction. Children with difficulties may feel rejected and relatively friendless. Tasks tap the ability to understand the complex grammar in sentences, follow complex directions, generate sentences flexibly, and find the correct words in response to picture stimuli (word retrieval). Younger children are assessed for their awareness that sentences are composed of words, and that words consist of specific sounds and sound patterns—building blocks for reading.

D.   *Large-Muscle Skills*:   Coordination abilities have an important bearing on the formation of self-esteem and body image. Tasks involving balance, eye/hand coordination, and the capacity to maintain rhythmic sequences are checked knowing that humiliation in play may justify intervention to help a child participate more effectively in recreation and social activities.

E.   *Temporal/Sequential Organization:* Taps a child's awareness of time sequences and serial order since these relationships influence intellectual development and information processing.

F.   *Visual Processing:* Checks the ability to focus on, analyze, store and retrieve data processed visually. These skills remain important for tasks requiring visual attention to detail, scanning, and efficiency of processing—even though the language system plays a larger role in learning to read.

Throughout the above, there is continuous opportunity and sufficient time to observe patterns of impulsivity, distractibility, deterioration during the task, superficial attention to detail or levels of over-activity. In addition, several laboratory tests contribute more data based on the direct measurement of a child's performance. Continuous performance tasks (C.P.T.) note a child's attention efficiency in recognizing particular patterns on a screen.   The Gordon Diagnostic System (G.D.S.), an electronic microprocessing device, can present tasks of continuous performance measuring sustained attention/impulsivity; a delay task measures the capacity to use self-control and delay in a context where delay is important to success. The Matching Familiar Figures Test (M.F.F.T.) is another performance task to study impulsivity in ADHD children. The Gardner Steadiness Test is an electronic measure of motor persistence and attention efficiency. When laboratory tasks reported to measure attention efficiency are used as part of a total evaluation or to assist in monitoring medication effect, parents should remember that these tests are not infallible and must be used in the context of other school, home and test information. Nevertheless, the effort to directly measure components of attention efficiency rather than to rely solely on the observations of others is of great benefit and will undoubtedly lead to further refinements. (For information on the tests mentioned, see Appendix 5.)

G. *Academic Performance Screening:* While neither a psychologist nor educational expert, the M.D. may appropriately use abbreviated measures of intelligence and academic performance to determine if further assessment is warranted.

The Interpretive Conference

After integrating all of the above, an understandable interpretive conference is scheduled for family and child. This should permit time for careful discussion, feedback, review of a written summary as well as constructive recommendations. Ideally, the physician would like to avoid diagnostic labels that contribute to risk. However, when specific diagnostic criteria are fulfilled, diagnosis permits the disciplined collection of clinical information by many research centers, rational assessment of interventions, helps insure equal protection under the law, and provides (when appropriate) insurance reimbursement for documented medical conditions. Parents should remember that the formulation of a diagnosis accurately encapsulates a child's condition at this point in time, but that circumstances may change. The length of time the disability has been present, pervasiveness, severity with which the condition (i.e., ADHD) interferes with family, social and academic functions, emotions and the likelihood of increased complications without treatment, are the main driving factors influencing the scope and intensity of intervention strategies.

The assessment process, whether orchestrated by a developmentally trained pediatrician or alternative team member, must carefully document developmental problems, consider the context, note contributing factors, and rule out conditions that can be confused with ADHD. ADHD is understood as a neurologically- based, long-term developmentally handicapping condition with very significant social and educational consequences. "Multi-modal" treatment is the accepted and effective management course. Responsible treatment means the coordination of medication, educational and psychological services, enhancement of parenting strategies, and continued orchestration of success experiences to vigorously protect self-esteem. To the extent that a child believes he no longer has worth or competence, the best programs will fail.

While traditional psychotherapy has not proven helpful with the core ADHD symptoms of impulsivity, inattention and restlessness, the secondary consequences of chronic success deprivation can create a state of demoralization: a sense of helplessness, inability to cope, self-blame, feelings of worthlessness, hopelessness, and alienation. This state of affairs is often benefitted by the inclusion of psychotherapy.

Medication use requires responsible follow-up on a regular basis in the context of a therapeutic alliance. Fifty years of research have contributed substantial data. Ritalin and Dexedrine are medicines of first choice and have been proven to impressively decrease activity levels and to improve attention, vigilance, reaction time, motor coordination and handwriting skills, but long-term academic gains are more uncertain. Antidepressants may be appropriate if adequate trials show that stimulants are not effective or contraindicated. A personal engagement of the child as an active participant and follow-up permits monitoring of medication effects and side effects, and also guards against inappropriate attribution of all progress to the medication at the expense of self-reliance. Explanatory guidance increases independence and self-advocacy. Target symptoms of inattention, impulsivity and hyperactivity are monitored together with school behavior, performance, emotional growth, peer relationships, leisure activities and family balance. Medication holidays with collaboration at school should be considered several times a year but not simultaneously with the confusion of field trips, holidays and birthdays when results are difficult to interpret.

A challenging role lies ahead for the developmental pediatrician as "demystifier," informed advocate, a community resource for assessment of scientific information, monitor of progress, and link with school as well as family ally.   As a collaborative partner, the physician is positioned to continually help the family accept reasonable goals and remind them that their child, no matter what the handicap, is still loved, and still valued . . . and fortunate to have them as parents. The focused energy of "parents supporting parents" will most certainly advance this process.

PART II

Medications: General Principles

*Shortly after I was told I had Attention
Deficit Disorder, I was faced with the
decision of taking medicine for it. Despite
overwhelming results in other people,
I was reluctant to take any foreign
substance that would not allow me
control over my actions.*

—16-year-old adolescent, 1985

5

The Role of Medication in Attention Deficit Disorders: Emotional and Social Issues

The most important information to surface from the last two decades of intensive investigation of attention disorders is that no treatment approach is successful alone—neither medical, behavioral, psychological nor educational intervention is, by itself, adequate. Rather, we must treat the *whole* person. We must treat every aspect of the child or adolescent—his neurophysiology, his social and psychological being, the development of self-discipline and responsibility and his educational needs—if we are to be truly successful.

Successful intervention, in my opinion, means that the benefits will continue not only during the time of treatment but will promote the necessary esteem, competence, organization, discipline and cooperative spirit which will ensure success for a lifetime. Our goals must transcend our desire for the child or adolescent to sit still in school, complete his work, and to make good grades. I truly believe every ADHD/ADD child or adolescent has the potential to become a competent, happy, fully-functioning adult who can be a productive, contributing member of our society.   This goal can be accomplished.   I have seen it happen far too many times in the last twenty years to have any doubt.

This book was written to assist in the understanding of one of the treatment options available.   It cannot be overstated that behavioral, psychological, social, educational and family interventions are considered equally important.   That medication alone is not enough has been shown repeatedly by research studies which have followed those treated with medication alone for several years in contrast to those who had the benefit of a multimodal intervention program.   For example, Dr. Jim Swanson, who has studied attention disorders for twenty years, found, in a major study of older adolescents, that those who received psychological and educational assistance in addition to medicine were significantly better adjusted than those who received medication alone.   The latter group was not significantly better adjusted than those not treated at all (Swanson, 1988). Likewise, the findings of Cantwell (1985) suggest that there are long-term benefits only from a multidisciplinary treatment program. Weiss et al. (1975) found, in a five-year follow-up study, that methylphenidate made ADHD children more manageable both at school and at home, but that they were not significantly different from non-treated ADHD children at the end of five years.   Hechtman et al. (1984) did report fewer accidents, less delinquency, better social skills, more self-esteem and better memories of childhood in a group they followed that had been treated successfully with medication for three years or longer.

Those who live and work with children and adolescents with attention disorders will find some interventions acceptable to them because they are consistent with their beliefs and lifestyles.   They can be expected to reject other therapeutic options which they find incompatible.   You, as a parent, teacher or professional, are encouraged to give each approach your careful and open-minded consideration.   Even if doubtful, you may wish to give each intervention a try.   Only then will you have sufficient data with which to make a decision about what is effective. The goal of this book is to help parents, teachers and professionals obtain adequate knowledge. I, like other professionals, respect each person's treatment decisions when they are based on accurate information. By contrast, it is painful to see children and adolescents denied the benefits of treatment when the choices of those making the decisions are the result of misinformation, fear or prejudice.

The medical interventions addressed in this chapter are for accurately diagnosed, physiologic attention deficit disorders as described previously.

ACCEPTING ADHD/ADD

Perhaps the first thing with which both child and parents must come to terms is that the child or adolescent has an attention disorder. Accepting that one's child, or oneself, has ADHD or ADD can be a painful experience. Each of us secretly hopes to have a perfect child and to be perfect ourselves. Accepting that our child has a problem is particularly hard, whether it be cancer, a learning disability, an emotional problem, or an attention disorder. Many times denial, anger, projection of blame, and grief accompany diagnosis. These feelings and emotions must be worked through if the child or adolescent is to succeed. On the other hand, many are relieved that the difficulties now have a medical name and that help is available. One no longer needs to blame oneself or the child for the difficult situations ADHD/ADD inevitably produce. Several resources are listed in Appendix 6 to assist parents with this grief process.

Secondly, one must grapple with and accept that ADHD and ADD are physiologic disorders. When one accepts this fact, it is a logical next step to think that they may require physiological intervention—i.e., medication. This is not to say that other physiological interventions are not needed. Rather, allergies, chemicals and toxins may also play important physiological roles. Meditation and biofeedback, which produce physiologic changes, have proven helpful to some as well. We must continue to investigate the impact of all possible factors until we have definitive answers. If stress relief, participation in support groups, and lifestyle changes result in major improvements in cancer, heart disease, arthritis, and diabetes, among others, it is not unrealistic to think they may, likewise, have the potential for producing improvements in those with attention disorders.

RELUCTANCE TO USE MEDICATIONS FOR ATTENTION DISORDERS

For at least fifty years, parents, teachers and pediatricians have been aware of this group of children and adolescents who are unmanageable at home and unsuccessful at school. For at least that long diverse treatment approaches have been tried and discarded. When one examines the medical literature, one is struck with the fact that one treatment approach appears consistently, for over fifty years, to have been helpful with this group, that is, the use of stimulant medications. From the vast array of research data at this time, one can safely say that medication is an appropriate and effective intervention for at least three-fourths of those diagnosed with physiologic ADHD/ADD. Recent researchers suggest that as many as 90% may be assisted (Calis et al., 1990).

Despite the impressive track record of medications, people are, nevertheless, uneasy about giving medication to children and adolescents, especially medicines which affect brain functioning. They are even more uneasy about giving it, presumably, *to control behavior*. Most do not understand the neurophysiology of ADHD/ ADD and thus do not realize that medication is not doing anything *to the child*, but rather acting as a normalizer of brain functioning, so that the child, adolescent or adult can function normally. How many parents would insist that a child simply cope with poor eyesight and berate him if he could not copy from the board? How many of us would deny the diabetic child insulin or the adolescent with hypothyroidism, thyroxin? Would physicians be allowed to continue to practice medicine if they denied antibiotics to a child with desensitization therapy for a child with life-threatening allergies an acceptable treatment option? Many of these medications have worse side effects than the most commonly used medications for attention disorders. They have not, however, caused the controversy and anxiety which surrounds the medical treatment of ADHD and ADD.

Concern about this area is not new. As suggested earlier, periodically people are alarmed by various groups and investigations are undertaken. Each time this constellation of difficulties and the treatments employed have been investigated, two findings typically emerge:

- This disorder is a very real one which requires ongoing treatment by physicians and other professionals and continued research into causes and solutions.

- Medication is an appropriate and necessary intervention, but one which must be utilized responsibly and with careful monitoring. These are the same safeguards that apply to all medical interventions for any disorder.

Healing is a matter of time, but it is sometimes also a matter of opportunity.
                                                    - Hippocrates

CONFUSION AND ANXIETY
ABOUT MEDICATION

In my opinion, there are several reasons for our current state of confusion and anxiety about medication:

1) The media have, unwittingly, presented much negative publicity about medication, especially in 1987 and part of 1988. As they have become more educated, however, the information presented to the public in newspapers and magazines, especially late in 1988 through the present, has been increasingly accurate and more supportive (Rosemond, 1989; Sterling, 1990; Bower, 1988; Stern, 1988; Gold, 1990; Segal & Segal, 1988; Wolkenberg, 1988). Parents, educators and professionals are urged to investigate carefully all sources of information which are affecting their decision-making. Only informed persons can make wise decisions.

2) ADHD and ADD have become catch-all categories for many difficulties which children are experiencing in school. When children are misidentified, or every problem is viewed as an attention deficit, people become confused about the true nature of the problem. Improper diagnosis leads, of course, to improper treatment.

3) Attentional difficulties are inadvertently being created, as discussed in Chapter 3, by some of our current educational, cultural, and parenting practices and goals, and are confused with physiologic ADHD/ADD. It is critical that these issues be addressed separately and not be confused with true, physiologic ADHD/ADD.

4) Children with attention disorders are, many times, being treated with medication alone. The results are less than satisfying since medicine alone is not adequate for long-term changes.

5) Medication is sometimes not properly monitored. Professionals must work together to establish protocols of treatment and follow-up typical of those followed with other disorders.

6) Parents often agree to treatment interventions without adequate education and emotional support. Compliance with the recommended treatment is often quite poor under these conditions.

7) Other causes for our current state of confusion and anxiety exist as well. These include concerns about long-term negative effects of medication, the relationship between early use of stimulant medication and later drug abuse, the possibility that medication will be used to control the child, or that medicine acts as an emotional straitjacket for the primary benefit of adults. These, and other concerns, will be addressed throughout this book.

A PERSONAL PHILOSOPHY OF TREATMENT

Before discussing the use of stimulant and other medicines as a treatment for attention deficit disorders, I would like to state my philosophy of treatment. It is my personal philosophy only. Each professional has a somewhat different approach for treating the problems of attention deficit disorder based on his or her particular experiences, education and interests.

True ADHD and ADD are physiological disorders and many times must be treated medically. However, there are usually many other variables which contribute to the difficulties even when the symptoms represent physiologic ADHD or ADD. Therefore, unless the child is in crisis and the school requires that something be done immediately, or the family is desperate, I believe it is very important to try nonmedication interventions first. These include education of the parents and child; behavior management strategies which will be required even if medication is used; organization and structure both at home and at school; a careful assessment of other medical problems, such as allergies or hyperthyroidism; investigation of potential environmental toxins; and psychological interventions. Assessment of the child's appropriate placement in both the grade he is in and the school he attends is also part of the initial intervention, as well determination of the child's learning strengths and weaknesses, and any learning disabilities or gaps in his acquisition of knowledge. Appropriate classroom modifications, as well as other educational interventions are, likewise, critical.

After two or three weeks of intensive educational, behavioral and psychological assistance, it is reasonably apparent how much benefit can be obtained from these interventions alone. If they are not adequate, and usually they are not, medication is considered. While medication is the most widely used treatment for ADHD and ADD and is certainly an appropriate one under most conditions, there are some problems inherent in trying it first.

RATIONALE FOR NOT UTILIZING
MEDICATION AS A FIRST OPTION

1) When medicine is successful, there is often little incentive to implement other interventions which are necessary for the long-term benefit of the child but require more investment of time and energy from both parents and teachers. For parents these include learning new ways of interacting with the child; learning organization and planning skills so that parents can manage both their own lives and their child's more effectively; adopting behavioral principles to promote change; and embracing new eating habits among others. Parents are usually grateful for the changes once implemented, but they are less likely to invest the considerable energy required if problems are not acute or if a solution appears to have been found.

2) While medicine is successful in alleviating many of the symptoms of ADHD/ADD, especially in school, research previously reported has found that those children treated with medicine alone had no better outcome by late adolescence than those who were not treated at all.

3)   Sometimes the amount of medication needed can be reduced after allergies are treated; stress is reduced; organization, structure and routine are implemented; and behavior management approaches are effectively utilized.

4)   Parents are much more content with medication after they have exhausted other alternatives and continue to need intervention.   Only parents at peace with giving the medicine will comply with the regimen recommended.

5)   Those children who may have been misdiagnosed or who will not need medication are usually very apparent after a few weeks of other interventions.

6)   Parents and teachers who may want an easy way out may be inpatient with this approach.   Instead of capitulating to their immediate stress, the are encouraged to consider options other than what some have called "the magic bullet."   Often it is the more impulsive or frustrated parent or teacher who wants medication on the first visit.   It is this same person who may most need assistance with nonmedical strategies as well. Delaying medication insures adequate time to utilize other interventions while the situation is still pressing.

7)   Medicine is less likely to be over-utilized or abused if safeguards are followed.   If medication is not given judiciously and within carefully monitored guidelines, there is a risk that the use of stimulant medication will become so controversial that it may not be available to those who truly need it.   The Drug Enforcement Agency (DEA) is, in fact, so carefully monitoring stimulant medications that many physicians are either uneasy about or unwilling to prescribe them.   Physicians usually need documentation from the school or a professional, as well as parents, to satisfy both their own and regulatory agencies' needs for an accurate diagnosis, thereby insuring appropriate medical intervention.   This safeguard is a necessary one and should encourage careful assessment and

documentation. It is sincerely hoped that it will not discourage the use of medication when it is appropriate. This requirement for documentation by the physician is often frustrating to parents who may wish to try medicine without going through an evaluation process. Testing *per se* is not always necessary, but, at the very least, behavior checklists completed by parents and teachers, and the results of behavioral interventions already tried should be available to the physician before his own comprehensive assessment.

School Assistance

Schools can assist both parents and physicians tremendously by addressing attention disorders early, completing behavioral and learning checklists, making appropriate classroom accommodations, and implementing behavioral interventions before psychological testing is recommended. The school's role in identifying and assisting in both the evaluation and treatment process is outlined in detail in *Attention Without Tension: The Teacher's Handbook on Attention Disorders* (Copeland & Love, 1990) and the school in-service videoprogram, *Attention Disorders: The School's Vital Role* (Copeland, 1990, 1994).

Teachers perform a critical role in the evaluation process before formal testing. Their role is especially important since waiting for the school to provide testing can delay treatment, unnecessarily, for months because of the backlog experienced by most school districts. Many students will require psychological/ psychoeducational evaluation to determine the presence of problems coexisting with the attention disorder. Such an assessment may follow the initiation of medical treatment if the managing physician is aware of, and is kept informed on, the behavior, learning and classroom intervention strategies, and their results, which have been tried.

SUMMARY

The treatment of attention disorders with medication is logical and empirically supported, but, nevertheless, remains socially controversial and emotionally difficult. Many of these problematic issues can be avoided if medication is viewed as it should be—not as a solution to the problem of ADHD/ADD or as a controller of behavior, but rather as an integral part of a carefully planned, systematically monitored, wholistic treatment plan. When medication is used as one part of a comprehensive intervention program, not the intervention itself, parents and, indeed, the culture as a whole, will be able to accept it more readily as a valuable tool in the treatment of attention disorders.

*We know the drugs work—they're very effective
—but we don't know how they work.*

—Josephine Elia, M.D., NIMH, 1989

6

Mechanisms and Goals of Medications for ADHD and ADD

Despite the relatively limited knowledge of the public about this disorder, it has received unprecedented research attention for the past ten years. Hundreds of investigations have been undertaken. The majority have studied the effects of various treatment approaches on ADHD/ADD. The use of medicine, especially stimulant medication, has been thoroughly researched. For those who question the helpfulness of stimulant medication, one has only to review the medical literature. The data from diverse institutions and investigators have resoundingly established the ability of medicine to alter the symptoms of attention deficit disorders. However, most have also shown that, for maximum effectiveness of medical management, psychological, behavioral, social, and educational interventions are necessary as well. It appears that *medicine enables the child to benefit from interventions which are ineffective without it.* As in many other disorders of neurochemical origin, the best solution is the one uniformly recommended by experts in the field, i.e., a multimodal intervention program that includes a combination of drug management and psychological/behavioral/educational assistance.

General Mechanism of Medications
For ADHD/ADD

The use of medication, especially stimulant medication, is the most common treatment for children, adolescents and adults with ADHD and ADD. Approximately one million school-age children and adolescents take medication annually for management of their attention deficit symptoms. Given the conservative estimate that 3-5% or more of our school-age children have ADHD/ADD, then less than one-third of those with attention disorders are currently being medically treated. Much of the stimulant medication prescribed at this time is utilized for older adolescents and adults, and for the treatment of *narcolepsy,* a neurological disorder characterized by excessive sleepiness. (Narcolepsy will be addressed in Chapter 13.)

As stated previously, attention deficit disorders are thought to result from deficiencies or imbalances in neurotransmitters or brain chemicals that affect the prefrontal cortex, the premotor cortex, the frontal lobes, the reticular formation, the limbic system, and other attention centers. When the attention system is not stimulated properly, the brain is not at an optimum level of performance and efficiency. All medications used for ADHD/ADD alter, in some way, the availability and absorption of the various neurotransmitters involved, resulting in improvement in the entire attention network.

Some estimate that as many as 80-90% of those correctly diagnosed with physiologic ADHD/ADD can be helped with stimulant medications (Calis et al., 1990). These medicines include Ritalin, Dexedrine and Cylert. For those who do not respond to the stimulants, tricyclic antidepressants, including Tofranil, Norpramin and Prozac, among others, are often helpful. Catapres is frequently used with over-focused

ADD children, those with a concomitant tic disorder, or those with aggressive symptoms, while Tegretol, an anticonvulsant, is utilized with ADHD/ADD children who are also explosive or have complex partial seizures. Major tranquilizers, such as Thorazine and Mellaril, are used with those who have ADD-like symptoms but whose primary problem is an emotional or psychiatric disorder. Haldol is frequently utilized as part of the medical intervention for Tourette Syndrome.

WHAT MEDICATIONS FOR ADHD/ADD CAN DO

Medication is designed to alter deficiencies and/or imbalances of the neurotransmitters which are problematic in attention disorders. When it does, there is simultaneous improvement in a person's ability to attend and in his impulse control, behavior, cooperativeness, reasonableness, and sensitivity to social cues and expectations. A positive change in alertness is noted in the underactive, daydreaming ADD child, adolescent or adult, while increased attention and decreased activity and restlessness are noted in those with overactive ADHD. Improvement in school is almost always noted, as well as improved vigilance, short-term memory, behavior, peer relations and family interactions. Sports, music and other nonacademic activities are also positively affected. To those who have worked with hyperactive and ADD children before and after medication is begun, no other treatment can produce such dramatic improvement in so short a time.

The goal of all medications used to treat ADHD and ADD is the normalization of attention, focusing and behavior, just as glasses normalize vision. Contrary to some people's fears, it is not to change the child or adolescent's consciousness or freedom of expression. Those treated with medication are simply better able to accomplish what they want to do. The treatment does not force a child or adolescent to be good or to act in a particular way. He will simply accomplish whatever his goals are more successfully on medication than off. Those goals usually become very positive ones. Our experience shows that most

ADHD/ADD children and adolescents desperately want to be like everyone else. To be unable to function efficiently and effectively much of the time is devastating to their internal sense of stability, predictability, self-control and confidence. They, like all of us, want to be successful and to maximize their inherent potential.

In addition to these general benefits, medication also has very specific benefits for the typical symptoms of attention disorders and hyperactivity.

Improved Attention and Concentration/ Decreased Distractibility

Off-task behavior and the inability to complete assignments at school and requests at home are among the most frustrating symptoms for all who live and work with children and adolescents with attention disorders, both ADHD and ADD. Assignments half done, the garbage almost to the street ... but not quite, chores abandoned midstream, and the teen's mind in never-never land while driving a car are situations which frustrate and frighten even the most patient and understanding adults.

Medications for attention disorders fortunately address these problems in most children and teens. Stimulant medications are especially effective in improving attentional abilities. Research data from many investigators and institutions strongly support their ability to improve attention in at least 70-80% of those studied. Pelham and others (1985), for example, found that stimulant medication effectively increased on-task behavior. The medicated children in their study maintained attention and missed fewer targets than non-medicated ADHD children. The effects became most pronounced during the latter part of the task.

This finding corresponds with every parent and teacher's experiences with ADHD/ADD children and adolescents, i.e., at the beginning of a new task they are alert and motivated. However, the initial interest wanes quickly as the task loses its novelty and becomes, in their favorite word, "boring." The ability to persevere with tasks that are not necessarily interesting, but which must be done, i.e., self-discipline, is the characteristic most lacking in ADHD/ADD children, but the one most necessary for success in adulthood. The increased availability of the requisite neurotransmitters results in a significant improvement in the attention spans of those receiving medical treatment. This improved attention is noted in almost every aspect of the child or adolescent's life. It has special implications for his performance at school. Medicine's effect on cognition, learning and academic performance will be discussed in detail in a later section of this chapter.

Adults with attention disorders, likewise, complain of poor concentration and the inability to accomplish tasks without becoming distracted as their most worrisome difficulties. Preliminary data strongly suggest that increased ability to attend and to stay on task and decreased distractibility and disorganization are major benefits of medication in adults as well as children.

At this time, thousands of children treated for symptoms of inattention and distractibility have been followed. Most investigators have found that more than three-quarters of those studied showed significant improvement on medication (Pelham, 1987; Pelham, et al., 1985; Barkley & Cunningham, 1979b; Barkley, 1977b). Medicine appears quite successful in alleviating inattention and distractibility, core symptoms of both ADHD and ADD.

Children express their pain and the effect of medication somewhat differently:

>*Sometimes I cry because I'm sad.*
>*I do naughty things, but I'm not bad.*
>*I'm just creative, and I like to dream.*
>*I need to let off lots of steam.*

When I'm in school, I can't sit still
Ritalin helps, that's a little pill.
I take it to calm my busy brain
And keep my mom and teachers sane.

—From *Busy Brain* by Mary Daum
ADD—ONS, Frankfurt, IL.

Decreased Impulsivity

Impulsivity is a second major characteristic of attention deficit disorders and one which has, perhaps, the most significant long-term negative effects for both the child or adolescent and those around him. Talking without raising one's hand, impulsively throwing a rock, recklessly riding a Big Wheel down a steep hill, or trying marijuana without a thought of its legal implications ... these are the things which cause parents and teachers countless sleepless nights.

Acting without thinking and ongoing poor judgment create not only problems at school, at home and in social activities, but in adolescence and adulthood they can result in increased experimentation with drugs and alcohol, more driving citations and accidents, and frequent skirmishes with the law. For those who know the long-term outcome of untreated attention disorders, this characteristic alone is an incentive for obtaining treatment if no other one seems adequately compelling. Educated parents, likewise, perceive the need to harness this lack of inhibition. A classic 15-year study of hyperactive children, conducted at McGill University, revealed that, when hyperactive children grew up, problems with impulsivity continued to be the most serious and long-lasting of their difficulties (Weiss & Hechtman, 1986).

Research data on the effectiveness of medication for moderating impulsivity and inappropriate behavior are encouraging. While the necessity for developing cognitive control over the child or adolescent's impulses through specific cognitive training cannot be overstated, medications for attention disorders do improve their ability to think before acting, to tolerate delay, and to consider the consequences of their behavior.

Impulsivity is often associated with low frustration tolerance. It is noteworthy that those hyperactive children and adolescents on medication are both perceived as, and do indeed respond with, less intensity and more thoughtfulness (Henker, et al., 1986). Stimulant medication was also found to reduce gross-motor movements, vocalization and disruption in hyperactive boys (Gittelman-Klein & Feingold, 1983); to reduce disruptive and anti-social behaviors in ADHD adolescents (Barkley, McMurray, et al., 1989); to normalize the classroom behavior of elementary children (Abikoff & Gittelman, 1985); and to improve the off-task behavior and compliance of preschoolers with adults (Barkley, 1988). Medication appears more helpful in the early years when strict behavior management programs and cognitive strategies have a better chance of augmenting the effects of medication for more long-lasting benefit.

Disorganization, notorious in those with ADHD/ADD, is also improved with medication. This trait, however, cannot be overcome entirely with medicine. Organization, structure, planning ahead and goal-setting must be consciously taught as well. With medication and much perseverance on the part of teachers and parents, these skills can, nonetheless, be taught quite successfully.

Decreased Activity Level in ADHD

Activity level, too, is an ADHD/ADD characteristic which is especially responsive to medication effects. In general, the excessive levels of activity characteristic of ADHD are positively affected by medication. The findings of Porrino and his associates (1983) also suggest that a reduction in activity occurs not all the time, but specifically during those times when decreased activity level is beneficial for the situation at hand. They found, for example, that activity levels during structured academic activities decreased, while activity levels during play and sports actually increased. Rather than being a general dampener of activity level, medicine is, instead, a modulator of activity, helping the child respond differentially and appropriately to the demands of each situation.

This point is important, for children are sometimes described as "zombies" on medication. This effect is not an appropriate medication effect, but rather is the result of inaccurate diagnosis, the wrong medication, or excessive amounts of the appropriate one. It is not a side effect which should be tolerated because of a beneficial effect on attention and work completion. These improvements, instead, can be obtained without making the child lethargic or dull.

While diagnosis is not a primary concern of this book, it is important to emphasize that almost every ADHD and ADD child can exhibit a normal activity level and behave appropriately in some situations. They are notably those encounters which are novel, interactive and involve one-on-one attention. A visit with the pediatrician or psychologist, of course, qualifies for this kind of setting. The child's behavior in the office, therefore, is usually not a good diagnostic indicator. Attention to Nintendo and TV are very poor indicators as well, since even the most hyperactive children can often attend to them for long periods. The more restrictive the environment and the more concentration required, the more likely the ADHD/ADD child is to exhibit symptoms of inappropriate activity level. Since school typifies these demands, both overactive and underactive children and adolescents encounter their greatest problems in the academic setting. Other situations which involve listening for long periods can also be difficult for them. ADHD/ADD adults also experience attention problems in similar situations.

Improvement in Underactive ADD

Most of the literature addresses the overactivity of the ADHD child. The improvement in energy level, focusing and accomplishment can be equally dramatic in the underactive, sluggish, slow-processing ADD person. Those on this end of the spectrum go unrecognized much of the time and are often relegated to lives of inefficiency, depression and underachievement. Drs. Shaywitz and Shaywitz (1988) described the identification of this group as representing only "the tip of the iceberg" and strongly advocated identification of and treatment for them. I certainly concur, for this is a group where minimal intervention can result in major improvements.

A recent study by Famularo and Fenton (1987) supports this view. Significant academic progress, as measured by school grades, was obtained in ten children diagnosed as ADD without hyperactivity, who were treated with Ritalin. Their grades declined equally significantly when the Ritalin was discontinued.

One of the goals of this book is to help people identify and treat subtle attention disorders, as well as the more blatant, hyperactive, unmanageable ADHD child or adolescent, so that we can maximize our human resources at a minimum of therapeutic and financial cost. At the present time, we are expending the greatest part of our treatment resources on a relatively small percentage of the ADHD/ADD population. While we certainly want to treat this group of severely affected children, we cannot afford not to treat those who would benefit so greatly from so little expenditure of our time and resources.

Improvement in Behavior

The ability of medication to decrease negative behavior and enhance positive, more appropriate behavior, both in the classroom and at home, has been demonstrated repeatedly. Children on medication, especially stimulant medication, are more cooperative; they talk out inappropriately in class less; they interact less aggressively with peers; they are less distracting to others; they obey class rules better; and clowning and attention-getting behaviors decrease (Pelham, et al., 1985; Barkley, McMurray et al., 1989).

George Still (1902), at the turn of the century, suggested that these children had a "defect in moral control" because they behaved so poorly. Barkley (1981) referred to their inability to conform to school and societal expectations as "a lack of rule-governed behavior." Most medications, and especially the stimulants, assist with compliance, enabling these children to benefit from social skills training and to engage in socially acceptable, rewarding interactions with others. Drs. Goldstein and Goldstein (1990) differentiate between *noncompliance* and *incompetence*. They state that "[incompetence] must be dealt with through education and skill building, while [noncompliance] is dealt with through punishment." Medication, when paired with behavior management and skill-development programs, is usually successful in assisting both. Positive reinforcement, substituted for punishment, also greatly benefits this process.

Adam, a second grader referred for severe ADHD, exemplifies the problems of behavior in overactive children. The following are the Conner's Teacher and Parent Rating Scales completed at the time of the intake evaluation:

Teacher's Questionnaire

	Not at all	Just a little	Pretty much	Very much
1. Restless in the "squirmy" sense.			✓	✓
2. Makes inappropriate noises when he shouldn't.				✓
3. Demands must be met immediately.				✓
4. Acts "smart" (impudent or sassy).			✓	
5. Temper outbursts and unpredictable behavior.				✓
6. Overly sensitive to criticism.				✓
7. Distractibility or attention span a problem.				✓
8. Disturbs other children.				✓
9. Daydreams.		✓		
10. Pouts and sulks.		✓		
11. Mood changes quickly and drastically.				✓
12. Quarrelsome.				✓
13. Submissive attitude toward authority.	✓			
14. Restless, always "up and on the go."				✓
15. Excitable, impulsive.				✓
16. Excessive demands for teacher's attention.				✓
17. Appears to be unaccepted by group.				✓
18. Appears to be easily led by other children.	✓			
19. No sense of fair play.		✓		
20. Appears to lack leadership.		✓		
21. Fails to finish things that he starts.				✓
22. Childish and immature.				✓
23. Denies mistakes or blames others.				✓
24. Does not get along well with other children.				✓
25. Uncooperative with classmates.			✓	
26. Easily frustrated in efforts.				✓
27. Uncooperative with teacher.			✓	
28. Difficulty in learning.	✓			

Adam cannot control himself at all! He is having a terrible time in school. I hope you can help him.

27

Adam's Parent Rating score

Parent's Questionnaire	Not at all	Just a little	Pretty much	Very much
1. Picks at things (nails, fingers, hair, clothing).		✓		
2. Sassy to grown-ups.				✓
3. Problems with making or keeping friends.				✓
4. Excitable, impulsive.				✓
5. Wants to run things.				✓
6. Sucks or chews (thumb; clothing; blankets).		✓		
7. Cries easily or often.	✓			
8. Carries a chip on his shoulder.	✓			
9. Daydreams.	✓			
10. Difficulty in learning.	✓			
11. Restless in the "squirmy" sense.			✓	
12. Fearful (of new situations; new people or places; going to school).	✓			
13. Restless, always up and on the go.				✓
14. Destructive.		✓		
15. Tells lies or stories that aren't true.		✓		
16. Shy.	✓			
17. Gets into more trouble than others same age. *at times*				✓
18. Speaks differently from others same age (baby talk; stuttering; hard to understand).				✓
19. Denies mistakes or blames others.				✓
20. Quarrelsome.				✓
21. Pouts and sulks.	✓			
22. Steals.	✓			
23. Disobedient or obeys but resentfully.				✓
24. Worries more than others (about being alone; illness or death).	✓			
25. Fails to finish things.				✓
26. Feelings easily hurt.				✓
27. Bullies others.				✓
28. Unable to stop a repetitive activity.	✓			
29. Cruel.	✓			
30. Childish or immature (wants help he shouldn't need; clings; needs constant reassurance).				✓
31. Distractibility or attention span a problem.				✓
32. Headaches.		✓		
33. Mood changes quickly and drastically.				✓
34. Doesn't like or doesn't follow rules or restrictions.				✓
35. Fights constantly.			✓	
36. Doesn't get along well with brothers or sisters.				✓
37. Easily frustrated in efforts.				✓
38. Disturbs other children.				✓
39. Basically an unhappy child.		✓		
40. Problems with eating (poor appetite; up between bites).		✓		
41. Stomach aches.		✓		
42. Problems with sleep (can't fall asleep; up too early; up in the night).				✓
43. Other aches and pains.	✓			
44. Vomiting or nausea.	✓			
45. Feels cheated in family circle.				✓
46. Boasts and brags.				✓
47. Lets self be pushed around.	✓			
48. Bowel problems (frequently loose; irregular habits; constipation).	✓			

Medication, in conjunction with a multimodal treatment approach, was very successful in assisting with Adam's behavior. He was treated for six weeks after which some areas were reassessed. The following is the Conner's Abbreviated Teacher Questionnaire completed by his classroom teacher.

ABBREVIATED TEACHER QUESTIONNAIRE

NAME *Adam*

TIME OF DAY OBSERVED *8:00 - 2:15*

TIME OF DAY COMPLETED *2:15*

TEACHER OBSERVATIONS

Information obtained 9   27   90   by *E. S.*
              Month Day Year
                     thurs

	Degree of Activity			
	Not at all	Just a little	Pretty much	Very much
1. Restless or overactive	✓			
2. Excitable, impulsive	✓			
3. Disturbs other children	✓			
4. Fails to finish things he starts – short attention span	✓			
5. Constantly fidgeting	✓			
6. Inattentive, easily distracted	✓			
7. Demands must be met immediately – easily frustrated	✓			
8. Cries often and easily	✓			
9. Mood changes quickly and drastically	✓			
10. Temper outbursts, explosive and unpredictable behavior	✓			

Comments: *Great Day !*

Reassessment revealed the following:

Writing and fine-motor control had improved dramatically. Likewise, his cooperativeness, reasonableness and self-esteem were markedly improved. Measurements of attention, concentration, impulse control, activity, compliance, and attention-getting behavior were significantly better as well.

A report to Adam's parents also included this information:

Adam is clearly a child with a severe attention disorder who is responding well to a multimodal treatment program. However, some difficulties continue at school. P.E. remains a problem. Adam is easily overstimulated, and the medication appears to wear off at about that time. The medication has been changed to Ritalin-Sustained Release (SR), which should help. He has also been removed from P.E. temporarily and is assisting kindergarten children as a peer tutor to enhance his self-esteem.

The effect of the medication wearing off before P.E. is clearly seen from the Conner's Abbreviated Teacher Questionnaire completed by his P.E. teacher the same day the "perfect" questionnaire was completed by his regular classroom teacher:

P.E. Teacher isn't There. "He wants problem". needs self-control."

ABBREVIATED TEACHER QUESTIONNAIRE

NAME _Adam_

TIME OF DAY OBSERVED _10:35_   _P.E._

TIME OF DAY COMPLETED _11:00_

TEACHER OBSERVATIONS

Information obtained _10 - 3 - 90_   by _CJ_
                     Month Day Year

		Degree of Activity			
		Not at all	Just a little	Pretty much	Very much
1.	Restless or overactive				✓
2.	Excitable, impulsive				✓
3.	Disturbs other children			✓	
4.	Fails to finish things he starts - short attention span				
5.	Constantly fidgeting				✓
6.	Inattentive, easily distracted				
7.	Demands must be met immediately - easily frustrated				
8.	Cries often and easily				
9.	Mood changes quickly and drastically			✓	
10.	Temper outbursts, explosive and unpredictable behavior				✓

Comments: _Deliberately ignored teachers' request to get a laugh from other students. Blamed another student for his talking. Rolling on the ground making noises and not paying attention to teacher directions._

As a result of the re-evaluation, the following recommendations were made, among others:

> The large classes, intense noise level, potential for overstimulation, and the relatively reduced level of structure necessitate close monitoring and modifications as needed to insure success in this class. Indefinite removal is not a long-term solution. The teachers should be aware of Adam's tendency to become overexcited and lose control, and to assign a teacher or student buddy to use signals, touch cueing and reminders to maintain control. If Adam feels he is losing control, he should have a quiet place he can go to regain his composure.

Following these modifications and additional changes in medication and the administration of it, Adam performed well. No one in his school can believe the difference. They marvel at his improvement and no longer consider him a problem student. Rather, they now appreciate his giftedness, humor and sensitivity to others' needs.

In working with ADHD/ADD children and adolescents, one must have a basic philosophy about their motives. If one believes they are inherently good and problems beyond their control are causing their misbehaviors, they can be a challenge, but also a joy. On the other hand, if they perceive you as thinking they have malevolent intent, you will have little positive impact on them. No amount of medication or education or social skills programs will be successful. Children become what we believe them to be. Each ADHD/ADD child or adolescent needs teachers, parents and professionals in his corner believing in him. When Weiss and Hechtman (1986), in their study of hyperactive adults who had grown up successfully before the advent of treatment, asked these adults, "What made the difference?" Almost all stated, "Someone who believed in me." Sometimes that person was a parent, sometimes a teacher, and sometimes another interested person.

The faith of others in children has profound and far-reaching effects. Perhaps medicine simply makes it a little easier, for those of us less hardy souls, to believe.

Effect on Cognition and Learning

The effect of medication on cognitive functioning and the ability to learn has been the subject of much controversy. Many consider attention deficit disorders to be learning disabilities. Likewise, *dyslexia*, as defined by the Orton-Gillingham Society, is very reminiscent of descriptions of attention disorders. The overlap of and confusion between these areas may account for the lack of consistent findings among those who have investigated cognition and learning.

I would like to stress that learning disabilities and attention deficit disorders are *not* the same, as previously addressed in Chapter 2.[1] It is important to determine very specifically what portion of a child's difficulties are ADD-related and what problems have resulted from learning disabilities.

When academic problems and school failure are primarily the result of an attention deficit disorder, medication can be expected to improve the student's accomplishments significantly. Many investigators have found that non-learning-disabled ADHD and ADD children on stimulant medication improved dramatically in their academic performance in reading and spelling (Rapoport, et al., 1986; Stevenson, et al., 1984), mathematical computation (Douglas et al., 1986), and tasks involving memory. These effects are especially noteworthy if treatment is begun early in the child's academic career before he has developed delays and gaps in his acquisition of knowledge. Once such deficiencies are present, medication will assist only to the degree that the gaps and delays are addressed through additional instruction by the teacher, the

---

[1]A child or adolescent may have a pure learning disability, a pure attention deficit disorder, or a combination of the two.

parents, or a tutor.

True reading disorders and learning disabilities are not believed to be substantially improved by medication. They require, instead, specific learning disabilities remediation and teaching strategies which maximize the child's best learning modalities. For those with attention deficit disorders, whether with or without learning disabilities, treatment with medication unquestionably aids academic achievement via more efficient and careful performance when the child's other learning needs are simultaneously addressed. As a primary and single intervention for academic problems, medication is, in my opinion, notably unsuccessful despite there being areas of improvement.

At the same time, I do not wish to minimize the positive effect medication can have on the learning capacities of learning-disabled children who have coexisting attention disorders. Their improvement in a program which addresses both can be immense.

Improved School Performance

While medication may or may not impact learning disabilities *per se*, it usually does improve school performance. The changes are, in fact, quite dramatic much of the time.

Work Completion

Improved attention and efficiency, as already suggested, have many positive effects on the child's performance at school. The amount of work completed by the student is typically increased dramatically. The overactive child, who usually rushes through his work, settles into a more manageable pace with notable improvement in neatness and accuracy. For some children, medication may solve their work-completion problems altogether. Slow-processing ADD children usually respond with an increase in speed. More compulsive children may have difficulty even on medication, and may get worse if their diagnosis is really *overfocused disorder* rather than underactive ADD. These children, even though working more quickly, may still require modifications in the amount of written work required if they are to be successful. The overfocused disorder is addressed in Chapter 10 in conjunction with the use of clonidine.

Handwriting

One of the most immediate and dramatic changes frequently noticed when ADHD children begin taking medication is an improvement in their fine-motor skills, especially handwriting. Handwriting samples before and after medication provide dramatic examples of the medication effect. The following handwriting sample of an eight-year-old off medication one day and on medication the next graphically illustrates this point.

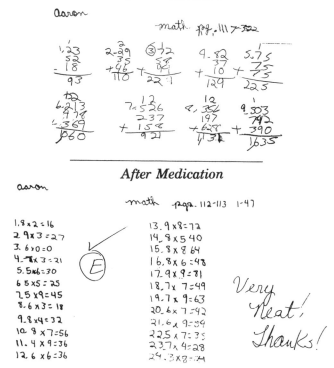

Before Medication

After Medication

Perhaps a more vivid example is that of a seven-year-old child, Edward, who wrote his letters and numbers first while experiencing the full effects of the medication:

The next sample shows Edward losing control as the medicine (5 mg. Ritalin) wore off. The loss of fine-motor and impulse control was dramatic:

Handwriting frequently improves in the treated ADHD child for three reasons: (1) he has more impulse control; (2) he can now pay more attention to his penmanship; and (3) his work rate becomes more consistent with the demands of his teacher. Those who formerly rushed through their written work are now more careful, while those who previously plodded through, daydreaming much of the time, work more efficiently.

While improvement in handwriting may occur, it may not—even with medication. Those students who continue to experience frustration, fatigue and impatience with handwriting can have major problems in school because they will write as little as possible to get by. The difference in their verbal and written performance can be close to unbelievable. The following is an example of a story written by a 13-year-old gifted student in response to a request to write a story to a sequence of scenes given him as part of a psychological/ psychoeducational evaluation:

When his handwriting difficulties became apparent, he was asked to dictate a story to the same three scenes. It is as follows:

Once upon a time there were some people on a far, faraway planet who knew their planet was about to explode. So they all jumped in their space buggy and went off to a planet called Tripton. Tripton was a yellow planet that had little machines all over it. They didn't know what robots were, so they figured it out and called them Scott. What they didn't know were that these Scotts were killer robots and they were going to kill them. So they started playing with them, and they were in favor of the little robots called the Scotts. Scott started liking them except for their leader. He didn't like them. He wanted to kill them. So he pulled out his big gun and he shot Bob. Bob was the oldest one. He was fixing to die anyway, so it didn't really matter. They were all upset. So they made a day honoring Bob. Every year they'd honor Bob by dancing around until they got tired of honoring Bob, so they quit. Sue had another little baby. They called her Avery. Avery was a cute little baby with blue eyes and yellow hair. Soon they figured out this planet was about to explode, too, so they all jumped in their space craft and forgot to put gas in it, so they rode off and they stopped in the middle of space. They were just going along, and they had to shut the engine out. They're still going because nothing was going to stop them. Pretty soon they stopped in the middle of space, no food, and they ran out of oxygen and died.

The difference in both quality, quantity, thematic maturity, style, and use of vocabulary is dramatic. This student is one who will require modifications in his written-work requirements, especially the use of a word-processor, to insure academic performance consistent with his potential.

Following Directions

Understanding directions and following them accurately are also greatly improved by the child's increased attention to the demands of the classroom, especially the teacher's instructions. Students, who formerly jumped the gun and started assignments before they really knew what their teachers wanted, can patiently sit through their explanations. Those with subtle auditory processing problems seem infinitely more able to understand language to which they have paid close attention. Research has demonstrated a positive, dose-related effect on language processing ability in reading-disabled, ADHD children, even though medication had no discernible effect on the speed or accuracy of their oral reading or reading comprehension (Ballinger, et al., 1984; Riddle & Rapoport, 1976). Both clinical experience and research consistently reveal improvement in listening and language processing. Those students who formerly became internally distracted in the middle of instructions can now stay tuned in. This ability to hear, understand and remember greatly increases the student's ability to achieve in school.

Neatness, Accuracy and Organization

Another noticeable medication effect is the child or teen's improved attention to detail and increased accuracy and neatness. Errors decrease dramatically in math and written language assignments. Internal organizational ability is enhanced to assist the student plan his work more carefully, thus enabling him to be more successful.

Concern about school performance is usually one of the primary reasons professional assistance is sought. From the above descriptions of the improvements which occur in work completion, handwriting, following directions, neatness, accuracy and organization, we can unequivocally say that medication can greatly enhance the child's success in school. When trying to decide whether to use medication and, later, in assessing its benefits, these areas should be carefully considered.

Memory/Concentration

Auditory short-term memory is significantly impaired in many with ADHD and ADD. In fact, measures of memory are part of most psychological/psychoeducational batteries assessing attention disorders. Visual short-term memory is less likely to be impaired but is affected in some children.

Adam, our bright second-grade, severely ADHD, student referred to previously, exemplifies the problem. Unlike most ADHD students, his auditory memory scores were close to age level. However, they were dramatically impaired for ability level.

Detroit Test of Learning Aptitude-Revised (DTLA-2)
Subtests

Before Medication

	Age Score	Difference From C.A.*
(C.A. = 7-5)		
Auditory Attention Span for Unrelated Words[2]	7-6	+1 mo.
Auditory Attention Span for Related Syllables[3]	7-0	-5 mos.
Oral Directions[4]	9-0 to 9-3	+1 yr., 7 mos. to +1 yr., 10 mos.

*C.A. = Chronological Age

---

[2]Memory for nonmeaningful, rote material (words, numbers, etc.).
[3]Memory for meaningful material (sentences, etc.).
[4]Auditory and visual memory utilized simultaneously. Part of the original DTLA.

Detroit Test of Learning Aptitude-Revised (DTLA-R)
Subtests

After Medication

(C.A. = 7-6)	Age Score	Difference From C.A.	Improvement after 6 weeks on medication
Auditory Attention Span for Unrelated Words	9-0	+1 yr., 6 mos.	+1 yr., 5 mos.
Auditory Attention Span for Related Syllables	8-6	+1 yr., 0 mos.	+1 yr., 5 mos.
Oral Directions	10-0 to 10-3	+2 yrs., 6 mos.	+11 mos.

Brian, a 13 1/2 year-old seventh grader, obtained scores very typical of the undiagnosed, older, severely affected student:

Detroit Test of Learning Aptitude-Revised (DTLA-2)
Subtests

Before Medication

(C.A. = 13-6)	Age Score	Difference From C.A.*
Auditory Attention Span for Unrelated Words	7-9	— 5 yrs., 9 mos.
Auditory Attention Span for Related Syllables	11-6	— 2 yrs., 0 mos.
Visual Attention Span for Letters[5]	9-6 to 9-9	— 4 yrs.
Oral Directions	6-0	—7 yrs., 6 mos.

---

[5]Rote memory for sequences of letters.

Concentration problems, distractibility and poor short-term memory problems contribute significantly to a measure often utilized in the assessment of attention deficit disorders, i.e., the Freedom From Distractibility Quotient (FFD) on the Wechsler Intelligence Scale for Children, Revised (WISC-R) and the WISC-III.

I.Q. or Ability Measures

While some measures of intellectual ability are relatively resilient to the effects of ADHD/ADD, others are not. On the Wechsler Scales, the most commonly administered individual tests of I.Q., the following are those areas affected and those relatively unaffected:

WECHSLER INTELLIGENCE SCALES
FOR PRESCHOOL, CHILD/ADOLESCENT AND ADULT

Verbal Scores	Performance Scores
• Information	•• Picture Completion
++ Similarities	++ Picture Arrangement
+ Arithmetic	•• Block Design
• Vocabulary	•• Object Assembly
++ Comprehension	+•• Coding
+ Digit Span	•• Mazes

+   Very affected by the attention disorder. Scores are usually much lower than other scaled scores. (Make up FFD score.)

++   Usually unaffected. These scaled scores give estimates of true potential.

•   Scores often lowered by reduced interest in reading and ability to retain academic information, although they may not be. More affected at older ages.

••   Scores may be lowered by impulsivity or an excessively slow work rate.

The following are Brian's test scores at the time of initial testing and before treatment of the ADHD, with tests very affected indicated (*).

INTELLECTUAL EVALUATION (WISC-R)

VERBAL TESTS	Scaled Score**	Percentile	Range
Information	12	75	High Average
Similarities	13	84	High Average
*Arithmetic	7	16	Low Average
Vocabulary	11	63	Average
Comprehension	14	91	Superior
*Digit Span	9	37	Average

PERFORMANCE TESTS	Scaled Score	Percentile	Range
Picture Completion	15	95	Very Superior
Picture Arrangement	13	84	High Average
Block Design	9	37	Average
Object Assembly	13	84	High Average
*Coding	7	16	Low Average
Mazes	13	84	High Average

***Scaled Score: A statistical score. Average of 10 = 50%*

Verbal I.Q. Score	108	69	Average
Performance I.Q. Score	109	72	Average
Full Scale I.Q. Score	109	72	Average
*Distractibility Quotient (FFD)	85	16	Low Average
Potential I.Q. (Based on scores least affected by ADHD/ADD)	115-119	84-90	High Average

Discussion of Brian's Intellectual Assessment: Results of the intellectual evaluation indicated that Brian was functioning overall at the high end of the Average range of mental abilities. There was not a significant discrepancy between his language abilities and visual/ spatial abilities. There was, however, significant variability among the subtest scores. The pattern of scores reflects interference, as well as potential higher than the scores obtained. A distractibility quotient was computed. This is an I.Q. equivalency score which frequently predicts the child's level of academic achievement better than I.Q. scores. This score was 85 and indicates that Brian's short attention span, distractibility and impulsivity interfered with his performance of this test. Therefore, the I.Q. scores obtained should be considered underestimates of his true ability. Areas of comparative strength identified were his common-sense reasoning and judgment, alertness to visual detail, abstract verbal reasoning, and long-term visual memory. Areas of comparative weakness noted were his short-term auditory memory, mental computation, and concentration. Brian's speed and accuracy in executing visual-motor tasks was significantly delayed and suggests graphomotor problems and an excessively slow work rate. Brian also had a significant problem with internal distractibility. His distractibility quotient is noteworthy in that it is 24 points below his Full Scale I.Q. score and 30 points below his projected potential.

The WISC-R scores on page 121 are those of Adam, our ADHD second grader, before, and approximately six weeks after, medication.

WISC-R Test Scores Before and After Medication

VERBAL	Before Medication (8/21/90, Age 7-5) Standard Scores	%	After Medication (10/1/90, Age 7-6) Standard Scores	%
Information	16	98	--	--
Similarities	18	99.6	--	--
*Arithmetic	10	50	14	91
Vocabulary	18	99.6	--	--
Comprehension	17	99	--	--
*(Digit Span)[6]	(8)	(25)	(10)	(50)
Verbal I.Q. Score	137	99+	142	99+
PERFORMANCE	Scores	%	Scores	%
Picture Completion	9	37	15	95
Picture Arrangement	10	50	--	--
Block Design	13	84	--	--
Object Assembly	13	84	--	--
*Coding	8	25	13	84
Performance I.Q. Score =	104	60	120	91
Full Scale I.Q. Score =	123	93	135	99

*FFD Components

Following the evaluation, Adam had been placed on stimulant medication (Ritalin). A strict behavior management program was instituted both at home and at school, as well as a responsibility program and a program of organization and structure.

---

[6]Digit Span score not used in computation of I.Q. scores.

Adam responded well to the above interventions. As recommended to his parents, those subtests especially affected by distractibility, impulsivity and poor motor control were readministered. The significant impact medication can have on a child's ability to perform on a test of intelligence is illustrated in the re-test results. The changes can be even more striking after several months of treatment.

Academic Achievement in Content Areas (Reading, Math, Social Studies, etc.)

Children with attention disorders are frequently underachieving significantly by the end of third grade, if not before. Neither parents nor teachers may realize this, since group-administered tests of intelligence, such as the Otis-Lennon Test of Mental Ability, usually do not accurately reflect the true ability of the ADHD/ ADD student. These measures, unfortunately, are negatively affected by the same variables that impair performance in the classroom.   Thus, a student's achievement scores may be consistent with his group-measured ability level, but *both* may be decreased significantly by the ADHD/ADD.

Brian's achievement scores illustrate the negative effect of ADHD on achievement:

Brian, Age 13-6, Grade Level = 7.7

WRAT-R, LEVEL 2

	Standard Score	Percentile	Grade Equivalent[7]
Reading	80	9	4-E[8]
Spelling	86	18	5-E
Arithmetic	75	55	5-E

---

[7]Grade equivalent is the grade level at which a student is performing regardless of the grade he is in. [8]E = End.

Brian's achievement was consistent with his Distractibility Quotient (FFD=85), not his intellectual ability (potential I.Q. = 115-119). There was, in fact, a discrepancy of 23 to 34 points between ability and achievement in all three measures reported. While Brian qualified as learning disabled (LD) because he met the discrepancy requirements of more than 15 scaled- score points between obtained I.Q. (109) and academic achievement (75, 80 and 86), it was the Examiner's opinion that the problem was more ADHD than LD.

As reported previously, academic achievement improves significantly on medication when gaps and delays are remediated and learning strengths are enhanced. By contrast, even very bright ADHD/ADD students whose disorders go untreated usually do relatively poorly on the Scholastic Aptitude Test (SAT) or the American College Test (ACT) since these are measures of acquired information and not just ability. Matt's scores are typical. Tested very late, as a senior in high school, he obtained a Verbal I.Q. of 124, 94%, a Performance I.Q. score of 114, 83% and a Full Scale I.Q. score of 123, 93%. However, his SAT scores were below average: Verbal SAT, 415; Math SAT, 372.

Once a pattern of underachievement is begun, a student becomes trapped into a low level of accomplishment until the problems are identified and treatment is obtained. Matt did obtain treatment and has been successful as a freshman in college.

Many more adolescents and college students are currently being identified as having attention deficit disorders. They benefit enormously from treatment and are usually ecstatic over their newfound hope.

The importance of early identification cannot be overstated. The following are the results of an evaluation on Edward, whose handwriting samples on and off medication were shown on p. 112. Edward was first evaluated at age four years, eight months.

Wechsler Preschool and Primary Scale of Intelligence-Revised (WPPSI-R)

Before Treatment

Edward, age 4-8

VERBAL	Scaled Scores	Percentile	Range
Information	13	84	High Average
Vocabulary	15	95	Superior
Arithmetic	9	37	Average
Similarities	14	91	Superior
Comprehension	13	13	High Average
(Sentences)	(8)	(25)	Average (Low)

PERFORMANCE

Animal House	10	50	Average
Picture Completion	12	75	High Average
Mazes	8	25	Average (Low)
Geometric Design	11	63	Average
Block Design	11	63	Average
Verbal I.Q.	117	87	High Average
Performance I.Q.	103	58	Average
Full Scale I.Q.	110	77	High Average
Verbal Comprehension D.Q.*	121	92	Superior Range
Perceptual Organization D.Q.*	103	58	Average Range
Distractibility Quotient	93	30	Average Range

*D.Q. = Deviation Quotient

Edward was evaluated again at age 7 years, 3 months after a successful multimodal intervention program of behavior management, treatment for allergies, educational modifications, and medication.

Wechsler Intelligence Scale for Children-Revised (WISC-R)

On Medication

Edward (Reevaluation after
Treatment) Age 7-3

VERBAL	Scaled Scores	Percentile	Range
Information	19	99.9+	Gifted
Similarities	19	99.9+	Gifted
Arithmetic	13	84.0	High Average
Vocabulary	19	99.9+	Gifted
Comprehension	19	99.9+	Gifted
Digit Span	13	84*	High Average

PERFORMANCE

Picture Completion	14	91	Superior
Picture Arrangement	15	95	Superior
Block Design	13	84	High Average
Object Assembly	8	25	Average
Mazes	12	75	High Average

Verbal I.Q. Score	150	99.9	Gifted
Performance I.Q. Score	117	87	High Average
Full Scale I.Q. Score	139	99	Gifted
Distractibility Quotient	117	87	High Average

*Missed most backwards

The rest of the evaluation reveals Edward's progress after two and one-half years of intervention.

Visual-Motor Integration
(*Beery-Buktenica VMI Test*)
Age Score = 9-4   Differential = +2 yrs., 1 mo.

Emotional

Much happier, more cooperative
"Delightful" in school
Proficient in horseback and art

Speech and Language
Some articulation problems still present.   Enunciates everything precisely, giving speech somewhat stilted quality.

Language-gifted. Incredible knowledge for a child his age.

Memory
Detroit Test of Learning Aptitude-2 Subtests

Auditory Attention Span for Unrelated Words

Age 7-6   +3 mos.

Visual Attention Span for Objects

Age 10-0   +2 yrs., 9 mos.

Visual Attention Span for Letters

Age 7-3 to 7-6   0 to +3 mos.

Oral Directions

Age 7-6 to 7-9   +3 to 6 mos.

Achievement

a) Wide Range Achievement Test-Revised: Level 1

Subtest	Grade Equivalent
Reading	2.5
Word Identification	3.6
Word Attack	3.4

b) Woodcock Reading Mastery Test

Subtest	Grade Equivalent
Letter Identification	2.5
Word Identification	3.6
Word Attack	3.4

Writing

Despite age-appropriate short-term visual memory, Edward is still having significant problems retrieving letters from long-term memory to write (see page 112). Many reversals continue to be present despite excellent letter recognition and reading ability.

Attention, Concentration, Impulse Control

Doing very nicely. On 2.5 mg. of Ritalin for school only. Mother very pleased with allergic desensitization and the elimination of food intolerances. Behavior management and responsibility programs very successful.

Summary

Edward is performing extremely well in all areas except visual processing and visual retrieval. His true intellectual giftedness has blossomed, as have his academic skills. His small stature, remaining articulation difficulties, and ADD influenced Edward's parents to keep him in kindergarten for another year. He is in a very accelerated academic program and should do well with continued close monitoring of speech, medication, behavior management and parent counseling.

Improved Sports, Scouts, Extracurricular Activities

It is not surprising that medication can positively affect sports as well as academics. One of the most notable changes is seen on the baseball field. This sport is one of the more slow-moving, and thus one of the most problematic for these children. The overactive child seems always in trouble for kicking the dirt, shoving other children, or arguing with the coach. Underactive ADD children can be seen in the outfield where daisies and airplanes are far more interesting than the game itself. On medication, both the overactive and underactive attention-disordered child and adolescent can be far more successful.

Tennis, with its demands for constant attention, also reaps the benefits of medication for many children and teens. Very active sports such as football and basketball, which require more reactivity and spontaneity and less attention, may either benefit or be slightly impaired by medication. The child or adolescent playing the sport is often the best judge of what is most helpful. Parents, too, are astute observers of positive and negative changes and can assist in the decision-making process.

Karate is a sport which benefits from medication and is also of great benefit to most ADHD/ADD children. With its emphasis on kinesthetic learning, individual accomplishment, and self-discipline, it is ideal for this child. Other individual sports, including track and swimming among others, can likewise be very positive pursuits.

Improved Peer Relations

The ADHD child's social relationships are an area of intense concern to parents, teachers and professionals alike. It is disheartening to see a child actively rejected by his peers because he lacks social skills and an intuitive understanding of the rules of social behavior. The ADHD child's overactivity, impulsivity, low frustration tolerance, attention-getting behavior, and bossiness make him especially vulnerable to peer disdain. The underactive ADD child by contrast may relate well socially or he may become isolated and lonely. He is usually not actively rejected or avoided, as is the ADHD child.

While some studies have failed to document a positive effect of medication on peer interactions in a laboratory situation (Cunningham, et al., 1985; Pelham & Bender, 1982), others have found positive dose-related changes in social behavior in a "natural context" (Whalen et al., 1987). Both adult observers and peers appear quite sensitive to changes in a broad range of behaviors in children who are placed on medication.

The difference is often described as "dramatic" or "like day and night." Peers are usually more accepting once the child is placed on medication. This is true, however, only if his social interactions become more appropriate and if he has not become a scapegoat.

Both the positive and negative findings of the research are observable in real life. Many children relate much more appropriately and improve their peer relations significantly when treated. Others, even on medication, appear to lack social antennae and require specific training in appropriate interpersonal awareness and social behaviors. Some of these differences may relate more to personality and style than to attention disorders. Other people are believed to have a true social learning disability, called *dyssmia* (Norwicki & Duke, 1992). Given that positive peer relations represent one of the best predictors of long-term adjustment (Cowen et al., 1973), it is critical that we expend as much energy on social skills and cognitive training as is necessary to facilitate this aspect of the ADHD/ADD child/adolescent's development. Social skills training and cognitive therapy, which have been theoretically combined and are now known as *cognitive behavior modification (CBM)*, have not been as successful for children not on medication as for those who are (Whalen et al., 1985). Without medication, these attempts at training are often characterized by great frustration for the child and therapist alike.

Better Family Relations

Like peer relations, family interactions have been shown to improve significantly with medical treatment of the attention disorder. Schachar et al. (1987) found that the boys they studied, who were Ritalin-responsive, showed improved interactions with their siblings and mothers, increased affection from their mothers, and fewer negative encounters with all family members.

Decreases in negative behavior on the part of the child typically result in a concomitant decrease in parental criticism, control and negative behavior toward the child (Barkley, 1988; Barkley & Cunningham, 1979a). The ADHD/ADD child's natural ability to increase the stress in his home often brings out the worst in both his parents and his siblings. Medication, when taken for home benefit as well as school, modulates negative family interactions quite effectively.

The positive benefit for siblings is perhaps an equally important consideration as to what is best for the child. The siblings of overactive children are usually given less attention and feel much anger and resentment toward the child and often the parents as well. Many are embarrassed by their ADHD sibling's behavior in school and may be teased by peers who know them both.

The stress of the ADHD/ADD child on a marriage can be enormous. When considering treatment, benefits for the entire family system must be considered.

Given the increased potential for social learning and positive interactions between the ADHD/ADD's child and his family as a result of medication, one must carefully consider the issue of how often to administer medicine and what the target goals should be. Social skills, rather than academic accomplishment primarily, should perhaps be our number one priority since they appear most predictive of successful long-term adjustment. Giving a child medication for school only may be as unfair to him as having him wear his glasses exclusively when copying work from the board, or taking antibiotics just while he has a fever. The child belongs to a system; the entire family system must improve for his success to be assured.

Enhanced Self-Esteem

When the child's behavior and grades improve at school, when his peer relations turn positive, when family interactions become a source of comfort and camaraderie, and when the child becomes successful in extracurricular activities, it follows that his self-esteem will improve. Clinical observations, family and teacher reports, and research confirm this expectation. Medical intervention, when a part of a multimodal treatment program, has been found to improve significantly both general esteem and academic confidence after several months of treatment (Kelly, et al., 1989). In this study by Kelly, it is noteworthy that improvement did not occur after one month only; rather several months of successful intervention were necessary to increase esteem. Enhanced esteem is a secondary benefit of success in other areas.

The positive interaction effects are seen frequently in our practice. Just as negatives can snowball downward, so can positives build up momentum in an upward direction. Self-esteem, in my opinion, is absolutely dependent upon success in endeavors the child deems important, and the positive regard of others. Medication appears, once more, to set the stage so that the promise of other interventions can be fulfilled.

WHAT MEDICATIONS FOR ADHD/ADD CAN DO

SUMMARY

- Improve attention and concentration
- Decrease distractibility
- Decrease impulsivity
- Decrease activity level
- Increase alertness and energy of underactive ADD
- Improve behavior
- Improve acquisition of information
- Improve school performance
- Improve short- and long-term memory
- Improve ability (I.Q.) measures decreased by ADD effects
- Improve academic achievement
- Improve sports, scouts, extracurricular activities
- Increase peer acceptance
- Enhance family relationships

WHAT MEDICATIONS FOR
ADHD/ADD CANNOT DO

Medicine unquestionably can have very positive benefits for the great majority of those diagnosed with ADHD or ADD. Lest we become overly dependent on this as a primary treatment, however, it is important to again emphasize that medicine alone is not enough. The research documents conclusively that, while medication may have very dramatic, short-term positive effects when used without other supportive therapies, long-term benefit can be minimal and is often absent altogether.

What Medicine Cannot Do For
School-Related Problems

School has been described as the ADHD/ADD child and adolescent's worst affliction. Even with medication, it may continue to be so if the limitations of medication are not realized and remaining difficulties aggressively addressed. To expand on Drs. Shaywitz's (1988) comments, "Proper school placement, appropriate teaching methods, and educational accommodations represent perhaps the most critical factors in the success of pharmacotherapy since this therapy will most certainly be ineffective unless the child's educational environment is both appropriate and satisfactory." While medication is certainly helpful, there are many goals neurotransmitter regulation cannot accomplish:

1) Despite improving grades and academic performance significantly, medication does not appear to improve long-term academic achievement (Ballinger, et al., 1984; Klee, et al., 1986), nor more complex cognitive processing such as divergent thinking (Salanto & Wender, 1989). Likewise, while simple language processing tasks have benefitted from medication, no improvements in oral reading or reading comprehension have been found (Ballinger, et al., 1984; Riddle & Rapoport, 1976).

2) Medicine does not enable a child to learn through inappropriate teaching methods. Even on medication, a visual learner will not be able to learn effectively through primarily auditory instruction. An overactive, kinesthetic learner, often a great athlete, will continue to make A's on the playground and F's in reading, even with appropriate medical intervention.

3) Medicine does not alter the negative effects of overplacement or inappropriate placement in school. Only evaluation and appropriate placement in both the grade he is in and the school he attends will enable the child to perform satisfactorily.

4) While medication helps, it is usually not sufficient to override the typical ADHD/ADD student's lack of organization and his inability to break tasks into smaller units. Both parents and teachers need to understand that organizational ability is directly related to neurotransmitter functioning. Most ADHD/ADD students must have specific structure and organizational assistance, and usually some form of ongoing close supervision, if they are to be successful. While organization may not come naturally, it can be learned.

5) Medication does not effectively treat true, neurologically based, learning disabilities. Specific learning disability assistance by a specialist who understands both LD and ADHD/ADD will be required.

6) Medication does not remediate delays and gaps in the acquisition of academic information. Only tutoring and specific academic instruction can meet these needs.

7) Medication helps normalize brain chemistry but it does not overcome the neurologic immaturity of most students with attention disorders. Careful selection of maturational peers is crucial. Many students will require delayed school entrance or retention for maximum

overall benefit. More medication will not resolve these difficulties.

8)   Handwriting and work-rate problems are almost universal in these students. While medication can have a dramatic and positive effect on these in some students, others experience little or no benefit at all. Alternative methods, including typing and word processing, tape recorders, and verbal or visual methods of sharing what one knows, must be available, as well as other classroom accommodations for areas of continued difficulty. Reducing the amount of written work required is a *must* for many students with attention disorders, even on medication.

Other Things Medicine Cannot Do
... At Home and At School

1)   While medication does decrease impulsivity and inappropriate responding, it often does not remedy long-standing social-skill deficits so characteristic of these students. These must be systematically taught to the child or adolescent by a trained person, either at school by a concerned teacher or counselor, or by a therapist, if the student is to make a successful social adjustment.

2)   Medication does not teach cognitive strategies to assist with many of the symptoms of ADHD/ADD which will persist even with treatment. Learning to stop, look and listen; to think before acting; to assess the consequences of one's behavior; and to learn problem-solving skills are essential components of the therapeutic process.

3)   ADHD/ADD children and adolescents profit less from experience, even on medication, than their non-attention-disordered peers. Instead of the usual consequences, which are effective with other children, they require very systematic behavior management programs with predictable and consistent consequences for both positive and negative behaviors. The use of natural or logical consequences alone is

rarely effective, thus rendering parent training programs based on this model less than ideal. Since research reveals an unusually poor response to punishment in those with this disorder, behavioral programs should be as positively oriented as possible. Kløve's discussion of the neurophysiology of ADHD sheds interesting light on the poor response to punishment often observed in overactive, hard-to-manage children. He states: "A dysfunction in the septohippocampal system [in the brain] in ADHD predicts that these patients respond positively to reinforcement but not to aversive operant conditioning" (Kløve, 1984). When negative consequences must be implemented at home and at school, "time-out" procedures are much more effective if, and only if, emphasis is placed on cognitive understanding and future coping strategies in the debriefing sessions which should follow the administration of any disciplinary action. Those with attention disorders are notoriously unresponsive to any form of perceived coercion or force. The worst behavioral problems in these children occur when they are dealt with in a rigid, authoritarian, punitive manner, whether verbal or more physical.

What Medicine Cannot Do At Home

Since the benefit of medication is often experienced primarily at school, especially when the child is on stimulant medication taken only twice daily, strategies for effectively managing the symptoms of ADHD/ADD at home are especially critical. Even when on medication, these developmental goals are not addressed:

1) Medication does not teach responsibility and self-discipline. Nor does it teach the value of work and team effort. Programs designed to organize and teach the child and adolescent very systematically that he is responsible for himself and his belongings and that he must adhere to a schedule of activities and chores goes far in assisting him develop the skills so needed for a successful adult life. Unlike the child who comes into this world organized and responsible, he will require much

more effort and training on the part of parents to help him acquire these same skills.

2)   Medication assists the child in being more cooperative, but it does not teach him the philosophy and values of this approach to life. Only those who internalize such principles because of their perceived worth will follow them later.   Parents must spend much time teaching impulsive children values and then guiding them to the means of achieving them.

3)   Compliance, a major problem for ADHD/ADD children, is again assisted by medicine.   However, the most successful parenting programs are those which change attitudes, as well as behavior, through positive reinforcement and ongoing cognitive emphasis.   These strategies require parent and teacher knowledge and effort which extend far beyond the medicinal effect.

4)   Medication does not teach skills—how to cook, repair the car, plan a budget, earn money, take messages, mend clothes, and the many other tasks of daily living.   The more skills a person has, the more competent he feels. A very real danger for children with any kind of problem is that parents will feel sorry for them and decrease both their level of expectation and the knowledge they impart. If parents or teachers feel sorry for the ADHD/ADD child, he will feel sorry for himself. The ADHD/ADD child can be expected to become what adults expect of him. Belief in the child and perceiving his worth are, in the long run, perhaps the most critical gift adults can give this youngster.

5)   Consideration and respect are, likewise, values which are taught by caring adults.   They are not acquired through neurotransmitter regulation.

These examples represent only a few of the challenges facing those who understand the wholistic nature of the ADHD/ADD child or adolescent, and each parent's hopes for him, both currently and for his adult life. Medication is of tremendous assistance in this process. Perhaps its greatest benefit lies in its ability to enable the child to respond positively to and learn from the appropriate and helpful inter-actions of those who love him, care for him, and teach him.

Summary

For most children, adolescents, and adults with attention disorders, medication will prove to be the single most critical aspect of an effective treatment plan. It must be remembered, however, that medication cannot be the only aspect an intervention program and can be used successfully only in combination with other behavioral and educational interventions. Medications for ADHD/ADD should be seen, then, as a cornerstone of a long-term treatment program, but, in the same way that the cornerstone is but the beginning of the building, medications are but the first step in long-term solutions of attention disorders.

*People are usually more convinced by reasons
they discovered themselves than by those found
by others.*

— Blaise Pascal (1623-1662)

7

Medication Usage: Practical Issues

DECISION TO USE MEDICATION—
ASSESSING THE BENEFIT: RISK RATIO

To medicate ... or not to medicate? That is the question which haunts
parents the most and one which professionals must address repeatedly
until parents are as reconciled as they possibly can be to a difficult
situation where the treatment possibilities are somewhat limited. When
treating a medical problem, the options sometimes become "Which is the
least troublesome of the *negative* alternatives?" With ADHD/ADD, the
negative alternatives may be to give medicine and live with the potential
side-effects, or not give medicine and live with the almost certain
negative social, emotional and academic consequences.

Parents and physicians usually reach a decision about utilizing
medication by: (1) comparing the benefits of treatment with the risks of
treatment, i.e., assessing the benefit:risk ratio to see which is greater;
(2) comparing the benefit:risk ratio with the risks of no treatment at all;
and (3) comparing the benefit:risk ratio with alternative treatments.

The relative benefits and risks of each medication are detailed in Section III to enable parents, teachers, and professionals to understand both the positive and negative potentials of the medications used most often to treat attention disorders.

DECIDING WHICH MEDICATION IS BEST

Deciding on a particular medication can seem like a trial-and-error procedure to the uninitiated. There are, however, guidelines for the use of each. Those who have worked with ADHD/ADD children for a long time also often have an intuitive sense of what will be effective. Ritalin and Dexedrine are by far the most commonly used medications. Ritalin has traditionally been prescribed much more frequently than Dexedrine. Dexedrine has been used since 1937, while Ritalin was developed in the 1960's. Both are known to affect neurochemicals at synapses in the brain. Cylert is the most recent stimulant medication available. Approved for use in the U.S. in 1975, we have the least information on long-term effects of Cylert. However, fifteen years of usage suggests that it is reasonably safe. Both Ritalin and Dexedrine have been used for many years without notable long-term side effects.

Drs. Calis, Grothe and Elia (1990), of the National Institutes of Health and the National Institute of Mental Health (NIMH), state:

> In clinical practice it is generally recommended that each child be given an adequate trial of both dextroamphetamine [Dexedrine] and methylphenidate [Ritalin]. Careful records of the child's response to each medication should be noted. The medication that results in the greatest behavioral improvement with the fewest adverse effects should be selected. When a long-acting agent is desired or the adverse effects with dextroamphetamine or methylphenidate are too severe, pemoline [Cylert] should be considered as an alternate stimulant. Preliminary results from a three-year ongoing

National Institute of Mental Health (NIMH) study suggest that dextroamphetamine and methylphenidate are equally effective in the pharmacologic management of ADHD [and ADD] and that lack of response is rare when a trial of each drug is given using wide dosage ranges. In this study, 96% of children had an overall improvement when both drugs were tried and a wide range of doses was used, with some children responding preferentially to one drug over the other. Since methylphenidate and dextroamphetamine are equally effective, cost may be a consideration for some individuals....

For the rare child with documented ADHD [or ADD] who does not adequately respond to a thorough trial of the three stimulants or who is unable to tolerate their adverse effects, a trial of alternative methods may be useful. Second-line agents found to be of some value in the pharmacotherapy of ADHD [and ADD] include the tricyclic antidepressants, the monoamine oxidase inhibitors (MAOIs), and clonidine.

ADMINISTRATION OF MEDICATION

Having decided whether to use medication, and, subsequently, which medication is best, the next issue with which both parents and professionals must deal is the administration of the medicine: When? How much? For school only? Or for home and non-academic activities as well? What are the target symptoms? Who should benefit?

Before deciding on when medicine should be administered and how much should be given, one must decide on target symptoms. For the very hyperactive child who is experiencing severe behavioral problems both at school and at home, spending much of his day in "time-out" or in the principal's office, being suspended frequently, or threatening his peers, medication throughout the day seven days a week may be necessary to insure the child's ability to succeed socially and emotionally, as well as academically.

On the other hand, an underactive, daydreaming child, or a restless, inattentive, fidgety child or adolescent may need assistance primarily for school. His medication might be given only in the morning and at lunch (if Ritalin, for example), and only on school days. From the fourth or fifth grade on a third dose for homework and studying, as well as weekend doses, may be needed for the overall best effect academically, socially and emotionally.

In general, the optimal dose of medication and the best schedule is the one which produces, for the child, the greatest benefit for the greatest number of target goals with the fewest side effects. One may need to rank-order the target goals since an optimum dose for one symptom may not be the best for a different symptom. For example, high doses of Ritalin (1.0 mg/kg) produce the greatest improvement in activity level. However, doses at these levels result in poorer scores on memory and attentional tasks (Sprague & Sleator, 1977). Performance on both cognitive and behavioral tasks improves in dose-related fashion from 0.3 to 0.8 mg/kg (kg = 2.2 pounds). For a student to function best cognitively and behaviorally, one would have to adjust the medication being conscious of both target symptoms simultaneously.

Likewise, a child might perform beautifully academically and behaviorally at a certain level of medication but perceive himself as *too quiet* or *not funny*. Because this effect is often so negative to the child or adolescent, one must decrease the dose level, even if at some loss of attention and behavioral control. "Class clowns" can be especially troubled when they no longer feel they can attract attention and assure themselves a place with their peers in even this way.

It is important for parents, physician and the child to discuss and record all symptoms, rank-order them and decide which they will target most concertedly.

How Should Medicine Be Administered?

It is important that medicine, regardless of kind, be started at low doses and increased under the close supervision of a physician. If the medicine is initiated at too high a dose causing an adverse initial response, it can frighten both the parents and child, and they may discontinue the medicine prematurely without a chance to succeed. Many of the negative responses, especially those dramatized by the media, may have occurred because the dose was initially too high. Sensitive and allergic children are especially vulnerable to side-effect from medicine.

The stimulant medications, Ritalin and Dexedrine, do not build up in the blood stream and can, therefore, be increased fairly rapidly, while other medications, such as Cylert, the antidepressants, and clonidine, build up in the bloodstream gradually and take longer to reach maximum effectiveness.

While medicine may be given initially at doses which are too high, all too frequently the child or adolescent is started on low doses of medication, receives some benefit and the medicine is never increased to its optimum therapeutic level (Wender, 1987). Thus the child is helped some but not nearly to the degree that he might be. To obtain the best therapeutic benefit, the medicine is usually increased gradually with close monitoring of effect until the greatest assistance is achieved with the fewest side-effects possible. Specific administration guidelines will be discussed for each medication.

Children and adolescents with ADHD and ADD are extremely sensitive to changes in their lives and in their environments. It is, therefore, important that medication not be initiated with other changes if at all possible, so that the medical effect can be clearly determined. Starting medication at the same time the child changes schools or begins to receive resource assistance can be confusing in one's attempts to determine accurately the medicine's effects.

Monitoring of Medication

Second only in importance to the initial evaluation is the careful follow-up of a child once he has been placed on medication. Lack of adequate follow-up and the use of medication alone without the benefit of a multidisciplinary effort are the two major concerns of those who work in this field. A task force study on the use of Ritalin exemplifies these concerns:

> There is no evidence of widespread abuse or diversion .... The major abuses of the drug, however, appear to lie in its use without appropriate adjunctive measures, and in its prescription without an adequate interdisciplinary, differential diagnosis of ADHD or careful monitoring of children using the medicine over time. (Virginia DOE, 1991)

Not only must physicians and professionals understand the need for careful follow-up, but parents must as well. All too often parents perceive the follow-up visit as an unnecessary expense, especially when the child appears to be doing well. Many times we have seen children who were reported to be doing well, only to examine them and find them significantly over- or under-medicated. Or, with only a little questioning of the child, found the medication to be causing unnecessary side effects even though improvement had been significant. Office visits also determine the efficacy of other interventions and provide opportunities to make appropriate recommendations.

Neither parents nor teachers have the training to spot all the potential problems which can occur. Only with adequate information from those closely involved with the child, and a check-up by the physician on a regular basis, can children and adolescents receive optimum benefits from medical intervention.

Team Manager

The person responsible for coordinating the many professionals and interventions which comprise the multimodal intervention program may be the child's pediatrician, neurologist, or psychiatrist. Or it may be the psychologist who evaluated and diagnosed the child and continues to follow him and his family in treatment. Social workers, therapists, school counselors, and special education personnel may, likewise, assume the role of collecting data and communicating across disciplines the needed information. Working with ADHD/ADD children and adolescents is very time-intensive and requires considerable data collection and communication. Because the prescribing physician assumes major legal responsibility, he often designates a team leader if he will not be assuming this role himself. It is crucial that a team manager be designated. Otherwise, interventions tend to become fragmented and ineffective.

Monitoring Medication

In the beginning medicine should be monitored very closely with phone or office contact weekly or bi-monthly until the appropriate medication, dose level and schedule are determined. It is helpful to give both parents and teachers a schedule of the medication, a symptom checklist to be completed daily, and a side-effects checklist to be completed weekly. Examples of medication schedules, side-effects checklists and symptom checklists are found in Chapters 1 and 15, and in Appendix 4.

I have found that checklists save time and provide accurate feedback. Verbal feedback only can be unhelpful to misleading. "He's doing better," tells the physician or other professional little about the effect of the medicine on specific target symptoms. We have parents and teachers complete the *Copeland Symptom Checklist* as part of the initial evaluation. Problematic symptoms are circled and these are rated on a daily basis by parents and teachers until the maximum therapeutic benefit of the medicine, as well as other interventions, is achieved. The *Conners Parent and Teacher Questionnaires*, the *Achenbach Child Behavior Checklists*, the *ACTeRs*, the *Goldstein Behavioral Observation Checklist*, and *Barkley's Home Situations Questionnaire*, among others, are used as well.

It is helpful for the team manager to see the child at least once every two weeks until the appropriate level and regimen of medication are determined. Ideally, ongoing counseling of the child and/or parents is occurring simultaneously. The necessity of observing the child oneself was illustrated to me early in my ADD career when a mother kept insisting her child was "doing great." When I was finally able to persuade her to bring him in, he was the classic "zombie." The mother, well-intentioned but exhausted from years of hyperactivity, found this new behavior quite acceptable. Needless to say, we convinced her otherwise.

Once the therapeutic issues related to the medicine are resolved and the child or adolescent is doing well, follow-up with the prescribing physician every three to four months is recommended by the American Academy of Pediatrics and most ADHD/ADD experts. This visit should be preceded by obtaining behavior checklists from parents and teachers, a report of grades, and a side-effects checklist. These provide excellent data on the effects of medication and enable one to target remaining areas of difficulty which need intervention. Visits with the parent and/or child are not adequate by themselves to determine the appropriateness of the medication but are a necessary part of the monitoring program. One parent recently asked if there were a list for follow-up so she would know what should be done. One will be given for each of the medications discussed. Parents feel more comfortable using medication when there is close follow-up. They also have more confidence in the prescribing physician and other professionals working with their child or adolescent.

Reassessment

Since medications for attention disorders may be taken for many years, it is important that dosage be re-evaluated periodically. Parents and physicians are urged not to initiate these re-evaluations at the beginning of the school year. A bad beginning can mar the entire year. Periods off medication for evaluative purposes are far more effective after the child has successfully launched the school year. Teachers are most helpful when they know their students well. These re-evaluations should be undertaken with as much rigor as the initiation of medication, and appropriate before-and-after measures of effect on behavior, attention and academics should be obtained.

ISSUES IN MEDICATION ADMINISTRATION

Weekends and Evenings

Giving medication on weekends and in the evening is an important and somewhat controversial issue in the use of stimulant medications. Many physicians will prescribe medication only for school and believe that *less is better*. The child's symptoms after school, they reason, should be either managed or tolerated so that neither child nor parent becomes overly dependent on medication as a solution to the child's problems. The philosophical orientation that medication is necessary but basically undesirable characterizes their treatment protocols.

Other physicians view ADHD and ADD as neurotransmitter regulation problems which are *life* problems, not just academic problems. They believe that medication should be given for most of their patients' waking hours to maximize its normalizing effect on the attention and regulatory centers. They feel especially strongly about doing so for children and adolescents who are experiencing significant social and emotional difficulties because they disrupt the family with their excessive needs and inappropriate behaviors.

There is no right or wrong solution. Each decision must be made in the context of the child and family's total life, including their own views about medication, their lifestyles and their values. Only when all are acknowledged and considered can a treatment program be decided upon which will be effective and which will be one with which both parents and child will comply.

Holidays and Vacations

Since the child is not in school at these times, parents often do not give their children medication on holidays or when they take vacations. The results are often disastrous. Many a would-be happy occasion has ended with the child being punished and his parents embarrassed, frustrated and/or angry at their child's out-of-control behavior.

Holidays and vacations are notoriously unstructured, stimulating and frequently stressful. Any one of these conditions renders self-control and appropriate behavior more difficult. All three simultaneously place almost insurmountable odds against the child's behaving in an appropriate manner.

We have found that both the child and his family are generally better served by continuing the regular regimen of medication for these occasions. If it is an especially important event or one which will be excessively stimulating, such as a birthday party, the medication may be increased slightly. Parents usually become excellent judges of the best combinations of circumstances and medication dosage.

Summer

Giving or not giving medicine in the summer is a decision arrived at in a very similar manner as giving it on weekends and holidays. There are children who will need medicine every day, year round. Others may need it only once a day. Deciding upon one's objectives for the child will assist in determining when medication is administered. Children who are overactive and are attending camp or other structured activities often do need medication so that the social benefits can be obtained.

Drug Holidays

It is uniformly recommended in the ADHD/ADD literature that children and adolescents taking medications have *drug holidays*, i.e., times when the medication is discontinued. For non-buildup stimulants such as Ritalin and Dexedrine, these may be on the weekend as well as in the summer. For medications which require a blood level for maximum effectiveness (all except Ritalin and Dexedrine), such holidays are feasible primarily in the summer. Withdrawal from these medications should be a gradual process, as will be discussed in Section III.

If the child can function without major symptoms, loss of competency and decreased self-esteem, withdrawal from medication has positive benefit in that it allows the body to return to its non-drug, natural state. The relative benefits and risks of doing so should be assessed by all before the decision to do so is made.

Compliance

Compliance is a problem in the treatment program of any medical disorder. It is a major problem in the treatment of attention deficit disorders. Both parents and children frequently do not comply with the medication regime recommended. There are many reasons:

1) *Parents and children do not fully understand the disorder, the necessity of treatment and the availability of treatment options.* Treatment is far more effective when both parents and children/ adolescents are fully educated on both the disorder and the treatment options available. They can then actively decide which interventions they will support and which they will not. We have found through the years that parents will follow our recommendations only after we have listened to them and followed their wishes. It is, many times, a process of successive approximation. Interventions and combinations of interventions are tried until the most effective options, or the ones most agreeable with the child and his family, are determined. While this procedure is, of course, more time-consuming, it is, in the long run, the most effective. When one acknowledges that ADHD and ADD are lifelong disorders for many, it seems worthwhile to expend the necessary energy in the initial stages of treatment to insure long-term compliance and benefit. Those parents actively involved in support groups are usually the most knowledgeable, the most actively involved in the treatment process, and the most effective in implementing the interventions agreed upon.

2) *Parents and children forget.* It is helpful to establish a routine, such as taking the medication with breakfast or on the way to lunch at school, which becomes a part of daily life. Some have found it helpful to set multiple alarms on their watches to be reminded when schedules were too variable to be relied upon. High school and college students find alarms especially helpful. It is also an excellent way to assist the elementary child assume responsibility for his medicine.

3) *The medicine is not helping.* We have found through the years that children, and especially adolescents, will not take the medicine if they do not perceive it to be helpful. Close follow-up is critical to insure that benefit is actually received.

4) *The side effects are too troublesome.* When the side effects of medicine outweigh their benefit, compliance is extremely poor. It is crucial that the medicine be changed and adjusted until the child receives as much benefit as possible with few or no side effects. Often one must specifically go down the list of side effects with the child since these complaints are frequently not volunteered.

5) *Parents and children are embarrassed by the need for medicine.* When ADHD/ADD are not fully understood nor accepted as routine medical problems like near-sightedness or allergies, both parents and child can feel uneasy or ashamed. They may deal with their feelings by denying the disorder. One way they do this is by not taking the medicine. Education and counseling, to be discussed next, are critical to overcoming any sense of damage or inadequacy.

Sometimes children are teased at school about taking medicine. Or, without teasing, the child feels it makes him different. Adolescents are especially unwilling to do anything which singles them out in what they perceive to be a negative way. If the child or adolescent does not wish to take medication at school, or refuses to even consider taking it there, a long-acting form of stimulant should be utilized or another medication altogether. The psychological needs of both parent and child must be fully acknowledged and addressed if compliance is to be obtained.

IMPORTANCE OF EDUCATION
AND COUNSELING

Education and counseling for both children and their parents, whether accomplished in conference with a physician or psychologist, through sessions with a therapist, or in a support group, are essential to the successful treatment of attention disorders with medication. One of the greatest problems with medication, that of compliance, can often be overcome by such meetings.

What Parents Must Understand

To become an effective member of the multidisciplinary team designed to help their ADHD/ADD child or adolescent, parents must become informed consumers. In no area is this more true than in the use of medication. To be effective:

1) Parents must know as much as possible about

   - What the drug of choice is.
   - How it is expected to affect their child, both its potential positive benefits as well as its possible side effects.
   - Medical conditions the child has or other medications he is taking and how those might be affected by the medication chosen for the attention disorder.
   - Possible allergic reactions.

2) Parents must understand the nature of medication choice. While the mechanisms of medications utilized for attention disorders are reasonably understood, it is not possible to predict, with total accuracy, how a particular child will respond. Trials with several medications may be required before the optimal one and the optimum regimen are determined. Feedback from both parents and teachers will be essential, as well as close follow-up and supervision by the physician in the initial phase of treatment. There are usually no quick solutions—even with medicine.

3) Parents must understand how medicine is administered. It is usually begun at the lowest effective dose and usually requires incremental increases to arrive finally at the most effective amount.

Tolerance, i.e., the need for ever-increasing amounts of medication, is typically not a problem in children; therefore, the medication does not continually have to be increased. While confusing to parents, the dose needed for maximum benefit is usually not determined by the seriousness of the problem, but rather by the child's sensitivity to drugs and his metabolic rate.

4)   Parents must be patient. The selected medication, especially the tricyclic antidepressants and clonidine, may not be optimally effective for several weeks.   In addition, symptoms may worsen initially before improving.   Such knowledge enables parents to avoid disappointment and/or alarm and not discontinue medication prematurely.

5)   Parents must not look to medicine as *the* answer. Medicine is not the answer to all the ADHD/ADD child's or adolescent's problems, but it can be a partial solution for this complex disorder.

6)   Parents must become comfortable with, and confident that, the benefits of medication treatment far outweigh the risks.

Parent Requirements for Medication Success

- Knowledge of medicines and medical issues.
- Close monitoring of medicine and accurate reporting to physician.
- Adequate comfort level to administer medicine appropriately.
- Utilization of a multidisciplinary intervention program.
- Patience and optimism.

What Children Need to Know

There are many psychological aspects to giving and taking medication. Parents must come fully to terms with giving the medication if they expect the child to be able to accept it as well. The parents' lack of true understanding and acceptance of the medication is often revealed in their disguising it as a vitamin or as an allergy medication when discussing it with the child. "It's okay to have allergies, but it is not okay to have ADHD or ADD," may be part of their belief system. Parents are generally comfortable giving medicine to their children for obvious medical conditions. Giving their children medicine for attentional and behavioral problems, however, can create much confusion for both the parents and the child. Rarely does a parent in our practice initially *not* say, "I don't want to give *my* child drugs." Taking medication when he does not feel sick can be equally confusing to the child.

If medical intervention is to be successful, several goals with the child or adolescent must be achieved:

1)   He must understand why he is receiving medication. Children can often tell you exactly how the medication affects them. They are thus confused when a pill that helps them "be good" or "sit still" or "get class- and homework done" is called a vitamin. Openness, directness and trust are essential, for the child will be called upon many times to explain to others what the medicine is for and how it helps him. Several books which are helpful to the child or adolescent in understanding both attention disorders and medications are listed in Appendix 1 in the *Suggested Readings: Books for Children and Teens.*

2)   The child or adolescent must not interpret needing medicine as meaning that he is *bad, dumb,* or in some way *damaged.* It is helpful to explain that no one is perfect: some of us have allergies; some, ear infections; others wear glasses; and he has an attention disorder. An

exercise we encourage in classrooms is a round robin discussion of "I'm not totally okay, you're not totally okay, and that's okay." It is important to acknowledge the human condition—i.e., most of us have some aspect of our lives that is not perfect. How we deal with that lack of perfection is usually a key ingredient in our success or failure.

3)   The child or adolescent must not begin to attribute his good behavior to the medicine and his bad behavior to himself. This attribution of positive behavior to the medicine has been found by many. It is important for children to feel that medicine simply enables them to be in control of themselves and their lives. Teachers and parents often reinforce this attribution of goodness to the medicine by asking, any time the child misbehaves, "Did you take your medicine?"

4)   ADD must not become an excuse for negative behavior or lack of responsibility. As one of my favorite fourth grade ADHD patients is fond of telling his parents, "You know I can't do that ... I have ADD."

5)   The child must come to accept his ADHD or ADD as simply a manageable problem in his life. He must understand also that he, not the attention disorder, is the master of his fate. Once he does, he is well on his way to overcoming its effects successfully.

6)   Finally, while the difficulties associated with the attention disorders are addressed, it should be emphasized that there are also many positive traits in children, adolescents and adults with ADHD and ADD. Most ADHD people have a high energy level which, if channeled and organized, can be their best asset. Many accomplish far more than their non-ADHD peers. Organization, structure and planning are the keys.

In addition, most ADHD children, if not demoralized by continual negative feedback, are sociable and enjoyable. As young children they are described as "never meeting a stranger." When older, they enjoy social situations and function quite effectively. Many are highly successful in sales. They frequently win all the prizes in school selling contests. Later in life they are also among the top producers. Entrepreneurs abound among ADHD adults. If they have organized, detail-oriented assistants or spouses who will follow through on the details and planning which they may overlook, they can be exceptionally successful.

Perhaps as a function of their own hurt over the years, many ADHD/ADD children and adolescents are exquisitely sensitive. Mothers often describe this child as the one in the family who can be the most loving and caring and the most sensitive to her feelings and needs. Perhaps this accounts for the special bond that frequently develops between the mother and her ADHD child even as he is driving her wild. The ADD child is an unusually easy one with whom to be, especially if not meeting deadlines or having to march to someone else's drum.

Other positive traits are more unique to each child and adolescent. Those with attention disorders who received early assistance and intervention have become some of our most outstanding citizens.

SUMMARY

Now that the reader has a thorough understanding of attention disorders and the complex issues surrounding the use of medications to treat them, the specific medicines utilized to assist those with ADHD and ADD will be addressed. While getting to this point may have been lengthy, the issues addressed are far too important to be skimmed over. Medications are serious business. Concerned parents, teachers and professionals will insist on answers before committing their children, students and patients to this treatment approach. It is hoped that I have either provided answers to your questions or have guided you to resources which can. If previously unrecognized considerations have emerged, it is hoped that answers to those have also been forthcoming. Attention deficit disorders are complex problems which deserve a thoughtful and comprehensive response from all who live with, teach or work with those affected. Having raised the issues, I urge you to seek the best possible solutions which can be found, both to satisfy yourself and to assist those for whom you care.

PART III

Medications

Three psychostimulant medications—
dextroamphetamine sulfate [Dexedrine],
methylphenidate hydrochloride [Ritalin],
and pemoline [Cylert] — are considered
the drugs of first choice for management
of the behavioral manifestations of ADHD.

— Drs. Calis, Grothe and Elia
NIH and NIMH, 1990

8
Stimulant
Medications

Ritalin
Dexedrine
Cylert

Stimulant medication, officially termed *psychostimulant medications*, are in the words of Drs. Calis, Grothe and Elia (1990), of the National Institutes of Health, "the mainstay in the contemporary management of ADHD." Ritalin, Dexedrine and Cylert are currently the drugs of first choice for treating most children with attention deficit disorders. The efficacy and safety of these medications is "dramatic and powerful" (Donnelly & Rapoport, NIMH, 1985).

The general mechanism of stimulant medications was first thought to be that of increasing norepinephrine release on the presynaptic neuron so that more was available at the synaptic cleft. The greater availability of norepinephrine throughout the attention/impulse/motor network was thought to improve the behavioral and attentional symptoms of ADHD and ADD. Increasing evidence accumulates that stimulant medications affect dopamine systems as well and that dopamine may be the more important neurotransmitter in attention disorders.

Each medication acts somewhat differently and affects somewhat different parts of the brain. The tricyclic antidepressants, for example, prevent the reuptake of norepinephrine leaving more available at the synapse. Zametkin's research demonstrated that many areas of the brains of hyperactive adults had decreased rates of glucose metabolism, presumably because of decreased effectiveness of neurotransmission. He stated in an address to the Second Annual National CH.A.D.D. Conference, 1990, "Stimulants are all very different drugs. People respond differently on each medication because each affects the brain and nervous system differently." The current challenge of physicians, neurophysiologists, and psychopharmacologists is to determine which areas cause specific symptoms and to define more precisely the effects of the different medications on each area of the brain and on each of the neurotransmitter systems involved in that area of the brain.

Hans Lou's (1989) findings that methylphenidate increased blood flow to particular areas of the brain and improved symptoms, likewise, suggest that stimulant medications increase the availability of neuro-transmitters, in turn facilitating the transmission of both excitatory and inhibitory messages within the brain. Many different and specific areas of the brain have, likewise, been implicated for the diverse symptoms associated with ADHD/ADD by Jensen and Garfinkel (1988).

A more in-depth discussion of the hypotheses regarding the neurophysiology of ADHD/ADD is beyond the scope of this book. The interested reader is referred to Appendix 2 for excellent review articles. Research data at present strongly support the view that ADHD and ADD are the result of central nervous system dysfunctions and that both norepinephrine and dopamine deficiencies appear to contribute to these symptom complexes.

DEFINITION OF TERMS

Two terms that appear often in discussions of the mechanisms of medication are pharmacokinetics and pharmacodynamics. *Pharmacokinetics* is defined as the relationship between the dose of medication administered and the concentration in the blood, while *pharmacodynamics* refers to the relationship between a specific drug dose and the patient's response.

Each person has a unique response to medication which is dependent upon his unique physiological makeup. Such wide variability in response has led to attempts to determine what the pharmacodynamics are. It is very helpful when therapeutic blood levels, called *therapeutic windows*, can be determined. A patient's best response usually occurs when his blood level is within the window of the established therapeutic range. Specific therapeutic blood levels have been established for many medications including anticonvulsants, tricyclic antidepressants, and lithium, among others. Ritalin and Dexedrine are short-acting medicines which metabolize completely and have virtually no build-up in the blood stream. Therapeutic blood levels are, therefore, not available to assist the physician determine appropriate dosage requirements. It is thus largely a matter of successive approximation based on behavioral/attentional response. The lack of build-up has one major advantage, that is, it precludes addiction. Neither Ritalin nor Dexedrine is physiologically addictive. Likewise, neither requires successive increases to maintain a consistent level of effectiveness.

RITALIN
(Methylphenidate Hydrochloride)

Description

Ritalin, *methylphenidate hydrochloride*, is the most commonly used medication for attention disorders, the one most frequently tried first, and the one generally considered the safest. Approximately 70-80% of those diagnosed with physiologic ADHD or ADD find it effective. First synthesized in 1954, methylphenidate is manufactured by CIBA Pharmaceutical Company as *Ritalin*. It is available in generic form from Rugby Laboratories, Inc. in 5 mg., 10 mg. and 20 mg. tablets as methylphenidate HCL.

Classification

Methylphenidate is classified as a Schedule II controlled substance with legal restrictions on usage and prescription renewal. It is, therefore, carefully monitored by physicians as well as drug enforcement agencies. A written prescription is necessary from the physician. Thus, the medication cannot be called into the pharmacy. Parents who do not know this fact can be frustrated by insufficient planning ahead for refills. The mandated requirement for a written refill of the medication has positive benefit in that it insures greater supervision and control, both of the medication and other treatments as well, by the prescribing physician.

Clinical Pharmacology

The *Physician's Desk Reference (PDR)* states that "Ritalin is a mild central nervous system stimulant. The mode of action in man is not completely understood, but Ritalin presumably activates the brain stem arousal system and cortex to produce its stimulating effect" (1994, p. 835). Recent research indicates that Ritalin and other stimulants enhance the release of neurotransmitters on the presynaptic neuron at the synaptic cleft, making more available for neurotransmission. Both dopamine and norepinephrine are thought to be involved. The mechanism of action for norepinephrine is as follows:

MECHANISM OF ACTION:
NEUROTRANSMITTERS

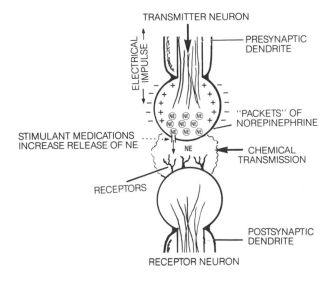

This figure portrays a transmitter neuron attempting to send messages across a synapse to a receptor neuron using norepinephrine (NE) as the model. Norepinephrine is stored in tiny sacs or "packets" inside the messenger neurons. When a stimulus sends a command to fire and release norepinephrine, the *synaptic vesicles*, packets of neurotransmitters, open and release norepinephrine out into the synapse. This released norepinephrine travels across the synaptic cleft to norepinephrine receptor sites to send its message on.

In ADHD and ADD, norepinephrine and dopamine are thought to be released in deficient quantities, thus impeding the transmission of impulses important for attention, concentration, impulse control, appropriate activity level and the many other activities involved in successful focusing, but deficient in those with attention disorders. Different functions are controlled, of course, by different areas of the brain.

All of the stimulant medications, including Ritalin, act to increase the availability of neurotransmitters, dopamine and norepinephrine in particular, thereby normalizing brain functioning. Antidepressants prevent the re-uptake of norepinephrine, while MAO inhibitors prevent the breakdown, or metabolism, of norepinephrine at the synapse. All three classes of medicines achieve the same end result, i.e., they increase the availability of neurotransmitters at the synaptic cleft, thereby increasing neurotransmitter efficiency. Dr. Larry Silver, in his address to the 1991 National LDA Conference, "Attention Deficit Hyperactivity Disorder: If It's For Real, Why All the Confusion?", used the analogy of a lake. The stimulants put more water (neurotransmitters) into the lake (synaptic cleft), while the antidepressants and MAOI's serve as a dam to keep the water in the lake. While their mechanisms are different, their end goals are much the same.

In summary, ADHD/ADD are believed to be a result of dopamine and norepinephrine deficiencies. Ritalin acts to enhance the availability of the neurotransmitters, thus normalizing brain functioning. In the future, it is likely to be found that Ritalin acts on the neurons in specific areas of the brain, while other medicines, Dexedrine, for example, affect neurotransmission elsewhere in the brain. Determination of appropriateness and efficacy of a particular medicine for a particular person and purpose remains somewhat of a trial-and-error procedure.

Availability and Duration of Effect

Ritalin is available in a short-acting tablet which lasts approximately three to five hours, most commonly four hours, depending upon individual metabolism. The short-acting form is the easiest to adjust dosage, or *titrate,* because it comes in three sizes: 5 mg., 10 mg. and 20 mg. tablets. Ritalin is also available in a long-acting, sustained-release

20 mg. tablet, *Ritalin-SR*, that lasts approximately seven to ten hours. It was designed to be the equivalent of a 10 mg. tablet taken twice daily.

All of the Ritalin tablets are quite small and usually present no problem swallowing. For those children who cannot swallow even tiny pills, ingesting it with yogurt or apple sauce is usually effective.

Short-Acting Form   **Long-Acting Form**

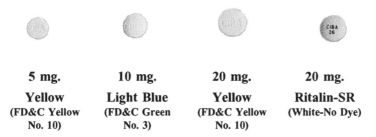

5 mg.	10 mg.	20 mg.	20 mg.
Yellow	Light Blue	Yellow	Ritalin-SR
(FD&C Yellow No. 10)	(FD&C Green No. 3)	(FD&C Yellow No. 10)	(White-No Dye)

Although not scored, the 5 mg. tablet may be split with a sharp knife for even smaller doses which may be needed for some children, especially those who are very sensitive to medications of any kind. The ability to split the 5 mg. tablet is also helpful when one is increasing the dosage. Some children, for example, are undermedicated on 5 mg. of Ritalin and are overmedicated on 10 mg., with 7.5 mg. being the optimal dosage. The more precisely dosage correlates with need, the more successful are the benefits.

It is important to be aware of the dyes in the Ritalin tablets. Those children who are dye-sensitive, especially to yellow dyes, may experience adverse effects ranging from irritability or bedwetting to increased hyperactivity from the FD&C Yellow No. 10 dye in the 5 mg. and 20 mg. tablets. An adverse response to the dye may be mistaken for a negative response to the Ritalin itself. To rule out such a possibility in an allergic or dye-intolerant child, parents can give the child, upon awakening, a glass of water with 1/4 teaspoon of yellow dye added. Allow 30 minutes to elapse before anything else is eaten or drunk. If there is not a negative response within that time, one can be reasonably assured that there will not be a dye effect. While yellow-dye sensitivity is not a frequent occurrence, it does happen often enough to rule it out in allergic and sensitive children. The FD&C Green No. 3 dye in the 10 mg. tablet is less problematic in our experience.

Indications and Usage

Ritalin is used primarily for the treatment of attention deficit disorders. The PDR (1990) stresses that "Ritalin is indicated as an integral part of a total treatment program which typically includes other remedial measures (psychological, educational, social) ...." Ritalin is also used in the treatment of narcolepsy.

Contraindications

A careful differential diagnosis of ADHD/ADD is crucial. Anxiety, tension, depression, agitation, hypertension, thought disturbance, and other symptoms which mimic attention disorders are usually made worse by Ritalin. Ritalin is also contraindicated in patients with glaucoma; those who are hypersensitive to the medication; and those who have an allergic response to Ritalin, which is rare. Patients with motor tics and anyone with a family history or diagnosis of Tourette Syndrome must be assessed carefully and the risk:benefit ratio judiciously considered. Stimulant medications do not cause, but can precipitate, a latent, genetic predisposition to TS. While caution is utilized, many with TS nevertheless take stimulant medications for control of their ADHD/ADD symptoms.

Warnings

Ritalin is a medication which must be used with care. There are situations where even more special attention is warranted:

Children Under Six

The safety and effectiveness of Ritalin has not been established for children under six years of age although clinically it has been utilized by many for children as young as age five. Dexedrine tablets have been approved for ages 3 to 5 for the young child who requires medical intervention. Dexedrine elixir is no longer available for young children.

Children and Adolescents Receiving
Long-Term Treatment

Those taking medication for a long time should be carefully monitored since sufficient data on long-term safety and efficacy are not available. Clinical data have thus far not revealed long-term negative effects and thousands of children have been on Ritalin for years. Of primary concern, long-term, has been the possible suppression of growth, which will be discussed under side-effects.

Seizures

There has been anecdotal clinical evidence suggesting Ritalin may lower the seizure threshold. While the manufactures state that it should not be used in patients with seizures, clinical practice often differs from this policy. Clinical and research data indicate that stimulant and seizure medications are often utilized together under the watchful eye of a neurologist. In general, physicians attempt to overcome as many interfering symptoms as possible with the fewest adverse effects, a goal which may at times require using more than one medicine simultaneously. This practice, called *polypharmacy*, requires caution and conservative measures. However, as knowledge in a subspecialty health area increases, the use of multiple medicines is often a concomitant occurrence.

Hypertension/Increased Heart Rate

Ritalin may cause a mild increase in heart rate. It is important to determine whether this is a side effect for your child. When it does occur, it is often a minor increase and does not warrant discontinuation of medication. However, there have been a few cases in which it necessitated a different therapeutic intervention.

Heart rate and blood pressure have been studied in children treated with stimulant medications. They have yielded conflicting and inconclusive results. An Emory University research study worthy of note is one which measured the blood pressure of black male adolescents taking methylphenidate. They found a significant increase in diastolic blood pressure (Brown & Sexson, 1989). Thus, it is especially important to carefully monitor this group of adolescents when they are taking Ritalin.

Ritalin should also be used cautiously in patients with hypertension. It is recommended that blood pressure be monitored at appropriate intervals in all patients taking Ritalin, and especially those with hypertension. Clonidine, an antihypertensive which has been found effective for some with attention disorders, may be the drug of choice for those with elevated blood pressure.

Drug Interactions

Drug interactions do occur with Ritalin. Of special concern are its effects on MAO inhibitors, anticonvulsants, tricyclic antidepressants and anticoagulants. The interaction of Ritalin with any drug a person is taking, or is going to take, should be carefully investigated by the prescribing physician.

Potential for Abuse

Any medication can be abused. Ritalin should be given cautiously to anyone with a perceived potential for abuse. For those who have abused drugs in the past, other medications, such as the antidepressants or MAOI's, may be preferred over the stimulant medications. However, Ritalin is increasingly utilized with success for those with addictive disorders. Caution and good judgement are critical to appropriate selection of interventions. A Virginia task force studying the use of methylphenidate in their Commonwealth stated:

> Recent reports in the controlled substance literature confirm that primary care physicians, including pediatricians, underestimate the abuse potential of methylphenidate. The drug is often used in combination with other licit and illicit substances (especially cocaine). Intravenous injection of Ritalin is associated with greater system toxicity than other similar drugs. Twenty milligram tablets, referred to as "poor man's cocaine" are the preferred form. (Virginia DOE, 1991)

Ritalin is also being used by students and truck drivers to stay awake. "Doctor shopping" by parents to obtain more Ritalin, presumably for themselves, has also occurred. Many parents of ADHD children, in particular, recognize the same symptoms in themselves and attempt to both self-diagnose and self-medicate. Careful computer monitoring of medication usage by regulatory agencies can hopefully prevent the abuse of Ritalin and other stimulants from becoming a widespread problem.

While the potential for abuse is present, the Virginia Task Force mirrors the opinion of most experts in the field:

> It is emphasized that the needs of patients for appropriate medication constitute the foremost consideration in designing

and implementing any drug monitoring system. Although restraint is recommended in prescribing any controlled substance, this restraint should not inhibit treatment with methylphenidate when psychostimulant medication is clearly indicated. (Virginia DOE, 1991)

Dosage and Administration

After deciding upon the medication itself, the most important factors contributing to successful medical treatment of attention disorders are determining the appropriate dosage and administering it at optimal time intervals.

Time of Administration

Ritalin is often given at or after meals to avoid its potentially adverse effect on appetite and the occasional stomachaches or headaches reported. Early research suggested that gastric juices interfered with metabolism, and it was recommended that the medication be given 30 to 45 minutes before meals. Recent research, however, has failed to confirm a negative effect of eating on the metabolism of the medication (Swanson et al., 1983), and most ADHD/ADD experts currently recommend giving it at times that are convenient and/or minimize side effects.

The Ritalin tablet generally requires about 30 minutes to become effective, with peak effectiveness at 1.9 hours with a range of 0.3-4.4 and gradually diminishing effectiveness the last hour. The time period of benefit varies widely among children, adolescents and adults with three to five hours being most typical. Determining the time of duration of effectiveness is crucial to proper administration. For example, a child who metabolizes the medicine in three and a half hours can be expected to have difficulty from approximately 11 a.m. to 12:30 p.m. if the medicine is given at 7:30 a.m. and 12:00 noon. Since lunch and unstructured activities at school generally occur around the noon hour, the child can continue to experience significant difficulty because of improper time intervals established. Adam, our gifted second grader, experienced this problem. As discussed previously, despite a good response to the medication, P.E. continued to be a problem because the effect of the medication had worn off by 11.00. Another child, who metabolizes the medicine more slowly, could be overmedicated from 12:00 noon to 1:00 p.m., for example, on this same schedule.

The Ritalin-SR requires approximately 45 to 60 minutes to become effective, peaking in children at 4.7 hours (1.3-8.2). It lasts approximately 7-10 hours with effectiveness diminishing over the last hour much more gradually than the short-acting form, thus avoiding a major rebound effect. Some children take a long-acting tablet with a "booster" of the short-acting. Others may take a Ritalin-SR in the morning and again approximately 6-7 hours later for all-day coverage.

Dosage

Ritalin is typically initiated in small doses, usually at 5 mg. A very sensitive, allergic child may respond to as little as 2.5 mg. It is usually increased gradually. Since Ritalin does not build up in the blood stream, its effects are often observable from the first dose. The dosage can be increased every three to seven days, or more gradually, until the most therapeutic level of medication has been determined. We have found that increasing it more rapidly in 2.5 mg. increments to be very helpful. Ritalin-SR is often utilized after the therapeutic dose level has been determined by using the short-acting form since it is available only in one size, the 20 mg. tablet.

Parents rightfully worry about the amount of medication their child is taking. The dosage required depends on many variables. Allergic children, for example, are usually sensitive and require less than high-dose responders who may take more than 60 mg. per day or even more, without adequate control of symptoms. Body weight is not a good indicator of dosage required even though it is a helpful baseline parameter. For example, a two hundred pound father of one of our patients received immense benefit from 5 mgs. of Ritalin four times a day, while his forty-five pound hyperactive son required 10 mg. of Ritalin three times daily. Many adolescents and adults respond to the same dose levels as much younger children, and often require less.

Dr. Harvey Parker (1989), in *The ADD Hyperactivity Workbook for Parents, Teachers and Kids,* gives the following chart to help parents determine whether their child's dose level, when compared with other children, is in the low, medium or high range in relation to the child's body weight. *Dose* refers to the amount per administration, not the amount taken per day; *kg* = 2.2 pounds.

Standard Ritalin Dosage Chart

Child's Weight	Low Dosage .3 mg/kg	Medium Dosage .6 mg/kg	High Dosage 1.0 mg/kg
22 lbs.	3 mg	6 mg	10 mg
33 lbs.	5 mg	9 mg	15 mg
44 lbs.	6 mg	12 mg	20 mg
55 lbs.	8 mg	15 mg	25 mg
66 lbs.	9 mg	18 mg	30 mg
88 lbs.	12 mg	24 mg	40 mg

Transient side effects such as headaches, stomachaches, decreased appetite and sleep problems may occur but often subside if the medication is continued. Starting off with a small dose usually decreases the intensity of any side effects until the body has adjusted to the medication. Some side effects, to be discussed later, may persist. If so, one must decide whether the benefits outweigh the negative effects, or whether a trial of a different medication is warranted. As stated earlier, patience, perseverance and a willingness to try different medications at different dosage levels result in significant benefit the great majority of the time.

Frequency of Administration

The Ritalin short-acting tablet is most commonly given twice a day, in the morning and approximately three and one-half to four hours later, if benefit is desired primarily for school. Assistance at home requires a third dose approximately four hours after the noon dose. That dose is typically one-half to two-thirds of the morning or noon dose. Occasionally even a fourth dose is administered for the very overactive child. The third or fourth dose of medication may help the ADHD child settle into sleep, or it may cause insomnia instead.

The long-acting Ritalin-SR is usually given in the morning and often again six to eight hours later. When assistance with symptoms is needed in the late afternoon, the tablet form may be used instead of the long-acting form.

The use of medication on weekends and holidays was addressed in Chapter 7. Medication should, in my opinion, always be used for the greatest benefit of the child and his family. It has been noted by teachers, parents and clinicians alike that Monday is often the child's worst day when not receiving medication on the weekend. Giving at least one dose on Sunday seems to help smooth the transition to Monday's school requirements for those who wish to avoid weekend usage but still retain the best possible benefits for school.

All of the Ritalin tablets are bitter and are best taken whole. Since Ritalin-SR is a time-release medication, it must be swallowed intact and never chewed or crushed. Ritalin-SR is very difficult to adjust dosage levels because it comes in only one size and cutting it interferes with the designed formula for absorption.

Rebound

Some children, especially those with ADHD, experience increased hyperactivity when the medicine wears off. It is as though they have contained the energy all day and once the medicine wears off this pent-up energy explodes. This effect is called *rebound* and can be especially taxing to mothers who are usually with the child when it occurs. This effect is observed in a relatively small percentage of children who take Ritalin and can be managed by a third or fourth dose of medication at one-half the morning or noon dose.

While often reported in clinical practice, research has failed to document a significant rebound phenomenon for the majority of children (Johnston et al., 1988). It may be that parents forget what the behavior was like before medicine was begun. Rebound can cause sleep difficulties for the child who experiences it at bedtime. The overactive child usually falls asleep much more easily if the medication is still effective at bedtime.

Other children, adolescents and adults may experience increased sensitivity and moodiness when the medicine wears off. This effect is often not worth the benefit and suggests that the medication may not be the ideal one. Others experience a rebound fatigue when the medicine wears off. This effect is more typical of those with underactive, sluggish ADD than for those with ADHD. Rebound is usually quite manageable once this effect is accurately recognized.

Adverse Reactions/Side Effects

The most frequently reported adverse reactions in those taking stimulant medications are *anorexia* or decreased appetite; *insomnia*, or sleep disturbance; stomach pain; headaches; irritability; and weight loss. The possible negative effect on growth and the potential for precipitating motor tics and Tourette Syndrome have raised the greatest concerns, however.

Appetite Suppression and Weight Loss

Appetite suppression is the most frequent side effect cited for both Ritalin and Dexedrine. In general, it is transient and poses no major problem. Most children will experience decreased appetite initially, especially for the noon meal. They may experience some weight loss over the first few weeks, after which both appetite and weight usually return to a more normal level.

Despite its being somewhat bothersome, many parents have found that appetite suppression can be managed. Giving the child breakfast before he takes the medicine will generally cause the morning meal not to be affected. The noon meal, however, is more often a problem than not, even if the child/adolescent takes the second dose after lunch. It is important to encourage the child to eat something and mothers can assist by packing appealing items. If the child does not eat lunch, he is usually hungry, irritable and fatigued by 3:00 p.m. This negative effect of hunger is often mistaken for a rebound effect of the medication. While it certainly may be, a nutritious snack usually does much to improve the child's mood. Even a light lunch will avoid this negative effect. Both parents and children are usually cooperative in facilitating the child's eating of lunch when they understand the positive benefits of doing so.

In general, children and adolescents on stimulant medications are somewhat slimmer than their peers, but most, I have found, are exceptionally healthy—that is, after the early years of ear infections and allergic sensitivities. Since Americans often eat more than is optimal, the appetite-suppressing effect of Ritalin can be of secondary benefit. This has certainly been true for some of our patients who were overactive eaters and whose excessive weight contributed to their loss of self-esteem.

Many children experience a lack of appetite only when the medication reaches a certain level. Careful adjustment of dosage can maximize the benefits of the medication while minimizing the side effects. For the few children who experience continued significant loss of appetite and weight loss, a change of medications is usually indicated.

Sleep Disturbance

Many children and adolescents with attention disorders on the overactive end of the continuum have difficulty falling asleep. However, most are reported to sleep like logs once they do. They are often difficult to awaken the next morning, and many develop sleep deprivation fatigue which only complicates their attention disorder. The negative effects which result from chronic loss of sleep will be discussed in greater detail in Chapter 13.

Ritalin and Dexedrine may cause or increase difficulty falling asleep. Fine-tuning the medication regimen can usually avoid these problems when medication is the culprit.

One intervention that is extremely effective with many children who have difficulty concentrating and focusing long enough to go to sleep is to use a sleep machine. These are available in inexpensive models with only one noise, such as rainfall, to expensive ones with multiple noises and multiple volumes. I discovered the positive effect of sleep machines after noting repeatedly that many of our ADHD children wanted to sleep with fans on, even in the winter. It was not cool air they wanted, but rather the noise the fan made. Consistent noise also blocks out episodic distractions that can keep the child from succumbing to slumber. Very auditorially hypersensitive children may even require soft ear plugs to facilitate sleep.

The key to sleep appears to be stimulating the attention centers adequately to allow the calming necessary for sleep to occur. Otherwise, the body may be still, but the mind remains in high gear. Dr. Marcel Kinsbourne found, in his work with high-dose responders who were hospitalized as part of a research project, that a bedtime dose of medication was essential for sleep (Hospital for Sick Children, Toronto, Canada, 1980, personal visit).

Underactive ADD children and adolescents often sleep too much. Medication often alerts their attention centers so that they no longer sleep excessively, but instead require more normal amounts of sleep.

Narcolepsy, a neurological disorder, is characterized by an excessive need for sleep and falling asleep at inappropriate times. It, too, is treated successfully with Ritalin and Dexedrine.

Stomachaches and Headaches

Stomachaches and headaches are frequent complaints when a child, adolescent or adult begins medication. They can be minimized by initiating the stimulants at low doses and gradually increasing the amount as the side effects subside. Occasionally one stimulant will cause the symptoms while another will not. Laura, a fourth-grade student with whom we worked, for example, had been on Ritalin for two years at the time of our initial evaluation. Upon questioning, she acknowledged ongoing stomachaches. She was, however, unwilling to give up taking the medication because it helped her so much at school. Her medication was subsequently changed to Dexedrine which caused neither headaches nor stomachaches.

For very sensitive children, especially allergic children, many medications may have to be tried to determine the most effective and least problematic one. For a very few, medicine may not be a workable part of the treatment program.

Lethargy

Lethargy, depression, becoming "glassy-eyed" or a "zombie" are not symptoms or side effects of the medication. Rather, they indicate that the dosage of medication is too high, the child is on the wrong medication for the ADHD/ADD, or the diagnosis is incorrect. It is crucial that neither parents nor teachers believe that these are side effects which must be tolerated to gain the benefit of the medicine. Children and adolescents on appropriate medication neither have personality changes nor do they become depressed. Rather, they are very much themselves, but have the ability to concentrate, contain their impulses, and have a more appropriate activity level. Children and adolescents who have depression with attention disorder symptoms may respond better to antidepressants than to stimulants, however, or to a combination of the two.

Tics and Tourette Syndrome

A few children and adolescents will develop motor tics, or involuntary muscle movements such as eye-blinking or grimacing, when placed on stimulant medication. When this occurs, medication is usually reduced or discontinued, although it is not necessary to do so. There is considerable evidence that children with a family history of tics or TS are more likely to develop them. In these cases, use of stimulant medications should be approached judiciously and parents should be advised of their treatment options and the potential side effects of intervention.

Growth Suppression

The possibility that stimulant medication might affect growth, both height and weight, was first raised by Safer, Allen and Barr in 1972 and by Safer and Allen in 1973. Since that time, this potentially negative effect has caused much anxiety among parents and professionals alike. "Doesn't Ritalin cause growth problems?" is always one of the first questions asked at any program given on attention disorders where medication is discussed. While the early studies by Allen and his associates reported reduction in height and weight for children on Ritalin and Dexedrine, with a greater decrease for Dexedrine, later studies showed no significant effect when dosage levels were maintained within a range of 0.6 mg/kg to 0.8 mg/kg (McNutt et al., 1976; Kalachnik et al., 1982). The American Academy of Pediatrics, in its 1987 *Committee on Drugs Report*, attempted to reassure physicians and parents that no growth suppression occurred in doses of methylphenidate up to 0.8 mg/kg even over a prolonged period.

Drs. Klein and Manuzza (1988) compared the growth rate of young adults who were treated with methylphenidate in childhood because of hyperactivity. They found no difference in height between the group that was treated and the population in general. Interestingly, they found that if growth is slowed down at all during the time children are taking the medication, there appears to be a *growth rebound* effect that occurs after they stop taking the medicine.

The general consensus among professionals, based on scientific investigations over the last ten years, is that stimulant medications, especially Dexedrine, may cause a transient decrease in weight and a slight slowing of height lasting for a period of two to three years. However, there is believed to be little risk of a long-term negative effect on either height or weight. Those remaining on medication for over three years showed no negative long-term effect.

A common belief among those taking medication is that discontinuation of medication in the summer will enhance growth. Research suggests that discontinuation for this period of time has little effect on growth one way or the other. Since children often have growth spurts during the spring and summer, it was a logical, if erroneous conclusion, that being off the medicine caused the increase seen in height and weight in children during these times.

Despite the fairly limited real danger, most physicians check height and weight three to four times a year and obtain an annual CBC and chemical profile. If problems are noted, the stimulants are discontinued. Other medications are usually tried in their place if still needed.

In twenty years of practice we have had only one child who did not grow for a year. Even though he had *Constitutional Slow-Growth Syndrome*, his pediatrician, endocrinologist and the prescribing psychiatrist agreed to change from Ritalin to Norpramin. He still did not grow, but at least everyone felt assured that Ritalin was not a contributory factor.

Follow-Up

As suggested in Chapter 7, close monitoring of the medication is the key ingredient for success with the medical management of the multimodal intervention program. Until the medication, dose level and regimen are determined for optimum benefits and the side effects are minimized as much as possible, contact with the prescribing physician or team manager is necessary on a weekly, and occasionally daily, basis. Once the program has been well established, monitoring of the medication every three to four months is recommended.

The following checklist was requested by parents and can serve as a guide to the procedures and purposes of the follow-up visit with the prescribing physician.

MEDICATION FOLLOW-UP VISIT:
CHECKLIST FOR PHYSICIANS AND PARENTS

RITALIN/DEXEDRINE

Preceding the follow-up visit, these forms should be completed
by the parents or obtained from the teacher:

___ Copeland Medication Follow-Up Questionnaire (Teacher)
___ Grades and Academic Progress Reports
___ Copeland Medication Follow-up Questionnaire (Parent)
___ Side-Effects Checklist
___ Questions and Concerns

The above forms should be brought to the physician's office
at which time the following are obtained on every visit except
where noted:*

___ Height and weight.   Percentiles are compared to those
    obtained on previous visits.
___ *Differential platelets count (CBC) for prolonged therapy
    (yearly)
___ *Thyroid Functioning Tests (before medication)
___ *SMAC (Chemical profile before medication)
___ Blood pressure/heart rate
___ Visit with child to observe and to review progress, feelings
    about the medication, benefits and any side effects.
___ Conference with parents to review all data obtained, as
    well as their observations and concerns and to make
    recommendations regarding medication and other
    interventions.

SPECIAL ISSUES

Ritalin Sustained Release (Ritalin-SR)

Ritalin, in general, has been an excellent medication and provides good control of symptoms for the great majority of those with both ADHD and ADD. The four-hour half-life of methylphenidate, which requires frequent administration for effectiveness throughout the day, however, is inconvenient for all. For those children and adolescents who will not take it at school, the short half-life can be a major problem. It was for these reasons, plus the desire for a longer-acting, smoother effect without significant rebound that Ritalin-SR was developed. The manufacturer hoped it would be effective for at least eight hours and that it would require administration only once or twice daily.

Both scientific investigations and clinical experience have produced disappointing results. Most favor standard methylphenidate over the sustained release form of Ritalin (Pelham et al., 1987; Whitehouse, Shah & Palmer, 1980). For most, the effectiveness in the afternoon is approximately one-half of the expected level—observed both behaviorally and in plasma levels. Some appear to metabolize most of the SR tablet early in the day, resulting in an overmedicated response initially, followed by an undermedicated effect in the afternoon. If the tablet is chewed, this effect is still more dramatic. Another disadvantage for the SR is that it comes only in the 20 mg. form, which makes fine-tuning of the dosage extremely difficult.

On the positive side, there are some children and adolescents who respond quite well to the Ritalin SR—in fact, better than to standard Ritalin. A trial-and-error procedure is the only way to determine, conclusively, a particular person's response. The writing samples below are those of a ten-year-old boy who responded better to the SR than to the standard Ritalin, both clinically and as revealed by his performance on fine-motor tasks:

On Ritalin 10 mg. tablet

The Elfman

Once I met an Elfman.
He was smoking a cigar
and crossing his eyes.
I asked "How old are
you?". He said "25,729.
I'm the littlest kid
in Elfland."
I said "Wow! you're old.
He said "I'm not old!"

On Ritalin-SR

Afternoon   Afternoon
Apart   Apart
barnyard   barnyard
bedroom   bedroom
birthday   birthday
everybody   everybody
everything   everything
haircut   haircut
least   least

An additional advantage of Ritalin-SR is that it does not have the
rebound so characteristic of the short-acting form. Those who prescribe
medication a great deal often use a combination of the standard and the

SR to achieve maximum benefit. For others who need the benefits of a sustained release form, the physician may switch to Dexedrine Spansule, a more easily titrated, evenly released, long-acting medication. Close follow-up with ongoing titration and therapeutic trials is essential to arriving at the optimum medication(s) and regimen. Those who persist with this process are generally successful.

Generic Methylphenidate

Generic formulations of medications are usually less expensive than brand names. They are not always as effective, however, because the margin of error allowed on either side of the specific dosage level is greater than that allowed for brand names. Generic medicines have come under increased criticism and scrutiny by both the FDA and the public. Given the high cost of most medications, however, effective generic formulations are needed.

Throughout the country there have been a number of cases where the generic methylphenidate has been partially or totally ineffective. Parents and teachers often mistake this lack of effectiveness for psychological or behavioral problems as the symptoms return and academic accomplishment plummets. If a child or adolescent on a generic brand has been doing well and has a dramatic shift in response after obtaining a new prescription, the parents should be alert to the possibility that they may have a "bad batch" and notify their physician and/or pharmacist. Those unaware of this potential source of difficulty often encounter an unexplainable exacerbation of symptoms. When this occurs, the temptation is often to increase the level of medication rather than look for underlying causes. It is rare that we give a conference in which the problems with generic methylphenidate are discussed that someone does not have an "aha" experience, suddenly understanding what happened with their child or student at one time or another.

Those who wish to obtain the financial savings of generic medications can do so safely only if they are fully aware of the pitfalls and take action immediately if a lack of effectiveness is noted.

Drug Abuse

All parents worry about the potential for abuse of the medication itself, increased risk of later drug abuse, and the possibility that, as a society, we may be teaching children and adolescents that drugs are a solution to problems by giving them medication to control behavior and attention. These concerns are valid ones and are expressed by many parents, most in fact.

In assessing the risk, one most look at not only the benefit:risk ratio of treating this medical problem, but also the benefit:risk ratio of not treating the problem. The risk of not treating ADHD and ADD are, in my opinion, often greater than the risks of the medicines used to treat them. Dr. Josephine Elia (1980) at the National Institute of Mental Health, has reported that ADHD/ADD children and adolescents on stimulant therapy do not become addicted to stimulants. She stated, "They don't get the euphoric effect that abusers do, and they don't experience withdrawal symptoms when they stop taking the drug." Dr. Zametkin (1990) stated emphatically in his speech at the National CH.A.D.D. conference, "Ritalin is safer than Tylenol and is abused I.V. only." The Virginia Task Force Study (1990) cautioned, however, that the potential for abuse is significantly underestimated. On the other hand, they acknowledge that the abuse is either that of students and truck drivers taking it to stay awake, or that of drug addicts injecting the drug intravenously. Appropriate safeguards must clearly be utilized to diminish these abuses.

Many studies argue against increased risk for potential drug abuse. Most children and adolescents do not like taking medicine and may, in fact, have a decreased willingness to take or abuse other drugs (Collins, Whalen & Henker, 1980). It is important to emphasize to the child or adolescent that he, not the medication, is in control. There is a tendency for children to attribute good behavior to the medicine but claim negative behavior as their own.

Drug and alcohol abuse are believed more common in untreated ADHD/ADD adolescents and adults than in those properly treated by a physician.   Without effective intervention, they experience anger, frustration, intense feelings of failure and significant loss of esteem. These are the conditions most likely to lead to drug and alcohol abuse. Clinical experiences strongly suggest that hyperactive and ADD adolescents are at higher risk for developing substance abuse problems. Research has confirmed clinical judgment. DeMilio (1989) in a study of 57 adolescents (40 boys and 17 girls), who were referred to an inpatient facility for treatment of substance abuse, found that 21% of them had an attention deficit disorder, hyperactivity, or impulse disorder. Forty-two percent had conduct disorders.

Often adolescents and adults will experience some relief of symptoms when they try drugs and alcohol experimentally. They may then begin to self-medicate. They often take too much and they may use other medications to offset these effects. It is usually the *downers* (tranquilizers and sleeping medications) to which they become addicted, not the stimulants. Self-medicating is exceedingly dangerous for both adolescents and adults.

In assessing risk, it is also important to remember that ADHD and ADD are physiological problems and not behavioral or learning problems. The attention centers are not being stimulated properly and, thus, are not organizing and integrating information efficiently. Medication alerts the attention system so that it functions effectively. If medication is taken by a child, adolescent or adult without ADHD/ADD, it will overstimulate the attention system and produce tension and overfocused behavior, not pleasure and euphoria. To achieve pleasant effects one must use the drugs I.V. or escalate the dosage sometimes a hundred times as much as a normal dose to receive the "drug" effect.

Despite its relative safety, all who live and work with those with attention disorders must be ever mindful that Ritalin is a controlled substance and should be respected accordingly.

DEXEDRINE
(Dextroamphetamine Sulfate)

Many of our most important discoveries in medicine have been made by an astute person who observed an unexpected effect and explored its significance. Our odyssey in the use of stimulant medications to treat hyperactivity and attention disorders began in 1937 when Dr. Charles Bradley first noted the effect of the amphetamine, Benzedrine, on the inattentive and hyperactive behavior of emotionally disturbed children in a psychiatric hospital (Bradley, 1937). Their response to this medication was quite dramatic and spurred further investigation. Bradley later compared, in the 1950's, the effects of the chemically related amphetamines Benzedrine and dextroamphetamine and found no significant differences between the two medications. Children with hyperactivity have been treated successfully with psychostimulants since that time. Only more recently (1980's) have children with ADD without hyperactivity been treated with stimulants.

Despite its efficacy, dextroamphetamine is used much less frequently than methylphenidate. Estimates suggest that 4% to 6% of those on stimulant medication for attention disorders are taking this medication (Safer & Krager, 1988; Virginia DOE, 1990). The reasons are unclear but may relate to the earlier abuse of dexedrine for weight control and as the street drug, *Speed.* It is also much less readily available in pharmacies and less is produced, rendering it a difficult medication to obtain. It is, nevertheless, the medicine of choice for some children and adolescents, especially those unresponsive to Ritalin. It is the only psychostimulant approved for children under the age of six.

In our practice, we have found it an effective medication in many adolescents who were responsive to Ritalin as children, but who have become unresponsive to Ritalin as adolescents. It is also helpful for those who either refuse or forget to take a noon dose. Calis et al. (1990) reported positive results with Dexedrine and suggested that it may be the medication of choice if finances are a major consideration. However, its somewhat greater potential for abuse makes the benefit:risk ratio an even more critical consideration.

Description

Since the discovery of the benefits of amphetamine in the treatment of hyperactivity and ADD, many different ones have been tried. Dextroamphetamine has emerged as the preferred amphetamine and is the only one currently recommended for the treatment of ADHD and ADD. Dextroamphetamine sulfate is commercially available from Smith Kline Beecham Laboratories as *Dexedrine*.

Classification

Like methylphenidate, Dexedrine is a Class II controlled substance with the same legal restrictions on usage and prescription renewal. Unlike Ritalin, Dexedrine has a higher potential for abuse ... and some fear that prolonged use may lead to drug dependence but not to *physiologic* addiction. While such concerns are obviously warranted, the experience of those using it with children with ADHD/ADD has been positive when medication usage is carefully monitored. It becomes somewhat more problematic for adolescents and adults.

Clinical Pharmacology

Dexedrine is a "central nervous system stimulant which affects multiple neurotransmitter systems, especially dopamine and norepinephrine. The exact mechanism by which it reduces ADHD symptoms is not yet known. Dextroamphetamine's CNS stimulant qualities produce peripheral actions which include elevations of systolic and diastolic blood pressures and weak bronchodilator and respiratory stimulant action" (PDR, 1990).

Shaywitz, Shaywitz, Anderson, et al. (1988) suggest differences in the mechanism of action for Ritalin and Dexedrine. From their data they hypothesize that dextroamphetamine influences brain noradrenergic mechanisms, leaving more norepinephrine available by reducing the turnover of this neurotransmitter. Calis, et al. (1990) suggest that its effects are due to its ability to block the release and reuptake of dopamine and norepinephrine from central CNS systems. Higher doses may cause the release of dopamine in other parts of the brain.

As one reads the various hypotheses about the mechanisms of the stimulants, it becomes increasingly apparent that, while much is known, there is more that remains a mystery. Dr. Elia's statement in 1980, "We know the drugs work - they're very effective - but we don't know how they work," is still largely true today, ten years later. It does appear, however, that both the mechanisms and sites of action of different medications differ, so that a person unresponsive to one stimulant medication may well respond positively to another stimulant or to another class of medication.

Availability and Duration of Effect

Dexedrine is available in a short-acting, four-hour, tablet form only in a 5 mg. size. The sustained release form, *Dexedrine Spansule*, is available in 5 mg., 10 mg. and 15 mg. capsules. Dexedrine came in liquid form, *Dexedrine Elixir*, at one time but is no longer available.

Dexedrine is the only stimulant medication approved for children ages 3 to 6. Most clinicians and researchers strongly support the use of behavioral interventions in the early years when possible. When they are not effective, the use of Dexedrine has been found quite helpful (Speltz et al., 1988). As reported earlier, increasing awareness of the correlation, and possible causation, between attention disorders, language disorders, reading disorders and learning disabilities may cause us to reconsider this position and more aggressively treat attention disorders in the preschool years.

Like Ritalin, both the Dexedrine tablet and spansules are easy to swallow and should be taken whole for maximum effectiveness. They, too, have dyes which may cause allergic-type reactions in susceptible individuals. Those with aspirin sensitivity should be especially cautious.

Tablet	Spansule		
5 mg.	5 mg.	10 mg.	15 mg.
Orange	Clear/Brown		
(FD&C Yellow Nos. 5 & 6)	FD&C Yellow No. 5 and No. 6, FD&C Blue No. 1, and FD&C Red No. 40		

Indications and Usage

Dexedrine is utilized in the treatment of narcolepsy, ADHD/ADD, and exogenous obesity. Again, it should be used only as an integral part of a total treatment program.

Contraindications

A careful diagnosis of attention deficit disorder is crucial before the administration of Dexedrine. Other disorders, including anxiety, bipolar disorder, thought disorders, hyperthyroidism, and hypertension, among others, can be seriously exacerbated. Dexedrine is the second-choice stimulant for most physicians after Ritalin has been tried and has not been found effective.

Dexedrine is contraindicated for persons with cardiovascular disease, hypertension, hyperthyroidism, glaucoma, hypersensitivity, and agitation. It should not be used with anyone with a history of drug abuse or within 14 days following the administration of monoamine oxidase inhibitors (MAOI's). It should also be used cautiously with patients with motor tics, or those with a family history or diagnosis of Tourette Syndrome.

Warnings

Dexedrine should be used only with careful monitoring by a physician familiar with both its benefits and potential problems. Except for its use in children, specific warnings are the same as those for Ritalin, addressed on pp. 168-172. In addition, it should be noted that gastrointestinal acidifying agents, such as orange juice, or gastric juices, decrease the absorption of amphetamines. Dexedrine, as do Ritalin and Cylert, counteracts the sedative effect of antihistamines.

Dosage and Administration

Time of Administration

Dexedrine may be given after meals to reduce the potential for headaches and stomachaches, realizing that there is some decrease in its availability under these conditions. The Dexedrine tablet requires approximately 15-30 minutes to become effective, with maximum effectiveness at approximately 2 to 3 hours with gradually diminishing effectiveness the last hour. As with Ritalin, the time period of benefit varies widely, depending upon individual sensitivity and metabolism, with the average being 4 hours with a range from 2 to 6 hours. It must be monitored closely to determine the optimal time periods of administration.

Dexedrine Spansule requires 45-60 minutes to become effective. It lasts approximately 8 to 12 hours depending upon the individual. The spansules, which look like *Contac*, are formulated to release the active drug in a more gradual fashion than the standard formula. It, too, avoids the rebound effect sometimes experienced with the tablet form. The relatively longer half-life of Dexedrine Spansule has been observed clinically to sometimes cause a build-up which can result in irritability, tension and other overdose effects after several weeks of administration. Those taking Dexedrine Spansule do much better with at least one drug holiday per week. Parents of those taking Dexedrine Spansule should be alert to this possible effect.

Dosage

Dexedrine, like all psychostimulants, is initiated in small doses, usually at 5 mg. However, the equivalent dose of Dexedrine is about one-half to two-thirds of that of Ritalin. Thus, a sensitive child might well need a smaller dose such as 2.5 mg. initially. It is increased gradually in much the same manner as Ritalin until maximum therapeutic benefit has been achieved. The Spansule form is usually begun with the 5 mg. Spansule. It is more easily titrated than the 20 mg. Ritalin-SR and has generally been found very reliable in its systematic release. There have been no complaints of overmedication followed by an undermedicated response in the afternoon as for the long-acting Ritalin.

Frequency of Administration

The Spansule is usually taken only once daily with an occasional tablet booster for evening study. The tablet and elixir forms last approximately four hours and are administered based on need, with considerations essentially the same as those for Ritalin. The use of Dexedrine on weekends and holidays was addressed in Chapter 7. Considerations are similar to the suggestions given for Ritalin on page 175.

Rebound

Like Ritalin, a rebound from Dexedrine has been reported for the short-acting tablet. The Spansule's gradual release avoids this effect. Rebound from Dexedrine is managed in much the same way as Ritalin rebound.

Adverse Reactions/Side Effects

The side effects and adverse reactions of Dexedrine are almost identical to those of Ritalin. It negatively affects appetite somewhat more, however, and has been shown to temporarily slow growth slightly more than Ritalin. The abuse potential is somewhat greater. For that reason, it is typically not used with adolescents in psychiatric facilities, those with histories of drug experimentation, or with impulsive risk-taking teens or adults. Cylert is often the stimulant of choice where abuse is considered likely.

Follow-up

Close monitoring is an essential part of the medical management of Dexedrine and is similar to that of Ritalin. It is emphasized again that medication is helpful only as a part of a comprehensive, multimodal treatment program. A "Medication Follow-Up Checklist for Physicians and Parents" is provided on page 183.

While Dexedrine poses slightly more risk than Ritalin in the treatment of both ADHD and ADD, its benefits often outweigh its risks for those nonresponsive to other interventions. With careful monitoring, both the negative effects and the abuse potential can be minimized. Its more reasonable cost may become a greater consideration as increasing numbers of children and adolescents are identified and treated. For those who do not obtain treatment because they cannot afford the medicine, cost becomes a major concern.

DESOXYN
(Methamphetamine Hydrochloride)

Desoxyn, chemically similar to dextroamphetamine, is rarely used for the treatment of attention disorders because of its high potential for addiction and abuse. It is produced by Abbott Laboratories in 5 mg., 10 mg. and 15 mg. tablets.

CYLERT
(Pemoline)

Description

Cylert (pemoline) is the newest stimulant on the market. It was introduced into the United States in 1975 after several years of use in Europe. It is manufactured by Abbott Laboratories and is currently not available in generic form.

Its introduction into the U.S. was greeted with great enthusiasm, for it was the first stimulant to hold promise of round-the-clock control of symptoms because of its plasma build-up. However, both side effects, especially reports of liver dysfunction, and its lack of the degree of positive benefit achieved with Ritalin and Dexedrine make it a third or fourth choice medication for most physicians except in special circumstances.

A 1987 study of stimulant medication usage in a Baltimore school district suggested that it is used in 1% to 6% of elementary school students taking medication (Safer & Krager, 1988). The use of methylphenidate was 91%, while 4% were receiving dextroamphetamine. Only 2% were taking nonstimulant medications.

Classification

Cylert is a controlled substance subject to control under DEA Schedule IV. The potential for abuse is not nearly as great as for Schedule (class) II drugs, and prescriptions can be phoned into a pharmacy eliminating the need to plan ahead so carefully. It is not restricted to a 30-day supply, and refills can be obtained.

Clinical Pharmacology

Pemoline is a central nervous system stimulant which is structurally unlike dextroamphetamine and methylphenidate. It has a pharmacological activity similar to that of the stimulants but has minimal effects on the autonomic nervous system. Animal studies suggest that pemoline acts through dopaminergic mechanisms. However, neither the exact mechanism nor the site of action of Cylert in man is known. While the majority of studies comparing methylphenidate or dextroamphetamine with pemoline show a superiority of the traditional stimulants (Dykman et al., 1976), researchers believe that pemoline is superior to methylphenidate for some learning tasks (Stevenson, Pelham & Skinner, 1984) and is a better medication for a few children (Dykman, et al., 1976).

Availability and Duration of Effect

Pemoline is a white, tasteless, odorless powder. Cylert is supplied as tablets containing 18.75 mg., 37.5 mg. and 75 mg. of pemoline. It is also available as chewable tablets containing 37.5 mg. of pemoline.

While the 18.75 mg. and the 75 mg. tablets contain no dyes, the 37.5 mg. tablet and chewable forms have FD&C Yellow No. 6.

18.75 mg.	37.5 mg.	75 mg.	37.5 mg.
White	FD&C Yellow No. 6	White	Chewable FD&C Yellow No. 6

The tablets are small and easily swallowed. They are relatively insoluble, necessitating the chewable form for those who cannot swallow pills.

Cylert was formulated to be administered only once a day, with a half-life of seven to eight hours. It is rapidly absorbed from the gastrointestinal tract following oral administration and achieves peak plasma levels in two or three hours. Wide variability has been reported in pemoline metabolism, resulting in unpredictable reactions of children and adolescents at times. As much as two to three hundred percent variability in response has been reported. Physicians should be aware of the potential for such wide differences in metabolism when they prescribe the medicine.

While an observable effect is usually seen within one to three hours of administration, maximum therapeutic effectiveness may take three to four weeks in some children (Calis et al., 1990), and four to eight weeks in others (Conners & Taylor, 1980). When discontinued, the medication requires several weeks to fully dissipate from the bloodstream. Since it does have a build-up effect, it should be discontinued gradually, unlike Ritalin and Dexedrine, which can be fully discontinued at once.

Indications/Usage/Contraindications

Cylert is used only for the treatment of attention deficit disorders. It must be used with care and there are specific situations of special concern.

Children under Six

Cylert has neither been studied nor approved for use in children under six years of age.

Long-term Treatment

Those taking Cylert for a long time must be carefully monitored since sufficient data on long-term safety and effectiveness are not available.

Liver Disease or Damage

Cylert is contraindicated in those with liver disease or damage, or a family history of hepatic disorders. A blood test to rule out elevated serum liver enzymes is recommended before the initiation of medication. Liver dysfunction from Cylert use is discussed at length under *Adverse Reactions.*

Tics and Tourette Syndrome

Like other stimulant medications, Cylert is contraindicated in any one with motor tics or with a family history of Tourette Syndrome. The considerations are the same as those outlined in detail on page 180 in the discussion of Ritalin.

Seizures

Seizures have been reported with the use of Cylert. It is, therefore, usually contraindicated in those with seizure disorders. Decreased seizure threshold has also been reported in patients taking Cylert concurrently with anticonvulsant medication. However, some physicians believe that control of the ADHD/ADD symptoms in seizure patients is so important that it is worthwhile to increase the seizure medications slightly to overcome this disadvantage. These decisions should, of course, be made by the child or adolescent's neurologist.

Drug Interactions

The interaction of Cylert with other drugs has not been studied in humans. Patients taking Cylert concurrently with other drugs should be monitored carefully, especially if the drugs have CNS effects.

Potential for Abuse

Thus far Cylert has failed to demonstrate potential for abuse. However, given the similarity to other psychostimulants, caution is urged. There have been no reported cases either of abuse or of physical or psychological dependence. It is, therefore, the psychostimulant of choice for many physicians treating high-risk ADHD/ADD adolescents and adults for whom a stimulant is needed.

Dosage and Administration

Given its longer acting qualities, Cylert is administered somewhat differently than other psychostimulants.

Time of Administration

Cylert is usually administered in the morning. However, recent investigations suggest that Cylert may produce a better response on a morning and noon dosage schedule, as opposed to once daily (Collier, Soldin et al., 1985). In general, giving medication in divided doses appears most satisfactory for those medications which are not sustained-release preparations.

Unlike Ritalin and Dexedrine, Cylert must be given on weekends as well. Two days off the medication reduces serum levels and consequently its therapeutic benefit. In conferences for parents and teachers at least one person at each conference acknowledges having mistakenly assumed that the medication is administered only on school days as Ritalin and Dexedrine often are.

Dosage

The usual starting dose is 37.5 mg. given as a single dose in the morning. However, sensitive children and adolescents may need to start at a lower dose such as 18.75 mg. The advantage of a lower starting dose is that the side effects will be less intense.

The dose can be titrated upward in 18.75 mg. weekly increments to a maximum of 112.5 mg./day. As the dose is increased, divided doses are often more effective. The most typical therapeutic dose ranges from 56.25 mg./day to 75 mg./day for the average child (Calis et al., 1990). Adjusting the dosage downward may be necessary as the child matures to maintain the same level of effectiveness. As children mature, the medication actually seems to be more, rather than less, effective.

Rebound

Because of its gradually increasing serum level and its longer half-life, rebound has not been a problem with Cylert use.

Adverse Reactions/Side Effects

Insomnia

Insomnia is the most frequently reported side effect of Cylert. It usually occurs early in therapy and subsides with continued use. Adjusting dosage to take care of this effect is usually all that is necessary to overcome it once some time has elapsed.

Liver Damage

Many studies have shown that Cylert may cause liver damage or failure. The PDR (1990) warns that "There have been reports of hepatic dysfunction, including elevated liver enzymes, hepatitis and jaundice in patients taking Cylert." This possibility necessitates blood tests which include liver function tests (LFT's), notably those measuring liver enzymes (SGOT and SGPT). Blood tests are obtained before the administration of Cylert and at least every six months during treatment. Should elevated serum liver enzymes occur, the medication is discontinued. Discontinuation usually reverses the problem. Cylert is contraindicated in anyone with a personal or family history of any hepatic disorder or aplastic anemia.

Decreased Appetite and Growth Suppression

Anorexia and weight loss may occur during the first weeks of therapy. Stomachaches and/or nausea may also occur. These are usually transient side effects only. If they continue, another medication should be utilized.

Decrease in growth was an early concern for Cylert, just as it was for Ritalin and Dexedrine. However, researchers following children on pemoline for many years have shown that after 48 months of continuous treatment there are no observable differences in height and weight in those who have taken Cylert and those who have not, except an occasional increase in weight (Friedman et al., 1981). The American Academy of Pediatrics Committee on Drugs advised physicians that children treated with pemoline may experience short-term decreases in height and weight gain but assured them that there is little concern long term (*AAP Committee on Drugs*, 1987). The growth pattern effect of Cylert is very similar to that of other stimulant medications.

Hypertension/Increased Heart Rate

Cylert has not been found to affect heart rate or blood pressure. Thus, it appears safe for those with hypertension who may not be able to take Ritalin or Dexedrine but who need a stimulant medication.

Summary

Despite being the medication of choice for a few patients, the lack of equivalent effectiveness for most ADHD/ADD children and adolescents, the possibility of liver damage, and the necessity of frequent blood tests are significant disadvantages for Cylert and have rendered it relatively unpopular with patients and physicians alike. As more is learned, however, a specific superiority of Cylert may well surface, particularly for some children and for some learning tasks.

Follow-up

Like all medications, close monitoring is the key for maximum therapeutic benefit with the fewest adverse reactions and side effects. The relatively significant possibility of elevated serum liver enzymes and the potential for liver damage or even hepatic failure necessitate careful evaluation both before and during the initial phases of drug titration. Once a therapeutic regimen has been established, follow-up is recommended every three to four months with liver enzyme studies every six months.

The *Medication Follow-up Checklist* on page 205, similar to that for Ritalin and Dexedrine, can serve as a guide to the procedures and purposes of the follow-up visit with the prescribing physician.

MEDICATION FOLLOW-UP VISIT:
CHECKLIST FOR PHYSICIANS AND PARENTS

CYLERT

Preceding the follow-up visit, these forms should be completed
by the parents or obtained from the teacher:

___ Copeland Medication Follow-up Questionnaire (Teacher)
___ Grades and Academic Progress Reports
___ Copeland Medication Follow-up Questionnaire (Parent)
___ Side-Effects Checklist
___ Questions and Concerns

The above forms should be brought to the physician's office
at which time the following are obtained on every visit except
where noted:*

___ Height and weight. Percentiles are compared to those
obtained on previous visits.
___ *Differential platelets count (CBC) for prolonged therapy
(yearly).
___ *Liver functioning tests (SGOT, SGPT) (Initially and every
six months).
___ Blood pressure/Heart rate.
___ Visit with child to observe and to review with him his
progress, his perception of the medication, and any side
effects.
___ Conference with parents to review all data obtained, their
observations and concerns and to make recommendations
regarding medication and other interventions.

FENFLURAMINE
(Pondimin, Ponderax)

Fenfluramine Hydrochloride, marketed by A.H. Robins Company, Inc. in 20 mg. *Pondimin* tablets, is an analogue of amphetamine. It was developed as an antiobesity agent, but has been of much interest as a possible adjunctive treatment for infantile autism. Because of its structural similarity to the amphetamines, it has been suggested that it might offer potential benefit for the treatment of attention disorders.

The mechanism of action of Pondimin is uncertain but appears to be related to brain levels of serotonin rather than to norepinephrine or dopamine. It produces central nervous system depression, unlike the CNS stimulation produced by amphetamines and methylphenidate. While not studied extensively, the results of at least one clinical trial comparing Dexedrine with Pondimin has not shown this medication to be effective in treating ADHD (Donnelly & Rapoport, 1985). Aman and Kern (1989), in an extensive review article on fenfluramine in the treatment of developmental disabilities, reported that the research data suggest that fenfluramine may lessen hyperactivity in autistic children but not in attention deficit disordered children of normal I.Q. and socialization.

While fenfluramine may hold promise for developmental disorders, its effectiveness does not compare with the medications already widely used for attention disorders.

I hit bottom. I knew I could not go on. I saw a psychiatrist, a wonderful man, who became my therapist, my medicine man, my mentor and my friend. He diagnosed my ADD. Then together we sorted out the emotional baggage I had collected for thirty-five years.

— Successful ADHD adult, 1989

9

Antidepressants: Second-Line Medications

Tricyclic Antidepressants
Prozac
Monoamine Oxidase Inhibitors (MAOI's)

"Antidepressant" may be a misnomer for this group of medications used to treat a number of disorders involving neurotransmitters. The tricyclic antidepressants affect the availability of norepinephrine and dopamine, while Prozac and the MAO Inhibitors affect serotonin transmission. These antidepressants are used not only to treat depression, but also to treat bedwetting, migraine headaches, eating disorders, obsessive-compulsive disorders, and attention deficit disorders, among others.

Imipramine (Tofranil), the original tricyclic antidepressant, has been used since the mid-sixties to treat depression. It was also found to have a beneficial effect on enuresis, or bedwetting, and is utilized in children six years and older for this disorder.

Desipramine (Norpramin), a derivative of imipramine, acts much like its counterpart, but produces fewer side effects. While most psychiatrists are familiar with Norpramin and prescribe it more than

Tofranil, pediatricians and other physicians may be more comfortable prescribing Tofranil because of greater familiarity with it.

Prozac, introduced in 1987, was the first in a new class of antidepressants which decreases the availability of the neurotransmitter, serotonin. Prozac has taken the public by storm despite some controversy over its reported, but unproven, potential for precipitating aggression or hypomania in some people. Monoamine oxidase inhibitors (MOAIs) are also increasingly seen as having positive potential for treating some kinds of attention disorders.

The antidepressants, especially the tricyclic antidepressants, are considered by most to be a valuable second-line treatment to be used when the stimulants are either ineffective or contraindicated because of side effects or other medical reasons. In addition, the tricyclics, Prozac, and the MAOIs have some distinct advantages over the stimulants: their effects are longer lasting so that control of symptoms occurs consistently throughout the day and evening; they enhance sleep rather than increasing sleep disturbance; appetite is not suppressed; and there is usually a positive effect on mood and self-image concomitant with a decrease in irritability and lability. Since abuse is not a problem with antidepressants and, in fact, they are often utilized in treating addictive disorders, they are sometimes preferable to stimulant medications for those for whom abuse potential is present.

TOFRANIL
(Imipramine Hydrochloride)

Imipramine hydrochloride has been the most extensively utilized and the most thoroughly studied tricyclic antidepressant prescribed for the treatment of ADHD and ADD in children and adolescents. Pliszka provided an extensive review of its use in 1987. Biederman and associates (1989) reviewed its use in a research report on the efficacy of desipramine in 1989. First prescribed in 1965, its success rates have ranged from 45% to 85% (Wiener, 1985).

Imipramine hydrochloride is available from several manufacturers including Biocraft Laboratories, Inc.; Geneva Pharmaceuticals, Inc.; Par Pharmaceutical, Inc.; and Roxane Laboratories, Inc. It is available in Tofranil ampules, Tofranil tablets and *Tofranil pamoate* (the equivalent of imipramine hydrochloride) from Geigy Pharmaceuticals. The *Tofranil* brand of imipramine is the most commonly utilized and has been researched the most.

Classification

Tofranil is a not a Schedule II medication. While subject to the usual restrictions for drugs and prescription renewal, it is not controlled in the same manner as the stimulant medications. Prescriptions for it may be phoned to a pharmacy followed by a written prescription from an M.D. and refills can be ordered. It requires, nonetheless, careful supervision and ongoing monitoring.

Clinical Pharmacology

The exact mechanism of Tofranil is not definitively understood. Its action, however, is not primarily that of a CNS stimulant. Rather, research data suggests that it acts primarily by inhibiting the re-uptake of catecholamines, primarily norepinephrine, thus increasing the concentration of neurotransmitters at the synaptic cleft. More efficient transmission of nerve impulses is the desired goal. The mechanism of action is as follows:

MECHANISM OF ACTION:
NOREPINEPHRINE

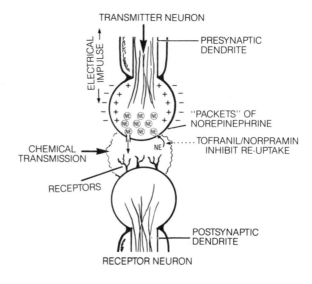

As described previously, in ADHD and ADD norepinephrine is thought to be secreted in deficient quantities, thus impeding the transmission of both excitatory and inhibitory impulses important for attention, concentration, impulse control and appropriate activity level and responding. While the stimulants increase the amount of dopamine and norepinephrine in the synaptic cleft by stimulating the release of more of this neurotransmitter from the presynaptic neuron, the tricyclic antidepressants—both Tofranil and Norpramin—increase the availability of norepinephrine by preventing its re-uptake after release into the synaptic cleft. While the mechanism is different, the net effect for nerve transmission is very similar to that of the stimulant medications.

Availability and Duration of Effect

Tofranil is utilized for the treatment of depression primarily and secondarily for attention disorders. However, it has not been approved for the latter.

For the treatment of ADHD/ADD Tofranil tablets of 10 mg., 25 mg., and 50 mg. are most frequently used. Tofranil-PM is available in capsules of 75 mg., 100 mg., 125 mg., and 150 mg. These, however, are never recommended for children of any age because of the increased potential for acute overdosage due to their high unit potency (PDR, 1994). All of the Tofranil tablets are quite small and are easily swallowed.

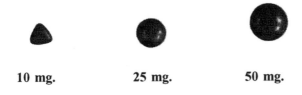

| 10 mg. | 25 mg. | 50 mg. |

Low doses of tricyclics (50 mg. per day, or doses less than 1 mg/kg/day) have not been effective in most children and adolescents according to the literature. Most studies have used a daily dose of 50 to 150 mg. or a 3 to 5 mg/kg weight-basis dosage. However, we have had several children, particularly younger children, whose symptoms became worse on stimulants, who have responded exceedingly well to sub-clinical doses of Tofranil taken at bedtime or in divided doses morning and noon. Others, too, have found lower doses useful in the treatment of the attention disorders of adolescents and adults as well.

Tofranil is a medication which requires plasma concentration for maximum effectiveness. However, improvement usually occurs within two or three days. By contrast, noticeable benefit in depression typically requires two to three weeks. The mechanisms of action appear different for ADHD/ADD, depression and enuresis, but hypothalamic involvement seems evident as one of the sites of action.

Indications and Usage

Tofranil was developed for use as an antidepressant initially. Its beneficial effect on enuresis was noted very quickly, and it continues to be utilized for childhood enuresis. Tofranil has been utilized as a second-line medication for the treatment of these disorders for twenty-five years and has been investigated fairly extensively. Calis and his associates (1990) at NIMH, following intensive investigation of medications for attention disorders, state, "The FDA has not yet approved the use of tricyclic antidepressants for the treatment of ADHD. There is, however, overwhelming scientific evidence to support their use for this condition."

Specific Benefits

Tofranil is especially helpful for children, adolescents and adults who are anxious, who have sleep problems, or who have a disturbance of mood or affect with their attention disorder. Those described as *irritable, moody* and *prone to highs and lows* may especially benefit. Likewise, those with a family history of depression or bipolar disorder may respond overall somewhat better to the tricyclic antidepressants than to the stimulant medications. Likewise, those who experience anger and aggressiveness appear to respond better to Tofranil. While one researcher has judged it superior to the stimulants for the treatment of attention disorders (Pliszka, 1987), most clinicians and researchers consider it a valuable second-line choice or a medication for special situations. Those treated with tricyclic antidepressants do show improvement on behavioral scales, in clinical assessment, and on objective measures of attention, impulse control and cognitive abilities (Huessey & Wright, 1970). Werry and his associates (1980) conducted a study in which ADHD children were treated with 0.4 mg/kg of methylphenidate, 1.0 mg/kg of imipramine, or 2.0 mg/kg of imipramine.

At both dose levels, imipramine had a positive effect on learning, motor performance and social relationships.

Many studies attest to the short-term effectiveness of the tricyclics. Long-term effectiveness remains much less certain (Wiener, 1985; Quinn & Rapoport, 1975). The problems with long-term effectiveness will be addressed at length in the section on adverse reactions.

Contraindications and Warnings

A major concern in the use of the tricyclics is their potential for exacerbating cardiac problems of any kind and their potential cardio-toxicity. Anyone with conduction defects, cardiac arrhythmias, a family history of heart disease, or heart problems of any kind whatever require cardiac surveillance at all dosage levels. While the manufacturer recommends electrocardiograms (ECGs) for those taking larger-than-usual doses, many physicians obtain an ECG prior to the initiation of medication and at appropriate intervals thereafter until steady state has been achieved. A dose of 2.5 mg/kg/day should never be exceeded in children.

Tofranil is also contraindicated with the concomitant use of monoamine oxidase inhibitors because of their combined potential for precipitating seizures.

Of importance, parents must be aware of the extreme danger of the antidepressants, especially imipramine and desipramine, should a child overdose. Tricyclic antidepressants can be fatal with as few as ten pills because of the cardiac arrhythmias caused by these medications. All medications should be kept in a safe and locked place. This is especially true when young children are in the household, or when a teenager or adult in the home is seriously depressed or has suicidal thoughts.

Tofranil may enhance the CNS depressant effect of alcohol, and both adolescents and adults should be warned not to drink while taking this medication. An ADHD teenager determined to drink beer, for example, would be unable to tolerate a tricyclic but might have an overall better response to the shorter-acting stimulants, especially Ritalin, for school days only.

Tofranil should be used with caution with those with renal or hepatic disorders. Decongestants, local anesthetics and any sympathomimetic amines (epinephrine, norepinephrine) should be avoided since they potentiate each other. Sunlight exposure should also be minimized while taking Tofranil, since there have been reports of photosensitization.

Dosage and Administration

For children and adolescents Tofranil should be initiated at low doses and increased gradually, noting carefully the clinical response and any evidence of intolerance. For children the dosage can range from 20 mg. to 60 mg. per day given in divided doses depending upon target symptoms. Adolescents usually begin at 30-40 mg. per day and usually do not exceed 100 mg. per day. A build-up occurs in two to three days and an effect is often observed from the first day of administration.

The effective dosage depends on many factors including an individual's particular responsivity to this class of medications, his general sensitivity and his metabolism, among other variables.

Tofranil's positive effect on sleep can be of great benefit when given in the evening. On the other hand, some children and adolescents report increased difficulty falling asleep if medication is taken after dinner. They usually find morning and noon dosing more satisfactory.

It has been noted clinically that some children and adolescents who will benefit from daytime administration are often difficult to awaken and sluggish from evening doses. It is crucial to monitor administration carefully since the best time for positive benefit is less predictable than for the stimulants.

Since the tricyclics build up in the bloodstream, they should be continued on weekends and holidays. If no medication is desired in the summer, it should be discontinued gradually over a two-week period. Immediate cessation of most medications after prolonged treatment will cause withdrawal symptoms. For Tofranil these include headache, malaise, and nausea.

Rebound

One of the benefits of the tricyclics is their improvement in symptoms around the clock. There is no rebound effect because the plasma concentration is achieved and maintained.

Adverse Reactions/Side Effects

Cardiac

Tofranil's major adverse reaction has been discussed previously, i.e., its cardiovascular effects and its potential for cardiotoxicity. It is contraindicated in anyone with heart disease or cardiac irregularities of any kind.

Anticholinergic

Anticholinergic side effects occur in varying degrees depending upon dose and individual sensitivity and may include dry mouth, blurred vision or urinary retention, among others. These effects are less pronounced in children whose most common side effects include nervousness, sleep disturbance, fatigue, and mild gastrointestinal disturbances. These effects are usually transient or managed with decreased dosage.

Long-Term Effects

While short-term effectiveness of the tricyclics has been demonstrated, their long-term effectiveness is questionable. Gittelman-Klein (1974) found that an initial positive response at 2 weeks was not maintained at 12 weeks. Quinn and Rapoport (1975), likewise, reported that more ADHD children had discontinued imipramine at one year follow-up than the stimulants despite an initial positive response. Since ADHD and ADD are long-term disorders, it will be important to determine whether the tricyclics will be beneficial on an ongoing basis.

Tics and Tourette Syndrome

Like the stimulants, Tofranil has been associated with the precipitation or exacerbation of tics and Tourette Syndrome. It should be avoided when possible, or used in the lowest effective dose to reduce this potential side effect. Weighing the benefits versus the risks is especially important when treating TS.

Other Side Effects

Tofranil has the potential to cause neurologic, psychiatric, allergic and endocrine side effects as well. The prescribing physician must carefully evaluate the child or adolescent for medical problems prior to initiation of this therapeutic option and be aware of the potential for negative reactions. The risks associated with antidepressants are greater than those for the stimulants.

Follow-Up

Close monitoring of the tricyclic antidepressants is critical. Both parents and children should be counseled regarding the benefits and advised as to the risks and how to successfully cope with them.

During the initial phase of treatment, weekly contact with the physician or team manager is essential. After the optimal dosage and regimen have been established, monitoring of the medication every three to four months is recommended. As with the stimulants, antidepressant medications are often the cornerstone which enables the other components of the multimodal treatment program to become effective.

The following checklist was designed to serve as a guide for the follow-up visits with the prescribing physician:

MEDICATION FOLLOW-UP VISIT:
CHECKLIST FOR PHYSICIANS AND PARENTS

TOFRANIL/NORPRAMIN

Preceding the follow-up visit, these forms should be completed
by the parents or obtained from the teacher:

___ Copeland Medication Follow-up Questionnaire (Teacher)
___ Grades and Academic Progress Reports
___ Copeland Medication Follow-up Questionnaire (Parent)
___ Side-Effects Checklist
___ Questions and Concerns

The above forms should be brought to the physician's office
at which time the following are obtained on every visit except
where noted:*

___ Height and weight. Percentiles are compared to those
obtained on previous visits.
___ *Differential platelet count (CBC) for prolonged therapy
(yearly).
___ *SMAC: Blood profile
___ Blood pressure/heart rate/pulse.
___ *Electrocardiogram (ECG). (Before initiation and
periodically until a maintenance dose has been established;
thereafter yearly.)
___ *Liver function tests (LFT). (Before initiation and
periodically as long as medication is continued)
___ Visit with child to observe and to review with him his
progress, his perception of the medication, and any side
effects.
___ Conference with parents to review all data obtained, their
observations and concerns and to make recommendations
regarding medication and other interventions.

NORPRAMIN
Desipramine Hydrochloride

Desipramine hydrochloride, the active metabolite of imipramine, had until the early 90's, received high marks as an alternative tricyclic antidepressant. Produced by Marion Merrell Dow Pharmaceuticals, Inc. as *Norpramin*, it had been found to be very effective in reducing symptoms of impulsivity, hyperactivity and distractibility in children with ADHD without causing or exacerbating tics (Riddle et al., 1988). It was also reported to have fewer side effects than imipramine. A recent review of three sudden deaths in children receiving Norpramin has cast some doubt on the potential promise of this relatively new medication in the ADHD armamentarium of therapeutic options in children under the age of twelve.

Description/Classification/Clinical Pharmacology

A metabolite of imipramine, desipramine is considered a secondary amine tricyclic antidepressant and is believed to have somewhat greater activity in blocking the reuptake of norepinephrine than imipramine, and thus a more rapid onset of effect. It is metabolized in the liver with the rate of metabolism varying widely among individuals. Up to a thirty-six fold difference in plasma level has been found between individuals taking the same dose of medication.

Desipramine is not a controlled drug. It has been approved for use in depression, but not yet in ADHD despite wide clinical use and much research on its effectiveness (Donnelly et al., 1986; Biederman et al., 1989a, 1989b). It has not been approved for use in children under the age of twelve. It has the same restriction on prescription requirements and renewal typical of most medicines.

Availability and Duration of Effect

Norpramin is available in 10 mg., 25 mg., 50 mg., 75 mg., 100 mg., and 150 mg. tablets. The smaller tablets are recommended for adolescents because of the potential for overdosage due to the high potency of the larger tablets. All of the tablets are relatively small and should be swallowed whole.

Desipramine typically requires administration for two to three weeks before benefit is achieved. However, in ADHD/ADD symptom improvement is often obtained within the first few days of administration, often even the first day. Plasma concentration is achieved, resulting in benefit around the clock.

Dosage and Administration

Despite the build-up effect obtained with desipramine, it has been clinically observed to be more effective for ADHD/ADD if given in divided doses, usually morning and later in the day. Some adolescents and adults respond better to evening administration.

Desipramine should be initiated at a low level and increased according to both clinical response and any adverse effects. Plasma concentration is achieved, although the therapeutic blood levels established for depression are not directly applicable for the treatment of attention disorders. Clinical response is the best determiner of benefit and dosage requirements. Once established, the therapeutic blood level can usually be maintained with a single daily dose, a time schedule which encourages compliance.

The usual adolescent dose of Norpramin is 25 mg. to 100 mg. daily. Doses over 150 mg. per day are not recommended for this age group. Like imipramine, desipramine builds up in the plasma for continuing round-the-clock effectiveness. It, likewise, should not be discontinued abruptly, but tapered over ten to fourteen days. Careful monitoring is essential.

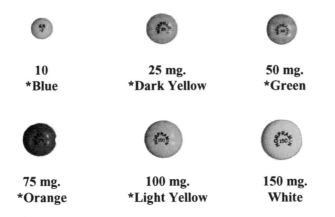

10 *Blue	25 mg. *Dark Yellow	50 mg. *Green
75 mg. *Orange	100 mg. *Light Yellow	150 mg. White

(*These medications have D&C Red No. 30, D&C Yellow No. 10, and/or FD&C Blue No. 1)

Indications and Usage

Norpramin was developed as an antidepressant primarily for the treatment of various depressive disorders, especially clinical or endogenous depression. Its use in ADHD, and especially ADD, has been determined through scientific investigation. It is considered a valuable second-line medication for ADD adolescents and adults who do not respond optimally to the psychostimulants (Biederman et al., 1989; Calis et al., 1990).

The tricyclics are often utilized along with the stimulant medications for those with anxiety and depression co-occurring with the ADD. Those with a primary diagnosis of anxiety or depression, however, are often misdiagnosed as undifferentiated ADD (McClellan et al., 1989). They obviously respond better to the antidepressants which target their primary diagnosis more specifically. Likewise, those diagnosed as depressed are often experiencing depression because of the failure and loss of esteem associated with ADD. Careful differential diagnosis is extremely important for appropriate treatment.

Specific Benefits

The benefits of desipramine are essentially the same as those for imipramine with fewer side effects.

Contraindications and Warnings

Contraindications for the use of desipramine are very similar to those of imipramine and include anyone with cardiovascular disease or a family history of cardiac difficulties; those with a history of urinary retention; patients with a history of glaucoma; patients with a history of thyroid disease or those taking thyroid medication; and those with a history of seizure disorders, among others. Desipramine should not be used within two weeks of MAO inhibitor drugs, in patients performing potentially hazardous tasks, and especially those with alcohol abuse potential. In desipramine usage, the benefit:risk ratio is weighted more heavily to the risk side. Thus a careful assessment of benefit with close monitoring of potential adverse reactions or side effects is essential. The following situations warrant special attention:

Children Under the Age of Twelve

Desipramine has not been approved for children under the age of twelve and is specifically cautioned against in the manufacturer's package inserts. On the other hand, skilled clinicians at NIMH (Calis et al., 1990) and Massachusetts General Hospital/Harvard Medical School (Biederman et al., 1989) have found it useful. As mentioned previously, cardiac toxicity in children under the age of twelve is a significant risk.

Since tricyclic medications are frequently prescribed in adolescents with attention deficit disorders, depression, and nocturnal enuresis, the deaths of three children taking Norpramin have raised serious concern among clinicians and researchers alike.

Dr. Riddle and his associates at Yale University School of Medicine reviewed the available data on the three children involved and made specific recommendations in the January, 1991 *Journal of the American Academy of Child and Adolescent Psychiatry.* The cases were as follows:

Case 1

a) March 1987: Eight-year-old boy collapsed at school.

b) 50 mg. Norpramin a day for approximately six months.

c) At age four he developed paroxysmal atrial tachycardia during a muscle biopsy procedure. There was also a family history of sudden cardiac death.

Case 2

a) October 1987: eight-year-old boy collapsed at home.

b) Treated for two years on Norpramin for hyperactive behavior disorder - dose unknown.

c) Cardiac and family history unavailable.

Case 3

a) (Based on newspaper accounts) Summer, 1988: nine-year-old boy collapsed at school after running laps.

b) Treated with Norpramin for one year for depression after an automobile accident in which he sustained a concussion and a broken leg.

c) Tests two months before death indicated no cardiac problems. Mother died of congestive heart failure three days after his birth.

Based on the information available, five hypotheses were proposed and the data to support each were reviewed as well as data on the cardiac effects of desipramine in children. They also reported on physiological changes which occurred in a child followed by them at the Yale Child Study Center where cardiac changes resulting from

Norpramin administration were carefully monitored and documented. Subsequently the following recommendations were made:

> Based on the authors' review of the three deaths and this recent clinical experience, increased caution is warranted in the use of desipramine and, perhaps, other tricyclic drugs in the treatment of prepubertal children. Although the limited information available does not provide an adequate basis for developing an informed recommendation, prudence suggests that an EKG with a rhythm strip obtained at baseline and during medication "loading" and steady state, with specific emphasis on measurement of the QT_c, may be helpful in identifying potentially vulnerable children. It may be contraindicated to administer tricyclic antidepressants to children who have prolonged QT_cs at baseline, and it may not be wise to continue the medication in any patient whose QT_c exceeds 0.425 to 0.450 seconds while on medication. If prolonged therapy is contemplated, a steady state drug plasma level would help assure that unusual pharmacokinetics are not present. A more comprehensive cardiac assessment may be indicated in children with a positive family history of cardiac conduction defects or sudden death. Clinicians should also be aware of the value of checking a patient's pulse during treatment with tricyclics. (Riddle et al., 1991, p. 106)

Riddle and his associates also recommended more research, stating that many fundamental questions remain regarding the use, in children, of tricyclics in general and desipramine in particular. For example, is the metabolite (desipramine) more toxic than the parent compound (imipramine), as the data suggest? They emphasized the broader issue in pediatric neuropsychopharmacology and drugs in general, that is, the need for the same rigorous, systematic investigation of the drugs utilized for children and adolescents that precedes their use in adults. Children are not physiologically, or in any other way, "little adults." Rather, they differ in significant ways in pharmacokinetics, developmental differences in a drug's impact of various bodily systems, efficacy and short- and long-term behavioral and biological side effects. This thoughtful article is recommended reading for all physicians and professionals who are daily juggling the demands of patient needs against the constraints of available treatments and our knowledge thereof.

Long-Term Effects

Little is known about the long-term effectiveness or side effects of desipramine.

Tics and Tourette Syndrome

Unlike the stimulants and imipramine, desipramine has not been found to precipitate or exacerbate tics or Tourette Syndrome. It has, in fact, been utilized with children with tic disorders to treat their ADHD and decrease the tics (Riddle et al., 1988).

Follow-Up

As emphasized repeatedly throughout this book, careful monitoring of clinical response, adverse reactions and side-effects is essential to the success of treatment. Such follow-up is crucial for this medication. The guidelines suggested on page 218 are recommended.

PROZAC
(Fluoxetine Hydrochloride)

Prozac, the nation's most prescribed antidepressant, was introduced in the United States in December, 1987. It immediately captured both the market and the public imagination. Easier to prescribe, with far fewer side effects, dramatically positive response and good press, it became an instant success. By 1990 an estimated 15 million Americans suffering from depression became hopeful as 650,000 Prozac prescriptions were written each month. More than four and a half million Americans had taken the drug by 1993 with the range of uses markedly versatile—from depression to obsessive compulsive disorders to social inhibition, among others.

Prozac is so widely used and so effective that some have raised the issue that the drug may be being utilized cosmetically rather than to treat serious medical conditions. The mnemonic of Peter Kramer, M.D., a psychiatrist, in *Listening to Prozac* (1993) is "cosmetic psychopharmacology." His book is a must for those interested in the medical/ethical/scientific dilemma of all who explore the implications of drugs that so effectively reshape temperament and behavior.

Prozac is currently being prescribed for some with attention deficit disorders. Its use in undifferentiated ADD has been described as quite effective, raising the question of accurate diagnosis of the ADD. At this time there is much clinical wisdom that suggests that this medication is very effective for the depression which often co-occurs with attention deficit disorders.

Description

Fluoxetine hydrochloride is a white crystalline solid manufactured at the present time only by Dista Products Company as *Prozac Pulvules*. Two sizes are available—a green and gray 10 mg. pulvule and a 20 mg. green and off-white pulvule. They contain FD&C Blue No. 1 with other inactive ingredients. A liquid oral solution is also available.

Classification

Prozac is not a strictly controlled medication. Long-term studies have not been undertaken to determine its potential for abuse, tolerance or physiologic dependency, although none has been reported at this time. It is a CNS-active drug and therefore has the potential, of course, to be abused by someone determined to do so. It does not appear to result in a withdrawal syndrome or any drug-seeking behavior which would promote addiction.

Clinical Pharmacology

In contrast with tricyclic antidepressants which increase the availability of norepinephrine, the antidepressant action of fluoxetine is linked to its inhibition of CNS neuronal uptake of serotonin. Serotonin has not been thought to be involved in the basic pathophysiology of ADHD because drugs that significantly influence serotonin metabolism have had only minimal effects on ADHD symptoms (Raskin et al., 1984; Zametkin et al., 1985). While this is true, our clinical experience, and that of others, has been that many depressed ADHD/ADD mothers of ADHD and ADD children have responded quite well to Prozac with improvement in their sense of well-being, their organization and their accomplishments. Fathers have, likewise, obtained benefit as have many other adults with whom we have worked. Optimum benefit necessitates treatment of the ADD as well.

Indications and Usage

Prozac was developed for the treatment of depression. Its efficacy was established in five- and six-week trials with depressed outpatients whose diagnoses most closely responded to the DSM-III category of Major

Depressive Disorder. It has also been utilized to treat anxiety, addictive disorders, bulimia, and obsessive-compulsive disorders. Research evidence, as well as clinical practice, suggests that it is effective in treating obsessive-compulsive disorders associated with Tourette Syndrome (Brunn, Cohen & Lechman, 1990).

Availability/Usage/Dosage/Administration

Prozac is available in both 10 mg. and 20 mg. Pulvules. Like other antidepressants, it requires plasma concentration for maximum effectiveness and is eliminated slowly from the body, with a half-life of two to three days. It is taken only once daily, aiding compliance. It typically takes three weeks to become effective. Blood monitoring is not required, and there is little risk of overdose. Prozac is expensive, costing twenty times as much as some generic antidepressants.

Contraindications and Warnings

MAOIs

Prozac should not be taken within two weeks of MAOIs. It is also contraindicated in those allergic to it.

Appetite and Weight

In clinical trials, approximately 9% of patients treated with Prozac experienced loss of appetite, and 13% experienced a significant weight loss, greater than 5% of their body weight. This anorectic effect is positive for some, while for others who are already underweight, this effect can be quite negative.

Seizures

Prozac has the same risk for the precipitation of seizures as other antidepressant medications—approximately 0.2%. It should be avoided or used with extreme caution in those with a history of seizure disorders.

Activation of Hypomania/Mania

During premarket testing, hypomania or mania occurred in approximately 1% of those treated. This effect has been observed in a small proportion of patients with Major Affective Disorder treated with other antidepressants as well.

While Prozac received glowing reports in 1988 through mid-1989 (Cowley et al., 1990), it became the focus of negative attention both in the media (*Newsweek*, April 1, 1991) and on talk shows in 1991. Some researchers and physicians questioned whether Prozac, unlike other antidepressants, could directly induce violent or suicidal thoughts in a person who did not have preexisting, underlying disturbance which merely surfaced as the person became less depressed. Several psychiatrists reported incidences of violent, suicidal or self-destructive thoughts or behavior after taking Prozac (Dr. Martin Teicher, Harvard Medical School; Drs. Robert King & Mark Riddle, Yale Medical School's Child Study Center). Drs. Riddle and King, who had researched ADHD extensively, suggested that by disrupting the availability of serotonin, Prozac might directly affect the brain's ability to regulate aggression.

At this time many of the issues raised by the Church of Scientology, as well as by clinicians and researchers, have been addressed. Prozac does not appear to increase violent or suicidal behavior. Given the millions who have received unprecedented reprieve from the disabling illness of depression, it is unlikely that its benefits will be discarded for the relatively few who may responded adversely. However, differential diagnosis becomes more critical and follow-up essential to assure that the benefits continue overwhelmingly to outweigh the risks. Depression can be so devastating to the millions of Americans afflicted that we must continue to search for solutions. Many of these depressed adults are those with residual ADHD or ADD, or those who have grown up with an attention disorder which has left them frustrated, unfulfilled, lacking in esteem, and eventually clinically depressed.

Drug Interactions

Prozac does interact negatively with a number of medications. Therefore, the prescribing physician should take a careful history of other medication usage and advise patients of those medicines which must be avoided while taking Prozac.

Adverse Reactions/Side Effects

The most common side effects of Prozac are headaches, nervousness, insomnia, weight loss, nausea, and diarrhea. Fifteen percent of the 4,000 patients in clinical trials discontinued the medication because of an adverse response. Nervousness, anxiety, and insomnia were the primary causes for discontinuation. These negative effects usually diminish with time.

Follow-up

Because Prozac is easy to administer, has few side effects, does not require blood tests and other laboratory tests before or during treatment, appears so safe, and the majority of prescriptions are written by physicians other than psychiatrists and neurologists, initial diagnosis and follow-up may be less than optimal. Patients should, however, be carefully diagnosed and then monitored initially as closely as one would monitor a patient on any other neuropsychiatric medication. Patients should also be advised to contact the prescribing physician if negative reactions occur, especially hypomania, suicidal impulses, or destructive thoughts or actions. While Prozac is not believed to cause these effects, the lifting of the depression may precipitate underlying tendencies toward them. Patients' families should also be advised since people tend to become unreasonable, uncooperative and unrealistic in hypomanic and manic episodes. They can also become overly sensitive and even paranoid, making effective intervention increasingly difficult.

While offering great promise, Prozac also appears to have risks. It must, therefore, be utilized both judiciously and conscientiously if its potentially negative effects do not render it so controversial that it will be removed from the market. Knowledgeable physicians and patients can have a major impact on utilizing it in the best possible manner with the least possible adverse effects.

MONOAMINE OXIDASE INHIBITORS
Nardil (Phenelzine Sulfate)
Parnate Tablets (Tranylcypromine Sulfate)

As our understanding of the distinctions in neuroanatomy and neurobiology associated with distinctive behavioral disorders, including ADHD, ADD, conduct disorder, depression and anxiety, among others improves, the investigation of medications other than the traditional stimulants continues unabated. At some point it is hoped that once a disorder has been very specifically and discretely diagnosed, an equally discrete and sensitive medication will be utilized to treat it (Zametkin, 1990). Our use of medications at this time might well be described as a "shot-gun" approach. What will become increasingly necessary is that we determine the "bullet" for each particular disorder. A similar phenomenon has already occurred for infectious diseases. Broad-spectrum antibiotics have been replaced by those targeted for a particular organism. The benefits, of course, increase with this approach while the side effects and adverse responses are reduced.

An interesting study by Dr. Bowden and his associates (1988) attempted to determine whether there were differences in platelet monoamine oxidase and dopamine beta-hydroxylase in boys with attention deficit disorder with unsocialized conduct disorder and those with ADHD without unsocialized conduct disorders. Differences in MAO were, in fact, found. Several other studies have found differences in platelet monamine oxidase in those with impulsivity, disruptive behavior, and undersocialized conduct disorder (Bowden et al., 1988; Stoff et al., 1989). Stoff and his associates found that a subgroup of boys with high MAO activity exhibited significantly more impulsivity than a subgroup of low MAO activity on laboratory tasks requiring response inhibition. Both Wender and his associates (1983) and Zametkin et al. (1985) showed significant improvement in ADHD boys when treated with MAO-A drugs which tend to inhibit noradrenaline (norepinephrine) and serotonin metabolism and MAO-B drugs which mainly inhibit dopamine. Since those with severe impulsivity and unsocialized conduct disorders are very resistant to both psychotherapy and many other medications, the potential benefit of the MAOIs for this group of behavior- disordered children and adolescents is promising and warrants continued investigation.

Monoamine oxidase inhibitors inhibit the enzymes termed *monoamine oxidases* which are important in the degradation of serotonin, dopamine and norepinephrine. Beneficial effects of the MAOIs appear related to mono-oxidase inhibition rather than to chronic changes in receptive function. In that sense they are like the stimulants whose clinical effect is related to their effects on central monoaminergic systems. Their mechanism of action on norepinephrine, for example, is illustrated on page 233.

MECHANISM OF ACTION:
MAOIs

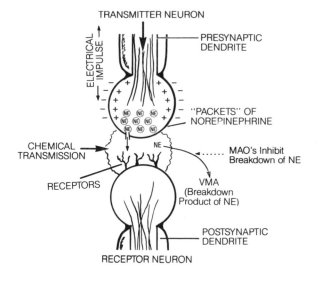

As mentioned previously, there are at least two types of monoamine oxidases in the blood. MAO-A acts primarily on serotonin and norepinephrine, and MAO-B acts primarily on phenylethylamine and dopamine. Current evidence suggests that clorgyline, an investigational MAOI specific for the MAO-A isoenzyme and tranylcypromine (Parnate), an inhibitor of both MAO-A and MAO-B, produce significant effects on sustained attention measured in the laboratory and on classroom behavior (Calis et al., 1990). The effects are comparable to those observed with amphetamine (Zametkin et al., 1985).

While MAOIs may have great potential benefit for some very impulsive ADHD children and adolescents, it is typically a medication of last resort. The primary reason for this is the acutely negative interaction with many other medications and with many foods. When an MAOI is taken in combination with foods and drugs containing tyramine or dopamine, a hypertensive crisis can occur and can be fatal. The foods to be avoided include pickled herring, liver, any kind of dried, pickled, fermented, aged, or smoked sausage or meat, or foods with any bacterial contamination. Patients must also avoid cheeses, beer, wine, yeast extract, and excessive amounts of caffeine and chocolate. Many medications, particularly those involving CNS depressant effects, must be avoided as well. This includes many over-the-counter medications as well as prescription drugs. Most medications and foods containing tyramine or dopamine must be avoided.

The MAOIs utilized the most frequently are Nardil (phenelzine sulfate) which is available in 15 mg. tablets from Parke-Davis, and Parnate tablets (tranylcypromine sulfate) available in 10 mg. tablets from Smith Kline Beecham. The initial starting dose of Nardil is one tablet three times a day. Dosage is typically increased to at least 60 mg/day at a fairly rapid pace consistent with patient tolerance and often to 90 mg/day to obtain sufficient MAO inhibition. It often takes four weeks to show clinical response. The usual effective dosage of Parnate is 30 mg/per day usually given in divided doses. The maximum is 60 mg/per day.

Nardil	Parnate Tablets
15 mg.	10 mg.
Orange	Melon
Phenelzine Sulfate	Tranylcypromine Sulfate

Side Effects

Side effects include headaches, pupillary dilation, weight loss and excessive sweating.

Follow-Up

Calis and his associates at NIMH recommend the following when prescribing an MAOI:

> Baseline monitoring should include an EEG, complete blood counts, LFTs, platelet counts, renal function tests and electrolyte measurements. Elevations in blood pressure and heart rate should be carefully checked as well. (Calis et al., 1990)

As can clearly be seen, the risks of the MAOIs outweigh their benefits except in very special situations when all other medications have been exhausted, or when one is treating a very responsible and disciplined patient. Anyone either prescribing or taking MAOIs should become thoroughly familiar with the package insert on the particular medication involved to avoid any possibility of precipitating a hypertensive or other medical crisis.

*If attention or activity were a steam engine, MPH
(Ritalin) increases the heat and applies the brakes;
clonidine turns down the heat.*

— Robert Hunt, M.D., 1988

10

Antihypertensives

Catapres

Clonidine, a medication that has been widely used as an antihypertensive agent in adults since the early 1970's and has been employed since 1980 to treat Tourette Syndrome, has been recently found to be very helpful in some children with attention disorders. Dr. Robert Hunt, formerly Director of Research and Training at Vanderbilt Child and Adolescent Psychiatric Hospital, was one of the pioneers in the treatment of ADHD/ADD with clonidine. He has successfully treated several hundred children with this medication and has authored many articles on its usefulness in child and adolescent psychiatry.

There are several subtypes of patients who appear to respond better to clonidine than to the stimulant medications:

1)   Highly aroused, overactive children who respond poorly to Ritalin or Dexedrine, or who have persistent side effects from the stimulants.

2)   Children who exhibit signs of conduct disorder, oppositional behavior, aggression and explosiveness.
3)   Poor responders to all other medications.
4)   Children who develop tics or Tourette Syndrome with the use of stimulant medications, whether over- or underactive.
5)   Overfocused children and adolescents.

OVERFOCUSED CHILDREN AND ADOLESCENTS

A problem that is often not addressed in the ADHD/ADD literature is that of the overfocused person. It is important to differentiate the overfocused child, adolescent or adult from the person with lethargic, slow-processing, underactive ADD. At the neurotransmitter level, very different processes are problematic and their treatments are quite different. Stimulants have an adverse effect on overfocused children, inhibiting an overinhibited system even more. Dr. Marcel Kinsbourne (1979) was the first to recognize overfocused children and addressed their dynamics in detail in *Children's Learning and Attention Problems*.

The overfocused child or adolescent, according to Kinsbourne, is at the extreme opposite end of the cognitive style continuum from the impulsive, hyperactive child. He is excessively deliberate, has difficulty changing activities, and can be quite compulsive and rigid as well.

Overfocused children prefer very traditional, highly structured situations where few decisions are required. Because they work so slowly and excessively check and recheck their work, they often have difficulty completing it on time. Overfocused children dislike distraction. They have great difficulty shifting to new activities even when it is something they prefer to what they are doing. They simply can't let go. They are very easy to discipline. In fact, they are too sensitive and responsive to limit-setting and become fearful and upset when faced with harshness or anger.

Overfocused children can be intense and shy; they often avoid others; and they become easily overwhelmed by cognitive or emotional stimulation. These children do best in bland, stable, non-demanding situations. Overfocused children are usually not recognized as having a problem because their careful, methodical, compliant style is very consistent with typical school expectations. Their biggest problem, both at home and at school, is their slowness in completing their work and other tasks.

The overfocused child's behavior is similar to that of normal children who are given stimulant medication or ADHD/ADD children are given too much medication. The excessive withdrawal and inhibition which can occur often frightens the parents of an ADHD/ADD child, and they may refuse to continue the medication, even when a lower dose would not produce these results and could be very effective.

Benefit has been achieved with overfocused children with behavior management strategies, education, and environmental manipulation. Clonidine has also been found useful. Stimulant medications, on the other hand, worsen their symptoms markedly. Although it is easy to overlook the overfocused child or adolescent because he is no trouble, it is important to recognize this individual as having a problem too . It is equally important to differentiate the overfocused child from the underactive, sluggish ADD child.

Like impulsive, overactive children, overfocused children suffer immensely. They both require and respond to therapeutic intervention greatly. Clonidine, as well as other medications for obsessive-compulsive disorder, can be quite useful.

Description of Clonidine

Clonidine is an antihypertensive agent which acts on the central nervous system. It is an odorless, bitter, white crystalline substance. It is available as *Catapres* for oral administration in three dosage strengths; 0.1 mg., 0.2 mg., and 0.3 mg., and it is manufactured by Boehringer Ingelheim

Pharmaceuticals, Inc. It is also available from several other manufacturers. Unique among medications for attention disorders, Catapres is also available in transdermal skin patches which are worn on the skin and release the medicine evenly all day. They are marketed as Catapres TTS 1, 2, or 3, and represent doses of 0.1, 0.2, and 0.3 mg/day, respectively. The patches can be cut to achieve intermediate dosages.

CATAPRES TABLETS

| 0.1 mg. | 0.2 mg. | 0.3 mg. |
| light grey | melon | Sand |

CATAPRES PATCHES
(Transdermal Therapeutic System)

TTS-1   TTS-2   TTS-3

Clinical Pharmacology/Mechanisms of Actions

In an article which offers a thorough review of clonidine as well as clinical guidelines, Dr. Hunt described its mechanism of action as follows:

In the central nervous system, clonidine treatment produces an immediate and persistent reduction in the firing of the locus coeruleus (LC). By reducing the release of norepinephrine, clonidine reduces the intensity of various behavioral expressions of excessive arousal, and may also provide an index of the role of noradrenergic locus coeruleus-based influences on certain behaviors. Norepinephrine appears to potentiate the response of certain receptors to their neurotransmitters. Central norepinephrine may affect the responsivity of various neurotransmitter systems and of many behavioral functions. Indirect effects may be seen in the serotonin and dopamine neurotransmitter systems (Antelman & Caggiula, 1977; Bunney & DeRiemer, 1982; Martin et al., 1984). Clonidine may exert widespread physiological effects on particular behaviors and responses by indirectly altering dopamine systems that may modulate attention in ADHD or control tic movements in Tourette's disorder, or by influencing serotonin systems that mediate the capacity to inhibit aggressive behaviors or thoughts. (Hunt et al., 1990)

Indications and Usage

Catapres was originally developed for the treatment of hypertension and continues to be widely prescribed as a hypertensive medication. In recent years it has also been found to be useful in several disorders that manifest symptoms of *high arousal.* These include manic episodes in adults with bipolar illness and aggressive outbursts in psychotic and agitated adults. Clonidine has also been utilized to alleviate anxiety, activity, hyperarousal associated with Post Traumatic Stress Disorder (PTSD), social phobia, and panic anxiety. Its effectiveness in Obsessive-Compulsive Disorder, particularly OCD associated with Tourette Syndrome, has been demonstrated. Clonidine is also very helpful for children with overfocused disorder. Hunt suggests that clonidine may be useful in ADHD, bipolar disorders in both children and adolescents, psychosis in adults, aggressiveness in agitated and psychotic adults and borderline personality disorder. Clonidine treats a number of disorders because of its presumed selective action on symptoms associated with hyperarousal.

Contraindications

Unlike most medications, and certainly those utilized for the treatment of attention disorders, Catapres has no known contraindications. It is not known to interact negatively with either foods or other drugs.

Dosage and Administration

Unlike the stimulants which act immediately and reach their therapeutic benefit in 30 minutes to one hour, the maximum benefit of clonidine may require one to two months of administration to be optimally effective. Clonidine is usually begun in very low doses. It is usually initiated at night in order to maximize its beneficial effect on sleep and to facilitate tolerance to the sedative effects. While Dr. Hunt recommends 0.05 mg., or 1/2 of a 0.1 mg. tablet once each day initially, we have found that many children can tolerate only 1/4 of a 0.1 mg. tablet at bedtime for three to four days, after which 1/4 of a 0.1 mg. tablet is added in the morning. This is especially true for allergic or sensitive children and adolescents. The medication is increased gradually to achieve its maximum therapeutic benefit. For children, the range is 0.15-0.3 mg/day, with a medium dose for an eight to twelve-year-old patient of 0.25-0.3 mg/day, and for adolescents, 0.3-0.4 mg/day. More than 0.5 mg/day is rarely necessary. While there is some build-up of plasma concentration of the medication when taken orally, resulting in greater constancy of benefit, the effects are still somewhat transient. Therefore, the tablet form of clonidine is most therapeutic if administered in divided doses three to four times daily.

Once the 0.1 mg. level is reached, the transdermal patch is available (Catapres-TTS 1, 2, or 3). Placed usually on the back, it is effective for five to seven days. This is an advantage for those situations where compliance is a problem.

Side Effects/Adverse Reactions

The most noticeable side effect of clonidine is drowsiness that occurs forty-five to ninety minutes after administration. Sleepiness and fatigue may last for several weeks and must be carefully assessed for their effect on school performance. When a child is unusually difficult to arouse in the morning, begins laying his head on his desk at school, or takes unaccustomed naps, one can be assured that the level of medication is too great and will need to be reduced temporarily, and increased more gradually. Getting through this period of sleepiness is often the most difficult aspect of clonidine treatment. In about 10% of children, this side effect results in discontinuation of the medication.

Hypotension and Cardiovascular Effects

Clonidine is an antihypertensive agent and usually produces hypotension. Since blood pressure is lowered, it must be carefully monitored, especially in children and adolescents. A 10% decrease in systolic pressure is often detected, but generally produces no significant symptoms or discomfort. In addition to its hypotensive effect, clonidine also diminishes cardiac output, lowers pulse and decreases peripheral vascular resistance, according to Dr. Hunt. No long-term negative effects are believed to occur. However, the medication will have to be discontinued in some patients because of low blood pressure.

Other Side Effects

Other transient side effects, including headaches, dizziness, stomach aches and nausea, may occur at the start of treatment. However, they are usually transient and subside if the medication is reduced but continued. Clonidine may also induce depression in children and adolescents who have a history of depressive symptoms or a family history of mood disorder. Clonidine has also been reported to produce orthostatic symptoms and cardiac dysrhythmia in adults. Given the concerns with desipramine and the awareness that the physiology of children is very different from that of adults, the use of clonidine in children and adolescents, when its effects on this age group have never been studied and approved, raises some concerns. It is an area which is worthy of investigation, particularly given the greatly increased use of clonidine as a treatment for attention deficit disorder. Much of the currently available knowledge has been obtained from information provided by independent researchers and by clinical experience shared by professionals.

Rebound Hypertension

Rebound hypertension has been noted after chronic treatment or sudden withdrawal of clonidine. It is a medication which should be withdrawn very gradually to avoid a potentially dangerous increase in blood pressure.

Specific Benefits

Clonidine appears to offer great benefit for a number of disorders involving hyperarousal. It has a major advantage in its stabilizing influence on the highly volatile arousal system of some ADHD/ADD children and adolescents as well as those with other disorders of hyperarousal. Clonidine appears also to have very beneficial effects on overfocused, obsessive-compulsive behaviors as well. Children taking clonidine are reported to be more cooperative and more emotionally stable. Parents, therefore, respond very favorably because Catapres, unlike Dexedrine and Ritalin, helps around the clock, alleviating much of the roller-coaster effect of the stimulants.

It has been noted that some children appear to have symptoms of the overfocused disorder and to be distractible and inattentive at the same time. While clonidine is effective in alleviating overfocused symptoms, as well as hyperarousal, it is not effective in alleviating symptoms of distractibility and inattentiveness. It may, therefore, be utilized in combination with stimulants with very positive results. Hunt's (1988) initial findings, as well as those of others, suggest that combined medications are safe when used conservatively and systematically.

Use in Tourette Syndrome

Clonidine has been used since 1979 in the treatment of Tourette Syndrome, although it is not considered as effective as either Haldol or Orap. It is generally better tolerated physically and thus more acceptable to patients because of its low incidence of side effects, especially tardive dyskinesia.

The benefit of clonidine for Tourette Syndrome is its reduction of simple motor and vocal symptoms with some improvement of attentional problems.

Dosage and administration of clonidine for TS is comparable to that for ADHD/ADD. It is initiated at low doses, usually 0.05 mg/day and slowly increased over several weeks to 0.15-0.30 mg/day. Some people do, however, receive benefit from very small doses. TS patients who are receiving benefit often experience a sense of anxiety, irritability or an increase in symptoms when the next dose is needed.

The benefit of clonidine is often gradual and goes through stages from a reduction in tension, then a decrease in motor tics and compulsions, followed by increased confidence, less irritability and fewer tics. The full benefit can take many months up to a year or more.

Follow-Up

As with all medications, close monitoring is essential. Since clonidine has been approved by the FDA only for use in hypertension, clinicians must be even more rigorous with follow-up if they choose to use it. Physicians can prescribe clonidine for other medical problems based on their own clinical judgement as long as they understand its use and fully inform the family of their rationale for using it.

With clonidine usage the essential ingredient for success is assessing the benefit while making certain that the patient's blood pressure does not drop precipitously. Titration of the medication also requires very close attention since the sedative effects, which may occur for several weeks, can be detrimental to the child's overall academic, social, and emotional adjustment. One very lethargic child with whom we worked, who developed tics on the stimulants, practically slept through the summer. However, once acclimated to the medication, he has responded extremely well to quite low doses. Given the degree of his academic difficulty and of the precipitation of tics by the stimulants, Catapres has truly been a life-saver for this child.

SUMMARY

Our current understanding of clonidine suggests that it holds significant promise in the treatment of a number of disorders including ADHD and ADD. Its relatively few side effects, its extremely low cost, its potential ease of administration, and its lack of abuse potential are major advantages for patients, physicians and the community alike. It is a medication worthy of intensive research investigation. Meanwhile, clinical use should continue in as scientific and thoughtful a manner as possible within the constraints of patient needs.

As with any therapy, there are risks. A carpenter whose only tool is a hammer is likely to perceive everything as a nail.

George Storm, M.D., 1983

11

Medications for Special Situations

Major Tranquilizers (Haldol, Thorazine, Mellaril) Tegretol, Lithium, Caffeine

MAJOR TRANQUILIZERS

The major medications used in the treatment of attention deficit disorders have been addressed at length, and the great majority of those with attention deficit disorders will have been found responsive to one of those medications or a combination of them. Nevertheless, there remain a few children, adolescents and adults who will experience serious difficulties for whom no treatment has yet been found effective. One group of medications occasionally used in the treatment of attention disorders is the class of medications known as the *major tranquilizers*. They are used primarily to control psychotic symptoms, and are rarely used as a primary treatment for attention disorders. Their major use in the field of attention disorders is in controlling hyperactivity undercontrolled by other medications, facilitating sleep, helping to manage aggressive ADHD children, or medicating ADHD/ADD children who also have other serious psychiatric problems. This group of *medications*, also called *psychotropic* medications, or *neuroleptics,* was first discovered to be beneficial for psychiatric problems about thirty years ago. Since that time they have been utilized in the treatment of serious psychiatric disturbance in adults and, to some extent, in children. When all other medications have been exhausted, these can sometimes be quite effective. There are many medications in this class and most are very similar chemically. Those most generally employed are Mellaril (thioridazine), Thorazine (chlorpromazine), Haldol (haloperidol), and Stellazine (trifluoperazine). These neuroleptic drugs have been used, with limited success, in the management of some with ADHD and ADD (Ross & Ross, 1982; Werry et al., 1975). Before the advent of stimulants and our understanding of ADHD/ADD, they were utilized far more often.

When considered appropriate by the prescribing physician, these drugs are effective in reducing excitement, hypermotility, abnormal initiative, affective tension and agitation through their inhibitory effect on psychomotor functions. It is often necessary to overcome these symptoms at the beginning phase of recovery in patients with severe psychiatric problems, especially those with major thought, mood or motor disturbance.

These drugs have also been utilized for the treatment of severe behavioral problems in children, especially those marked by combativeness or explosive, hyperexcitable behavior, and in the short-term treatment of hyperactive children who show excessive motor activity with accompanying conduct disorders. These medications are effective in decreasing impulsivity, aggressivity, mood lability, and poor frustration tolerance.

Contraindications and Warnings

The phenothiazines, the class to which all of these medications belong, are contraindicated in severe endogenous depression. Both hypertensive and hypotensive heart disease are also contraindications for usage.

Adverse Reactions

Involuntary Motor Movements (Tardive Dyskinesia)

Perhaps the worst potential side effect of the major tranquilizers is the ability of these medications to produce tardive dyskinesia, a movement disorder which often occurs with long-term use. These potentially irreversible, involuntary, uncoordinated movements may develop in any patient treated with neuroleptic drugs. The risk is believed to increase as the duration of treatment and the total cumulative dose of drug increases. However, it can develop after relatively brief periods of treatment and with low doses.

Other Side Effects

Other side effects with the major tranquilizers include stiffness, sedation, and possibly slower cognitive processing (Ross & Ross, 1982). Despite these very troublesome possibilities, the overall effects of these medications, especially their 24-hour benefit, have been viewed positively by the parents of ADHD children in some studies (Werry et al., 1975). In the past, they were utilized fairly often in the treatment of hyperactive children for the hyperaroused symptoms of the disorder. With our current state of knowledge, one would probably choose the stimulants or clonidine over the neuroleptics for hyperarousal since they have fewer side effects. On the other hand, their benefit for the short-term treatment of acute anxiety and acute mania or hyperactivity make them indispensable as medicinal options.

Haldol For Tourette Syndrome

An exception to the very conservative use of major tranquilizers is the use of haloperidol (Haldol) in Tourette Syndrome. Since the 1960's Haldol has been the primary treatment for TS. While the dosage was given at high levels initially, it is now generally accepted that Haldol is most effective at very low doses. Patients are generally started at 0.25-0.5 mg/day, and it is slowly increased every four to five days up to an average of 3-4 mg/day. Very impressive benefits have been obtained at very low doses and patients may have almost complete remission of the TS with few side effects. Some people benefit from as little as 1 mg/day or less.

Even though Haldol is often dramatically helpful, it is often not continued for an extended period of time because of its troublesome side effects. These include tardive dyskinesia, intellectual dulling, memory problems, personality changes, fatigue, weight gain, depression, loss of libido, and school or social phobias. To avoid the tardive dyskinesia, some patients are treated with anti-Parkinsonian agents, particularly benztropine. A very disabling side effect of Haldol in the treatment of TS is the development of school or social phobias. These may become so intense that they are totally disabling. When not recognized as side effects of the Haldol, they can continue for months. The intellectual dulling associated with all psychotropics leads to a marked decrease in cognitive and academic performance in school. The benefits of the medication are again often not worth the very negative side effects of dysphoria, poor grades, and social isolation.

Orap

Pemacide, or *Orap*, is chemically distinct from haloperidol and the other phenothiazines but has potent dopamine-blocking properties. It was approved for the treatment of TS in the United States in 1984 and is fairly commonly used. Its side effects are similar to those of haloperidol but may be less severe and impair fewer patients. In general it is better tolerated than haloperidol and is equally effective. While Orap is used for TS, it is not utilized in the treatment of attention disorders.

Dosage and Administration

The effective dosage level of major tranquilizers can vary considerably. For example, Mellaril is usually given in amounts ranging from 30-600 mg/day. Haldol, which is more potent, is usually given in ranges from .5-10 mg/day. As with the stimulant medications, it is difficult to predict how much medication a given child, adolescent or adult will require. Sometimes very active, larger people respond to comparatively small doses, while a smaller, quieter person may require much more. A person's general sensitivity and metabolism are far more important indicators of dose requirements than is size.

Major tranquilizers are build-up medications which require several weeks of administration for maximum effectiveness. They are most effective if given in divided doses, with more at bedtime to aid sleep. They must be discontinued gradually to avoid serious rebound effects.

Follow-Up

Close monitoring of major tranquilizers is obviously quite necessary. These medications can produce the most severe and most permanent side effects of any medications used for attention disorders. Tardive dyskinesia is not a disorder which can be viewed lightly. Neuroleptics are prescribed primarily by psychiatrists as part of an intensive treatment program which includes other therapies as well.

Summary

While major tranquilizers are usually medications of last resort, they can be very helpful, if closely monitored, for those who do, in fact, truly need them. While few with ADHD or ADD as a primary diagnosis will need major tranquilizers, they can be of benefit to a few at critical stress points in their lives. We must, therefore, continue to investigate their effects so as to optimize their benefits while reducing their risks.

TEGRETOL
(Carbamazepine)

Carbamazepine, an anticonvulsant, has been utilized successfully for many years in patients who presented with "psychiatric" symptoms of angry outbursts, hyperactivity, mania, irritability and impulsivity, who were subsequently found to have EEG irregularities associated with complex partial seizures. Tegretol is also utilized in combination with lithium in the treatment of bipolar disorders.

Tegretol has been suggested for the treatment of attention deficit disorders. Results have been mixed. Pleak et al. (1988) reported negative effects of Tegretol on the behavioral and neurological reactions of six boys treated with carbamazepine. In addition to other problems, they had a recurrence of absence seizures. Absence seizures, however, tend to be worsened by Tegretol, a factor which may have confounded the results. Others, probably those with undiagnosed complex partial seizures, responded well.

Careful differential diagnosis is of major importance in the use of Tegretol. This medication appears far superior to stimulants for ADHD-like symptoms which are the result of complex partial seizures and are *not* ADHD or ADD. Seizure disorders can easily be mistaken for ADHD and Tourette Syndrome, especially in adolescents. Complex partial seizures are addressed in more detail in Chapter 12.

LITHIUM

Attention deficit disorder, especially ADHD, versus *bipolar affective disorder*, or *mood disorder*, represents one of the most difficult diagnostic issues in child and adolescent psychiatry. Each disorder may occur independently or they may co-occur. For those unfamiliar with bipolar disorders, especially nonpsychiatrists, distinguishing between them may be especially difficult. All who work with attention disorders are encouraged to acquaint themselves with the symptoms of bipolar disorders and in the differential diagnosis of them.

According to Dr. Charles Popper of Harvard Medical School, ADHD and mood disorders share many characteristics (Popper, 1989).

- Both are characterized by inattention, impulsivity, excessive tension, high energy level, behavioral unpredictability, and emotional lability.
- Both may have co-occurring conduct disorders and oppositional defiant disorders.
- Both frequently have co-existing learning disorders.
- Both are characterized by a kind of *cognitive looseness* in which thought processes, both verbally and in written language, tend to be disorganized, tangential, and difficult to follow logically.
- Motor restlessness is seen in both disorders.
- Family psychiatric histories in both ADHD and bipolar illness frequently include mood disorders.
- Psychostimulants and antidepressants can be helpful in both disorders depending upon the particular phase of the bipolar disorder.

While the two disorders have many similarities, they also have distinct differences.   It is the differences which enable a correct diagnosis. These differences include:

- Psychotic symptoms occur in mood disorders, but rarely in ADHD unless the ADHD child is also psychotic.

- Poor reality testing is not typical of ADD children and adolescents, although they use a great deal of denial.

- ADHD children and adolescents, unlike those with bipolar disorders, do not typically have paranoid thinking or sadistic impulses.

- While children and adolescents with both disorders may be destructive, the destructiveness of ADHD children is more often a result of their poor impulse control and need to touch and handle things. ADHD children can become extremely angry and aggressive, but they do not tend to exhibit the raw and often somewhat violent aggression or rage the child or adolescent with a mood disorder, particularly in the manic phase, may exhibit.

- The length of time of the angry outburst also is different. ADHD children and adolescents typically calm down within 20-30 minutes. Those with bipolar disorder, by contrast, may continue to feel and act angry for several hours, and sometimes several days.

- The physical energy of the child, adolescent or adult with a mood disorder is extremely intense and would be exhausting to the average person, including the average ADHD child.

- During angry outbursts, bipolar children can become very disorganized in their thought processes, whereas such disorganization is rare in ADHD children.

- Sensory and emotional overstimulation are often the precipitating stresses for temper tantrums in ADHD children and adolescents. Bipolar children, by contrast, typically react negatively in response to limit-setting. They can become quite violent when their demands are not met.

- According to Popper, children and adolescents with both ADHD and mood disorders may experience quick mood changes. However, ADHD children are not as dissatisfied overall, nor as irritable as bipolar children and adolescents. Such irritability and discontent are especially notable in the morning when they are awakened. Those with mood disorders also seem to require several hours to overcome their irritability, general unhappiness and sluggish cognitive processing, while ADHD children awaken typically quite alert and ready to "take on the day." Those with mood disorders often experience headaches and stomachaches in the morning as well.

- Sleep patterns are also different. Both may have difficulty with sleep patterns during infancy. However, ADHD children typically have trouble settling into sleep, whereas those with mood disorders will experience nightmares, longer sleep latency, and have great difficulty establishing an overnight sleep pattern.

- Appetite and weight gain typically fluctuate a great deal in bipolar children and adolescents, whereas they remain fairly constant in ADHD children and adolescents.

- The cognitive abilities of these two groups also differ. ADHD children and adolescents tend to have more co-occurring specific learning disabilities, language disorders, and cortical function deficits. By contrast, learning in bipolar children and adolescents is often negatively affected by their dysphoria, lack of interest and seeming lack of motivation.

- In social settings, bipolar children tend to respond negatively and with rejection and hostility often from the first few moments of interaction. While ADHD children will be impulsive and overactive, they are typically more pleasant. Bipolar children are often very difficult to interact with, and can continue to be quite negative, whereas ADHD children respond with impulsivity, frustration and boredom, but are not overtly negative toward, or insulting of, another person.

- Bipolar children are much more intentionally aggressive and destructive. They will often look for fights and relish the power struggle. ADD children, on the other hand, often create problems and may frustrate authority, but they do not have the intense need to engage in power struggles.
- Bipolar children appear to enjoy danger and seek it out. Their high-risk behavior, sexual hyperawareness and daredevil behavior is often observed beginning in preschool and continues into adulthood.
- Needle phobia is often prevalent in bipolar disorders, but not typically in those with ADHD, although ADHD children and adolescents may not particularly enjoy injections either.

According to Dr. Popper, ADHD is "chronic and unremittingly continuous, but tends toward improvement." By contrast, children and adolescents with bipolar disorders tend to have increasingly more severe and problematic behaviors. As they get older, their difficult behavior becomes extremely hard to manage.

Lithium treatment typically is helpful for children, adolescents and adults with bipolar disorders. However, most researchers agree that lithium carbonate alone is not effective for the treatment of ADHD. It can be helpful when used with a psychostimulant in patients with co-existing bipolar disorders. They also suggest that it may be useful with patients with ADHD who have severe problems with temper, stress intolerance, impulsivity, and emotional lability (Carroll et al., 1987; Licamele & Goldberg, 1989).

A combination of stimulants plus lithium can be very helpful in treating co-occurring ADHD and bipolar disorder. There is some evidence that ADHD may be a precursor to the later development of a mood disorder

Dr. Popper suggests that in treating a child, adolescent, or adult with a co-existing mood and attention disorder, the mood disorder should be stabilized with lithium before the introduction of a stimulant, since stimulants can destabilize a bipolar patient and create the risk of a psychotic or manic episode. In treating those whose bipolar disorder mimics ADHD, lithium may in fact reduce the attention deficit symptoms. Those symptoms which persist after the use of lithium can be assisted with a lithium-plus-stimulant treatment regimen.

Since mood disorders and attention disorders are so difficult to differentiate, those working with attention disorders are encouraged to learn as much as possible about bipolar disorders so that they may clearly distinguish them from those with attention deficit disorders. For the most part, bipolar disorders are treated by child and adolescent psychiatrists, whereas attention disorders are managed by pediatricians, neurologists, family physicians, and general practitioners as well.

CAFFEINE

Caffeine, either in the form of coffee or caffeinated colas, has been reported by some parents to have a calming effect on their child. An equal number of parents report that it increases activity and the symptoms of ADHD/ADD. These contradictory findings occur in the research literature as well. Whether methylxanine caffeine should be considered an effective treatment for ADHD/ADD remains controversial. Early studies (Schnackenberg, 1973; Reichard & Elder, 1977) suggested that caffeine is effective. Later studies found no significant difference with caffeine intake. Conners (1979) and Garfinkel et al. (1987) found that low doses of caffeine were as effective as Ritalin in some children. By contrast, Schecter and Timmons (1985) utilized high doses of caffeine,

600 mg./day, and found them as effective as Dexedrine on continuous performance tasks and rating scales.

Caffeine may well be a substance to which people respond based on sensitivity. For a few it may be helpful. However, it appears unlikely to emerge as a treatment of clinical significance.

OTHER MEDICATIONS

Wellbutrin

Wellbutrin (bupropion hydrochloride) is a relatively new antidepressant which has been added to the medical options available to treat ADHD and ADD. Investigated by Casat and his associates (1987), they found thirty children diagnosed as ADHD in their study were clinically judged as improved and their activity scores significantly diminished on the Conner's Rating Scale after treatment with bupropion. Others have utilized Wellbutrin with mixed results.

Wellbutrin is available in 75 mg. and 100 mg. tablets from Burroughs Wellcome Company. While not approved by the FDA for the treatment of attention disorders, bupropion has been approved to treat depression. Its clinical use in the treatment of ADHD/ADD continues as research efforts are being undertaken to establish its efficacy.

Bupropion hydrochloride is chemically unrelated to the tricyclic, tetracyclic, or other known antidepressants. The neurochemical mechanism is not precisely known. However, it does not inhibit monoamine oxidase. It is a weak blocker of neuronal uptake of serotonin and norepinephrine, especially compared to the classic tricyclics. It also inhibits the neuronal reuptake of dopamine (PDR, 1994). Its effects are similar to a combination of an antidepressant and a longer-acting, less potent stimulant (Horachek, 1991).

Wellbutrin carries similar warnings and precautions as other antidepressants with one notable exception. Its potential for precipitating seizures is as much as four times that of other antidepressants when used in doses up to 450 mg/day. The estimate of potential seizures is up to ten times more between doses of 450 and 600 mg/day (PDR, 1994). It is contraindicated in patients with a prior or current diagnosis of bulimia or eating disorders because of its anorectic effect and its increased potential for seizures in these disorders.

Wellbutrin offers some benefits that other antidepressants do not. However, it should be utilized with caution with full awareness of its adverse effects and contraindications.

SUMMARY OF MEDICATIONS

This section of the book has attempted to acquaint the reader, in some detail, with the majority of the medications utilized for attention deficit disorders. Only when one has a full understanding of the neurophysiology of ADHD/ADD, the role of medications in normalizing neurotransmitter functioning, the potential benefits of medications, and the possible risks associated with them is it possible to arrive at thoughtful decisions with which one can be reasonably content. Knowledge of the practical issues of clinical pharmacology, classification, availability, duration of effect, contraindications, warnings, dosages, administration, rebound, adverse reactions and side effects should assist all who administer or take these medications to do so consistent with the latest available information and in the most helpful manner possible. These issues, however, are not addressed in the depth one needs in order to prescribe. Thus, readers must associate themselves with physicians who can prescribe and monitor within accepted practice guidelines and who follow the field closely to keep abreast of current changes. The study and treatment of both ADHD and ADD are so intensive and widespread that constant update is required of those who treat these disorders daily in their practices.

The benefits of medication for Adam, our gifted second-grade patient we have discussed throughout the book, enabled him to become an exemplary student. Once an angry, frustrated *tornado* of a child, he is now a happy, competent, delightful individual. Adam's parents too have blossomed as their faith and confidence, diminished but not daunted when they first arrived in our office, have been restored. Adam's mom shared with us his prize, shown on page 264, received after a successful multimodal treatment intervention program. He had been chosen for the *Principal's Award*, the highest recognition bestowed by his school and given to only two students each year.

ADAM'S AWARD

Principal's Award

To _____
Adam

For _____
being an "Outstanding Citizen"

Because of you our school is a better place to learn. You have proven to me by your actions that one person can make a difference. I applaud you for what you have accomplished and look forward to hearing even more great things about you in the future.

Given This ___28th___ day of ___January___ 19 _91_

CONGRATULATIONS AND BEST WISHES

Mrs. Dellinger
Principal

jostens
NATIONAL SCHOOL
STUDIOS INC.

Needless to say, Adam was extremely pleased and his parents were quite proud.   In fact, all of us who had had the opportunity to participate in this family's lives and their success were thrilled. Adam is on his way to becoming a productive, contributing and fulfilled citizen.

Adam's success is repeated daily as attention disorders are identified and treated.   We owe it to our children and to our nation to continue our efforts on behalf of those with attention deficit disorders as assertively and tirelessly as possible.

Other medical disorders frequently associated with ADHD/ADD are addressed in Section IV, followed by the School's Critical Role in Section V.

PART IV

Associated Neurological and Sleep Disorders

Do what you can, with what you have,
where you are.

—Theodore Roosevelt

12

Neurological
Disorders

Tourette Syndrome
Seizure Disorders

SIMPLE MOTOR TICS

A motor *tic* is an involuntary movement such as eye blinking or tossing one's head back as though to get one's hair out of one's eyes. Tics are, for the most part, unconscious movements. Bringing them to a person's attention often makes him uncomfortable and self-conscious. Because motor tics sometimes occur with the administration of stimulant medications, it is important to put them in proper perspective.

Childhood tics are common. About one-fourth of all children have them at one time or another, especially boys. They usually do not persist, however, and can be expected to disappear spontaneously within a year. Tourette Syndrome often begins with a simple motor tic. It then progresses to more extensive motor and vocal involvement. It is the potential for precipitating this disorder, though relatively rare, which creates so much anxiety among those involved with ADHD and ADD, whether parents, professionals or teachers. It is a possible negative effect of both the stimulant medications and Tofranil of which all should be aware. A tic should be identified as soon as it occurs and the child or adolescent's physician notified. If there is a family history of tics or Tourette Syndrome, stimulants may not be recommended. However, some physicians take issue with this approach, stating that one must treat the symptoms causing the most problems (Zametkin, 1990; Copps, 1992). If tics develop after the initiation of stimulant medication, the medicine may be reduced or discontinued, at which time most tics subside. On the other hand, stimulant medications are often used in combination with medications for Tourette Syndrome.

TOURETTE SYNDROME

Eye-blinking, head jerking, throat clearing, sniffing, touching things, an occasional outburst of an unacceptable word-these things occur in most children, adolescents and adults some of the time, so much so that they go unnoticed most of the time. When pronounced, however, they cannot be ignored. They are symptoms of Gilles de la Tourette Syndrome, usually shortened to Tourette Syndrome or TS, a neurologic disorder which involves dysfunction of cognitive, perceptual and motor skills. Its most obvious feature is abnormal movements and/or multiple habit spasms, or tics. When TS occurs, there are frequently coexisting attention disorders, learning disabilities and/or hyperactivity.

TS is frequently missed by those unfamiliar with this disorder. Instead, the symptoms are mistaken for attention disorders, behavior disorders, emotional problems or psychiatric illness. At times those with tics have been diagnosed as epileptic. At one time in history they were even considered possessed by devils and were treated with exorcism. Those with TS have suffered needless torment by those who do not understand.

Betsy was such a child. She was an extremely overactive child whose life had been frenetic since the day she was born—and long before. Even in the womb she kept a hectic pace. Betsy's parents had been concerned since infancy and had her evaluated before the first grade. *Attention-deficit hyperactivity disorder* was the not-so-surprising diagnosis.

Betsy was treated with both Ritalin and Dexedrine, neither of which was totally successful. She managed best on Dexedrine Spansule, however, to which Tofranil was later added in the evening to control bedwetting and to decrease her mood swings. Betsy's activity and academic work improved some but her constant sniffing and clearing her throat proved annoying to everyone. Increased levels of medication improved her behavior, but intensified the sniffing. Soon Betsy was not only sniffing her nose and clearing her throat, but was blinking her eyes and clicking her tongue. Betsy had Tourette Syndrome.

Betsy's medication was changed to Clonidine. While helpful with the tics, her hyperactivity and inattention were unmanageable, both at home and at school. Lower doses of Dexedrine were added in the medication regimen. Behavioral and educational accommodations were also introduced. While Betsy still occasionally sniffs when stressed, and clear her throat more than most, the tics are relatively well controlled. Her activity level and concentration are reasonably manageable as well. While there is not a perfect solution for all of Betsy's symptoms, she continues to make progress steadily, as all working with her understand her disorders and adjust their expectations accordingly. Betsy is really quite a happy fifth grader now.

Tourette Syndrome usually begins in early childhood, between the ages of two and fifteen, with the majority of cases occurring around age seven. It appears to be on a continuum from mild motor tics to complex motor and vocal tics, involving barking and cursing at the opposite extreme. The National Tourette Syndrome Association classifies two categories of tics with some common examples of each (Bronheim, 1990):

<u>Simple</u>

Motor: Eye blinking, head jerking, shoulder shrugging, and facial grimacing.

Vocal: Throat clearing, barking noises, sniffing, and tongue clicking.

<u>Complex</u>:

Motor: Jumping, touching other people or things, smelling, twirling about, and self-injurious actions including hitting or biting oneself.

Vocal: Uttering ordinary words or phrases, coprolalia (vocalizing socially unacceptable words), and echolalia (repeating a sound, word, or phrase just heard).

Tourette Syndrome occurs throughout the world. Accurate prevalence figures are not available, however, because it is often not diagnosed correctly. Some experts estimate that TS occurs in one in 2,000 persons with males outnumbering females three to one. Approximately 100,000 people in the U.S. are thought by a few to have the disorder (Zamula, 1988), while still other estimates are as high as 330,000 (Bower, 1990). Dr. David Comings, a geneticist who has studied Tourette Syndrome extensively and who has written an outstanding textbook on TS, found in a study of 3,304 elementary school students in southern California that one in 100 boys had some form of TS. This incidence is much greater than anyone has ever suspected. Girls, by contrast, were affected much less frequently—only one in 759 (Comings, 1990).

Tourette Syndrome, like other complex neurologic disorders, is believed to be the result of neurotransmitter abnormalities. These are thought to occur in the basal ganglia, a part of the brain which consists of four pairs of nerve cell clusters which help to coordinate physical movement by relaying information from the cerebral cortex to the brain stem and cerebellum. Early research in 1988 suggested that TS resulted from an excess of dopamine. More recent data suggest that a genetically caused scarcity of serotonin may be the culprit (Comings, 1990). This deficiency, it is postulated, interferes with communication between the limbic system, which controls behavior and initiates behavioral responses, and the frontal lobes, which integrate sensory data, organize them and are responsible for judgment, planning and foresight.

TS can be mild and interfere only minimally with a person's life, or it can be devastating. This is especially true for those with obsessive-compulsive behaviors or severe attention, learning and behavior disorders coexisting with the TS.

Children with this disorder frequently have severe problems in school because other children make fun of them or may even be afraid of them. They often use every ounce of their energy while in school controlling the TS symptoms, leaving little for academic tasks. Teachers may become impatient with their perseveration, or they may misinterpret their tics as misbehavior or attention-getting devices.

Parents, too, frequently do not realize that the behaviors they find so annoying are beyond the child's control. They may try all forms of both bribes and punishments to end the child's tic. They are frustrated by their lack of success and the child is devastated by his inability to control behaviors everyone says he should. Ass stress intensifies, so do the symptoms.

It is critical that those working with children and adolescents with attention disorders be cognizant of Tourette Syndrome and associated disorders. The TS Association describes the coexisting problems which may be present:

Obsessive-Compulsive Traits in which the person feels that something must be done over and over. Examples include touching an object with one hand after touching it with the other hand to *even things up* and repeatedly checking to see that the flame on the stove is turned off. Children sometimes beg their parents to repeat a sentence many times until it *sounds right.*

Hyperactivity and/or Attention Deficit Disorder (ADD) which occur in many people with TS. Often children will show signs of hyperactivity before TS symptoms appear. Indications of hyperactivity and ADD may include: difficulty in concentrating; failing to finish what is started; not seeming to listen; being easily distracted; often acting before thinking; shifting constantly from one activity to another; needing a great deal of supervision; and general fidgeting. Adults may have residual signs of ADD, such as overly impulsive behavior and concentration difficulties.

Learning disabilities such as dyslexia, arithmetic disorders, and perceptual difficulties.

Behavioral problems, which may result from obsessive-compulsive traits, attention problems, poor self-esteem due to TS symptoms, and poor school performance. There also appears to be a greater incidence of sexual acting out (such as exhibitionism) in TS.

Sleep disorders, which are fairly common among people with TS. These include walking or talking in one's sleep and frequent awakenings.

The concurrence of TS and ADHD/ADD has serious implications for those working with attention disorders. It has been shown fairly conclusively in studies reviewed by Dr. Gerald Golden in *Pediatric Annals* (1988) that all of the stimulant medications commonly used to treat ADHD and ADD can precipitate a tic response or exacerbate an already existing one. These medications are not thought to cause TS, however, and usually the tics subside with decrease or discontinuation of the stimulant. Similar findings of an increase in tics have been reported for Tofranil (Price et al., 1986), but not for Norpramin, which generally has fewer side effects than Tofranil (Hoge & Boedeman, 1986).

The learning disabilities which coexist in children and adolescents with Tourette Syndrome can be significant. The most striking disability is impairment of their visual-motor and grapho-motor skills. Writing and copying assignments can be a nightmare, as are those requiring organization and breaking large tasks into smaller units. The rote learning and written aspects of arithmetic can also be problematic, while reading and speaking abilities are much less affected.

Treatments for Tourette Syndrome include behavior management strategies, assistance with organization and structure, cognitive therapy, psychological counseling and modifications in educational requirements. Those with severe tics may require drug intervention. The drug most widely used historically has been Haldol (haloperidol). Clonidine (Catapres) is now being used successfully with some children with TS, especially if they have behavioral or attentional problems as well (Hunt, 1990). Two antidepressants that increase serotonin availability in the brain, Fluoxetine and Clomipramine, also show promise as TS treatments. Clomipramine has already proven effective in many cases of obsessive-compulsive disorder.

The Tourette Syndrome Association is a very active support network which provides an extensive list of publications, films and videotapes. In addition to support, it offers patient advocacy, discounts on medications for TS, and the latest information on research and treatment. While treatment of TS can be long and arduous, it is believed that, like ADHD/ADD, it can become a manageable problem in living when it is recognized early, accurately diagnosed and appropriately treated. A list of publications on TS and the address of the TS Association are in Appendix 7.

SEIZURE DISORDERS

One might wonder why seizure disorders are addressed in a book on attention deficit disorders. They are because children with subtle seizure disorders can easily be mistaken for those with attentional problems. This is especially true of absence seizures and complex partial seizures. *Strange* spells, especially in teens, or a child's continually seeming lost or confused, should alert one to these possibilities. Other seizure disorders present more compelling clinical features that are easily recognized as the neurologic problems they are.

Absence Seizures

Absence seizures, previously called *petit mal epilepsy*, are characterized by brief periods when the child "blanks out" or stares into space. These periods usually last less than 20 seconds. They are usually not associated with any type of precipitating stress, nor is there a noticeable post-seizure change in the child or adolescent. A child may have one or two seizures daily or, more characteristically, he may experience them continually. The adverse effect these seizures can have on academic performance, classroom alertness, understanding of expectations, and interactions with others can be profound. They can easily, however, be overlooked or misperceived as personality, behavioral or learning characteristics of the child.

Absence seizures require evaluation with an electroencephalogram (EEG) generally performed by a pediatric or general neurologist. They are associated with bilateral 2 to 4 Hz spike-and-slow-wave (spike-and-dome) complexes on the EEG.

An absence seizure disorder has its usual onset between the ages of four and twelve years. It is thought to be more common in girls and is typically an inherited condition. Absence seizures usually become less frequent in adolescence, although some may develop into grand mal seizures at that time. Approximately three-quarters of the patients who typically have onset between ages nine and ten will have a remission early in adulthood.

Typical absence seizures begin with an abrupt interruption of ongoing activity accompanied by staring or rhythmical eye blinking. Attentiveness, learning, perception and voluntary motor functions are all impaired, although their cessation is so brief that they may not be noticed. This is particularly true in the classroom where the child or adolescent's momentary loss of awareness, activity or motor control may become more of a frustration to those observing it than a diagnostic indicator. "Spacey" children may have underaroused ADD, narcolepsy, sleep apnea, or absence seizures. Lest we become too hasty with a diagnosis of *Attention Deficit Disorder*, it is important to be aware of the other very real possibilities.

The absence seizure usually ends as abruptly as it started: if the child is eating, she resumes; if he is listening to the teacher's lecture, he becomes more attentive; if he is reading, he continues. However, the seizure does interfere with the flow of activity and can create major learning problems. This is especially true for the child or adolescent who has multiple seizures per hour.

Seizure disorders are usually treated with anticonvulsant drugs. Stimulant medications are obviously inappropriate to treat absence seizures and may, in fact, lower the seizure threshold. On the other hand, those with both seizure disorders and attention deficit disorders may be treated with a combination of seizure and ADD medications. The treatment of children with multiple medical disorders requires a physician knowledgeable in all areas involved. Developmental pediatricians and neurologists typically manage these children and adolescents, often in consultation with the child's pediatrician or psychiatrist.

Complex Partial Seizures

Complex partial seizures, previously called *psychomotor* or *temporal lobe epilepsy*, usually last more than 30 seconds and are associated with a variety of *automatisms*. Automatisms are automatic motor movements not under the conscious control of the child or adolescent. They may include, but are not limited to, lip-smacking, hand-wringing, clicking sounds with the tongue, or repetitive hand movements. Strange or atypical behaviors preceding the episode are especially diagnostic.

Complex partial seizures are especially likely to occur during adolescence. They are often difficult to diagnose because the changes are typically viewed as behavioral and emotional symptoms. They include confusion, disturbances of mood or affect, ideational or unusual thought patterns, and behavior automatisms. Understandably, these symptoms are frequently diagnosed as psychiatric disorders. While school and clinical psychologists, counselors and therapists are often not familiar with this disorder, most psychiatrists are. Both neurologists and psychiatrists treat complex partial seizures.

Typical of most seizure disorders, these, too, are treated with anticonvulsant drug therapy. Carbamazepine (Tegretol) is typically the drug of choice because it is relatively free of side effects and does not produce drowsiness or ataxia in the doses routinely utilized. While Tegretol can cause aggressiveness in some, it reduces aggressive outbursts in many others.

Complex partial seizures are sometimes mistakenly diagnosed as Tourette Syndrome and vice versa. Both may need to be considered in the diagnostic process.

Narcolepsy

While narcolepsy is officially a neurologic disorder, it will be discussed in Chapter 13 under "Sleep Disorders" since most people associate it with falling asleep at inappropriate times.

THE IMPORTANCE OF CORRECT DIAGNOSIS

The importance of obtaining a correct diagnosis of the symptoms with which a child or adolescent presents cannot be overstated. Incorrect diagnosis leads, of course, to inappropriate treatment. In addition, many of these diagnoses carry serious implications. Any form of seizure, for example, has not only emotional and social consequences for the child and his family, but other limitations as well, including driving restrictions. All who work with children and adolescents must not only be caring and concerned, but must be knowledgeable and informed as well. Only then will our youth have a chance of not only fulfilling their potential but of realizing their dreams as well.

To sleep, perchance to dream...

—Shakespeare

13
Sleep Disorders

Sleep Apnea
Narcolepsy

Difficulty with sleeping is considered the second most common health complaint following the common cold. Problems range from transient insomnia to more severe forms of sleep disorders which include head banging, sleepwalking, nightmares, night terrors, sleep myoclonus (legs twitching and kicking), bruxism (teeth grinding), sudden infant death syndrome (SIDS), sleep apnea, narcolepsy and Ondine's Curse, an often fatal breathing disorder. There are over fifty sleep disorders which can render one's daytime hours inefficient and tedious.

SLEEP: GENERAL CONSIDERATIONS

Those who have worked with ADHD/ADD children and adolescents for many years are quite familiar with the symptoms of motor restlessness, inability to fall asleep, reduced need for sleep, teeth grinding, sleepwalking and night terrors which occur so frequently in our patients and clients.   Others have a biological clock, a Circadian pacemaker, which is out of sync with the typical schedule of work and school. *Night people* come to life in the late afternoon and evening, and struggle to arise by 7:00, 8:00, 9:00 or even 10:00 a.m. *Morning people*, by contrast, bounce out of bed at 5:00 or 6:00 a.m. smiling and ready for the day.

One adolescent with whom we worked was, in general, extremely sluggish. Awakening him had become a family crisis. He was failing in school because of frequently missed classes. His teachers were frustrated by, and impatient with, his presumed lack of motivation and disinterest. However, no amount of calling, threats, cajoling or harsh words aroused him. Multiple alarm clocks were put around his bedroom to no avail. John simply did not come to life until noon.

It finally became apparent that John's biological clock had to be respected. He was enrolled in a tutorial school where he could attend classes from noon to six p.m. His most productive period for study was 9:00 p.m. to 2:00 a.m. On this new schedule, he was quite efficient. John is now in college and continues to choose classes which fit his natural Circadian rhythm.

We saw John several years ago. Sleep disorders specialists now have a name for this sleep pattern. It is called *night-owl syndrome* or *delayed-sleep phase syndrome*, and treatment is available.   Sleep specialists can change the body rhythms of those out of phase with their environment with sessions of several hours of exposure to fluorescent lights interspersed with periods of darkness and sleep.

It has been shown conclusively that adequate sleep is necessary for efficiency and productivity, as well as physical and mental health. Neil B. Kavey, M.D., Director of the Sleep Disorders Center at Columbia Presbyterian Medical Center in New York City, likens sleep to a "regular body tune up. If we don't sleep, we don't function well. It's as simple as that" (Callahan, 1988). How long we sleep appears to be related to how long we live, with between 7 and 7.9 hours correlating best with longevity. Mood also depends on sleep. Both too little and too much sleep can be unhealthy. Restless sleep or *sleeping like a log*, so typical of those with attention disorders, is also problematic.

Many overactive ADHD children and adolescents are chronically sleep deprived, while those with sluggish ADD are underaroused and sleep too much. It is important that we address their sleep disorders as part of our intervention programs.

A second grader referred to us for ADD illustrates the need for careful assessment of sleep factors. Jane was a pleasant and cooperative child but drawn and fatigued. The 9:00 a.m. evaluation was obviously taxing to her. In our conversation during the evaluation her sleeping habits were questioned. She acknowledged problems falling asleep and indicated that she could do so only if she listened to an audiotape of her favorite songs. This revelation was not alarming until she reported that each thirty minutes when the tape clicked off she awakened and turned it over. She did this all night long. Needless to say, Jane exhibited classic sleep deprivation symptoms.

Many of our patients who sleep with a fan on summer and winter need the constant whirring noise to focus the attention centers and to block out episodic distracting stimuli so they can settle into sleep. This intervention can be a life-saver for sleep-deprived children.

Jane's sleep deprivation was *cured* with an inexpensive sleep machine that produced sounds of rainfall throughout the night. After a month of adequate sleep, she no longer experienced ADD symptoms. As suggested earlier, auditorially hypersensitive children who hear every noise may require not only sleep machines; soft ear plugs may be necessary as well.

Unlike Jane, who was only sleep deprived, many children have both ADHD or ADD and sleep deprivation. Medical intervention may surprisingly include small doses of stimulants given an hour before bedtime to facilitate sleep for those whose minds continue to race after their bodies are presumably still. Over-the-counter Benadryl can occasionally be helpful to reestablish the sleep cycle, especially for those with allergies, but it is not a long-term solution. Sleep machines, meditation, relaxation, or a warm cup of milk with its tryptophane, sleep-enhancing qualities, have been helpful to some with insomnia. A comforting back rub has been the solution for many a hyperactive child who needed the soothing strokes of loving hands to calm the overactive firing of the neurons in his brain.

SLEEP APNEA

Hyperactive, irritable, inattentive, forgetful and disinterested. . . or underactive, sluggish, and excessively drowsy. . . children and adolescents with these symptoms may have an attention deficit disorder—or they may have *sleep apnea.* The American Medical Association estimates that approximately 2.5 million Americans of all ages are affected by this disorder of which few have any knowledge. Sleep apnea is a significant problem and one which can be life-threatening in its more severe forms. Its symptoms frequently mimic those of ADD.

Sleep apnea, in its most common form, involves an obstruction of the upper airway during sleep. In children it is most frequently caused by enlarged tonsils and adenoids. In other cases, certain muscles and structures in the throat become flabby and cause blockages of the upper airway. Partial blockage produces snoring, while complete blockage produces apnea, or the absence of breathing. The inhaling of oxygen is blocked and the carbon dioxide level increases. It is this rising concentration of carbon dioxide in the blood which stimulates the breathing center in the brain, causing the person to respond by gasping for breath which, in turn, restores oxygen to the brain. The person then returns to a deeper sleep until the next occurrence.

Episodes of sleep apnea may occur from dozens to hundreds of times each night without any awareness on the part of the sufferer. Parents or spouses should be alert to sleep apnea if much snoring, grunting, gasping of breath, and restlessness during sleep occur and if there is pronounced daytime sleepiness and irritability. Teachers, too, should be alert if a student frequently sleeps in class or appears generally fatigued and inattentive. Young children often respond to the extreme fatigue with increased irritability, hyperactivity and behavioral problems. Frequent sore throats or ear infections are also clues. Those who are overweight appear more prone to the disorder. If your child or student is experiencing these symptoms, a careful assessment for a sleep disorder should be obtained before assuming that the problems are a result of ADD.

Sleep apnea is a serious disorder. It reduces productivity dramatically and impairs reflex responding. The resulting daytime drowsiness is believed to boost car accident rates by seven to ten times. It can also cause hypertension, heart disease, and even death from the cardiac arrhythmias that may occur during an episode.

Kelly, an eight-year-old, slightly overweight, third grade patient of ours, had experienced terrible difficulties in school. She was initially diagnosed as having underaroused ADD. Treatment with stimulant medication was moderately helpful, but she continued to be irritable and fatigued. After investigating her sleep patterns more thoroughly, she was referred to a sleep disorders clinic. Kelly did, indeed, have sleep apnea caused by enlarged tonsils and adenoids. After a tonsillectomy and adenoidectomy, she improved dramatically. With remediation for academic delays, school was no longer a problem. Her poor self-esteem and lack of confidence were aided by helping her develop social skills and athletic competence. Counseling and assistance with a weight-reduction program completed the therapeutic intervention.

Children, adolescents and adults who experience excessive daytime sleepiness without apparent cause, should have sleep apnea ruled out as a source of the difficulties. An armchair diagnosis is possible by sitting in the person's room and observing him during sleep or taping his sleep on a long-play tape recorder. As sleep begins, chest movement becomes irregular because of erratic breathing. As the oxygen levels drop, there is loud snoring or gasping for air. There may be a temporary cessation of breathing. If these symptoms occur, a physician should be consulted who can conduct an examination and make a referral to an accredited sleep disorders clinic if he concurs that such an action is appropriate.

Treatments for sleep apnea include surgery for enlarged tonsils and adenoids or surgery to remove part of the soft palate and dangling uvula at the back of the throat.   A new, noninvasive therapy supplies continuous positive airway pressure through a nose mask at night. Called Nasal CPAP, it blows the air passage open. While one may look like Darth Vader and find sleeping next to a whirring machine difficult, the alert and relaxed feeling one has upon awakening is usually worth the adjustment. The alternative to the surgeries mentioned and CPAP is a tracheotomy—a permanent surgical hole in the neck into which air is pumped at night. The tracheotomy thus bypasses blockages of the nose and throat.   This procedure is quite drastic and is becoming increasingly less common to treat sleep apnea.

This disorder is one of the most underdiagnosed in children and adolescents. It is worthy of the awareness and attention of parents, teachers and professionals alike.

In general, sleep problems in children, adolescents and adults are often not given adequate attention but instead are viewed as frustrating nuisances. They should, however, be addressed, for they can contribute significantly to the symptoms of attention disorders in many.

NARCOLEPSY

Narcolepsy, a distinct neuroleptic disorder characterized by excessive sleepiness and abnormal rapid-eye-movement (REM) sleep, has been described, in its extreme, as " . . . *a devil's brew of symptoms that includes sudden slumber, hallucinations at sleep onset and cataplexy—temporary paralysis while awake, most often provoked by laughter or emotion"* (Long, 1987). For most, however, its major symptom is excessive sleepiness or inappropriately falling asleep while involved in an activity.

This genetic disorder has a prevalency rate which varies from 1 in 500,000 in Israel to 1 in 600 in Japan. Its occurrence is estimated to be between 1 in 1,000 and 1 in 100,000 in Europe and the United States, respectively (Aldrich, 1990). It occurs equally in men and women. It can begin as early as age 10 or as late as age 50, but it usually begins quite gradually between 15 and 35 years of age.

Narcolepsy is often mistaken for other disorders, including sleep apnea, depression, and even psychiatric illness because of the hallucinations which can occur. The chronic underarousal characteristic of narcolepsy often produces symptoms of underaroused attention deficit disorder as well. Half of those with narcolepsy complain of memory problems, a significant finding in ADD. As in ADD, poor memory appears to be a factor of impaired attention and fluctuating levels of alertness.

Extreme drowsiness; *sleep attacks*; blurred or double vision; muscular weakness brought on by excitement, emotion or laughter; and/or hallucinations, especially visual hallucinations, should alert parents, teachers, and health professionals to this disorder. A diagnosis of narcolepsy can often be made on the basis of history alone, but most experts recommend laboratory studies as well. The most widely utilized, clinically useful test is the *Multiple Sleep Latency Test* which is usually performed by a sleep disorders specialist and requires the patient to sleep at two-hour intervals throughout the day. As reported by

Dr. Michael Aldrich in an excellent review article in the *New England Journal of Medicine* (1990), more than eighty percent of patients with narcolepsy have a mean sleep latency of less than five minutes and at least two REM periods at the onset of sleep, both of which differ markedly from the latency and REM sleep of normals.

Dr. Yutaka Honda, in Tokyo, pioneered the research which determined that narcolepsy is genetically based. Since it is a disorder of major significance in Japan, much scientific investigation has been carried out there. The essential deficit in narcolepsy appears to be a problem with HLA antigens which produces a lack of well-defined boundaries between the states of REM sleep, non-REM sleep and wakefulness due to impaired central regulation of the autonomic nervous system. The neurochemistry of narcolepsy parallels that of attention deficit disorders with its altered neurotransmitter activity.

Narcolepsy has been widely recognized and treated only within the last few years. Hundreds of thousands who suffer remain undiagnosed. Yet its symptoms wreak academic, economic, social and emotional havoc in its sufferers. As one person described his experience, *"I began to experience sleepiness when I was a teenager. Everyone told me I was just lazy ... no good. I went to extraordinary lengths to stay awake, pinching myself, walking around, drinking cokes. It was painful! Nothing helped. When I fell asleep in class, the teacher yelled at me and sent me home. My parents didn't understand either. I felt really stupid and inadequate."*

Many adults have trouble on the job for they can fall asleep mid-sentence. People who do not understand can be unsympathetic and harsh in their response. Productivity declines dramatically and accidents increase precipitously.

There are several treatments for narcolepsy. The most common is the use of stimulant medication, both Ritalin and Dexedrine. Cylert is occasionally used for those not responsive to the former two. Stimulants enhance the synaptic availability of norepinephrine in narcolepsy just as they do in attention disorders. Tricyclic antidepressants are often used when cataplexy and sleep paralysis are present as well. These medications inhibit the reuptake of norepinephrine and serotonin. MAO inhibitors are sometimes used as well. The increase in the diagnosis of narcolepsy accounts for much of the increased use of stimulant medication reported so alarmingly in earlier (1988-89) media coverage.

In addition to medication, patients may be encouraged to take naps as well. Dr. Jurgen Zulley, at the Max Planck Institute for Psychiatry in Munich, recommends a four-hour sleep-awake cycle with naps of 15-20 minutes at 9 a.m., 1 p.m. and 5 p.m. A short nap can dramatically improve alertness and reduce the need for medication. Perhaps we would all be well served by the once-traditional after-lunch siesta. Sleep researchers suggest: *"Don't fight sleep; instead use short naps to enhance your life. It is biologically correct"* (Long, 1987).

The ultimate solution for narcolepsy, as for other genetically-based disorders, may well be gene-replacement therapy. Until that time, the disorder will continue to be treated with medication and environmental accommodations.

PART V

The Educator's Important Role

*Based on our analysis of evidence, we find the
district violated Section 504 regulation by . . .
refusing to administer medication without a
waiver of liability and by failing to determine
[child's] needs for the administration of
medication and then administering it accordingly.*

    —Office of Civil Rights, 1990, Ref. 03901047
    U.S. DOE, Philadelphia, PA.

14

The Responsibility
of the School
Under Federal Law

Public schools, and private schools receiving federal funding, have been subject to increasing litigation and OCR[1] complaints because they are unaware of their obligations to students under Parts D and E of Section 504 of P.L. 93-112, and because they have failed to meet the educational needs of students with attention disorders, as required by federal law. Students with attention disorders are considered "handicapped" because their neurophysiologic impairments can interfere significantly with one of life's major activities guaranteed under P.L. 93-112, i.e., the civil right to learn.

Schools have been thrust into a new and difficult position. At the administrative and policy levels, there are no specific provisions for students with attention deficit disorders. Unlike learning *disabilities*,

---

[1] The Office of Civil Rights (OCR) was established to ensure compliance with P.L. 93-112, the "Rehabilitation Act of 1973," also known as "Civil Rights Legislation."

statistically defined by most states using various discrepancy criteria, there is no generally accepted *educational* definition of ADHD or ADD; there are no statistical criteria for ADHD/ADD the schools can utilize for the determination of services; there are no specific provisions for the training of teachers in attention disorders; and there is uncertainty regarding who should be responsible for these students (Special Education or Regular Education), where they should be educated (special classes or regular classes), what teaching methods are most appropriate, and what modifications should be implemented to assist them. Teachers are often not knowledgeable about attention disorders; they do not appropriately identify students exhibiting these symptoms; and they often feel overwhelmed by the excessive demands students with attention disorders can place on their already overburdened time and energy resources.

Historical Perspective

The current situation with ADHD/ADD is not unlike the confusion, frustration and increasingly litigious climates which have preceded most educational reforms. Major upheavals were a necessary precursor to each of the following educational policy shifts.

Compulsory Education

Compulsory education began its long judicial battle in 1852 when Massachusetts passed the first law requiring communities to establish public schools with the "Establishment of Schools Act." In *Dugan vs. State of New Hampshire* (1858), compulsory school attendance was challenged. However, it was ruled that the state can, in fact, compel school attendance. "The Enabling Acts of 1889" followed thirty-one years after compulsory education was required and resulted from intense lobbying to establish a free education. Through this legislation Congress required new states to establish free public schools. In 1924, in *Pierce vs. Society of Sisters (of the Holy Name of Jesus and Mary)*, the court allowed private education at the insistence of the people. However, it established governmental right to regulate and supervise all schools, including private ones. Both free public education and the right of government to regulate all schools were firmly established at this time and continue, at the present, unchallenged.

Segregation/Integration of Schools

This issue was likewise determined by court cases. *Plessy vs. Ferguson (1896)* established for public schools the doctrine of "separate but equal." There was increasing unhappiness with this doctrine, however, and in 1954 *Brown vs. Board of Education of Topeka* overturned the *Plessy vs. Ferguson* ruling and mandated the integration of all public schools under the Fourteenth Amendment Equal Protection Clause.

Rights of Handicapped Students to a
Free and Appropriate Education

Public Law 94-142, the current ruling law of the land regarding handicapped students' educational rights, was likewise a culmination of several court cases. In 1969 the court, in *Wolf vs. State of Utah*, ruled that mentally handicapped children were as entitled to a free public education as non-handicapped children. *PARC vs. Commonwealth of Pennsylvania* (1972) extended the *Wolf vs. State of Utah* decision and mandated not only a free public education but one appropriate to the student's needs. Parents of handicapped students became increasingly litigious. In that same year, 1972, the courts further ruled that alternative educational services for handicapped children must be appropriate to individual needs. Of particular interest, given the present situation with ADHD/ADD, is the fact that two of the seven litigant children were hyperactive. In 1973 the courts refused to allow schools to require parents to pay any additional expense of educating a handicapped child (In re *Downey*, 1973).

As a result of increasing unhappiness of parents with the educational services for their handicapped children and the resulting litigation, Congress passed Public Law 94-142 (EHA) in 1975. The changes emanated from a grass-roots effort very similar to that observed today for students with ADHD/ADD. A vehicle for complaint resolution was established with the Office of Civil Rights. This means of obtaining services is currently the primary means for dissatisfied parents to express their grievances and obtain what they believe to be an appropriate education for their children.

The numbers of complaints registered were so great between 1985 and 1990 that they compelled legislative action to decide the issue of ADHD/ ADD students' rights and by what means they should be guaranteed. In September, 1991 the Department of Education (DOE) issued the "Clarification of P.L. 94-142," which addressed the needs of students with attention deficit disorders under the *Other Health Impaired* (OHI) category if they met the discrepancy criteria of P.L. 94-142 and if not, under Section 504 of P.L. 93-112, *The Rehabilitation Act of 1973*.

From an historical perspective, it is clear that the needs of students with attention disorders made their way through the same evolutionary, revolutionary, judiciary, and finally the legislative process as other educational changes. Once mandated by law, the resulting educational and social consequences permeate the culture for decades. They often, in fact, have become historical turning points in the life of a nation.

Civil Rights, i.e. The Civil Right to Learn

A person's civil right to nondiscrimination on the basis of handicap was clearly established by the Rehabilitation Act of 1973, which provides that "No otherwise qualified handicapped individual in the United States ... shall, solely by reason of ... handicap, be excluded from the participation in, be denied benefits of, or be subjected to discrimination under any program or activity receiving federal financial assistance."

This regulation, adopted by the Department of Education on May 9, 1980, applies to all recipients of federal financial assistance for the Department of Education. Such recipients include all public, preschool, elementary and secondary school systems; colleges and universities; state education agencies; libraries; vocational schools; and state vocational rehabilitation agencies. It also includes any private school which receives federal grants for any purpose, including, for example, library grants or computer grants.

Section 504 was part of the original Rehabilitation Act of 1973 (P.L. 93-112), while the "Education of Handicapped Act", *EHA*, widely known in educational circles as P.L. 94-142, was a 1975 Amendment to the Rehabilitation Act of 1973. The name was changed to the "Individuals with Disabilities Education Act" (IDEA) when refunded in the summer of 1990 to reflect the more current view that individuals who have disabilities are not necessarily "handicapped" as the word has traditionally been used.

Guidelines for the Department of Education (DOE) were issued by Congress and published in the Federal Register May 9, 1980 (GPO, 1980). It is these guidelines with which schools must comply to continue to receive federal financial assistance. Some school districts have argued that the Department of Education alone has jurisdiction over the schools, not OCR. However, the courts ruled that OCR, as well as DOE, has jurisdiction over cases involving students with attention deficit disorders. Since EHA is simply one of the amendments to P.L. 93-112 for which OCR is responsible, OCR will continue to be responsible for the intent and purpose of the omnibus law—i.e., that all handicapped persons shall have full equality under the law.

Propelling the needs of ADHD/ADD students were parent groups active on behalf of their children (CH.A.D.D. and ADDA). They originally requested its specific inclusion under Paragraph 104.3(j)(i)(B) of Section 504. Congress and the DOE denied specific mention. Instead, it remained one of the disabilities covered under OHI.

Prior to 1991 ADHD and ADD were already, as neurologic disorders, included under the *Other Health Impaired* category of P.L. 94-142, and many states had accepted responsibility for these students and were assisting them as best they could. Others were not. While legal opinion consistently stated that ADHD and ADD were already included under federal law, and the problem was a lack of compliance, it was generally believed by those working in the field that specific inclusion of attention disorders would be necessary to bring about the fundamental educational changes necessary to assist these students adequately and appropriately. While not included as a separate disability category, the mandate for appropriate services and accommodations delineated in the 1991 Clarification of P.L. 94-142, has begun, several years later, to have a notable impact.

In educational conferences on attention disorders presented to school personnel prior to 1991 I found that the great majority of teachers and many administrators were unfamiliar with Section 504. Lack of knowledge of Section 504 is, itself, a violation of Section 504 (OCR Complaint #09-88-1072, 1989, Region IX, San Francisco, CA). Subsequent to Section 504 complaint resolutions, school districts were therefore required to conduct Section 504 workshops to present to educators their duties and responsibilities under the law. Most OCR offices were very willing to provide assistance upon request.

In the mid-nineties most educators—from superintendents to classroom teachers—are familiar with Section 504. Many, however, are lacking in knowledge regarding their full responsibilities and how to implement them effectively. Much research is currently underway to determine effective policies, procedures and teaching methods to accommodate the needs of students with attention deficit disorders.

The full text of the rules and regulations affecting preschool, elementary, secondary, and post-secondary education can be obtained by contacting the local OCR office, a list of which can be found in Appendix 8. It is emphasized that all schools receiving any federal financial assistance must meet these guidelines.

School Policies and Practices Which Have Resulted in Section 504 Complaints

Medication Policies and Medication Administration

While not the most problematic of the complaints the ten regional offices for the OCR have received, issues related to medication are most germane to this book and ones which have been included in other OCR complaints.

Requirement of Waiver of Liability

The desire to protect school personnel from personal liability which may be incurred in administering medication to students is an understandable motive and a very familiar one required for many medical services and procedures. Many school medication policies I have reviewed do, in fact, include a waiver of liability. An example is as follows:

Certificate of Authorization for
Administration of Prescribed Medication Only

With full knowledge of any emergencies, dangers, and risks related to the administration of such medication by the [ ] School's employees, officers, or agents, we, the undersigned, hereby waive all claims which might arise from said administration of medicine to said minor child. We hereby assume full responsibility for the administration of such medication to said minor child and the results thereof. We agree to indemnify and hold harmless [ ] School District, [ ] Board of Education, its members, officers, employees, and agents from any and all liability relative to the administration of such medication.

Requiring a waiver of liability as a condition of administering medication has been found a violation of Section 504:

> The Section 504 regulation, at 34 C.F.R. Section 204.33(a), requires that each recipient operating a public elementary or secondary education program provide a free appropriate public education to each qualified handicapped person within its jurisdiction. For this purpose, the regulation defines a qualified handicapped person to include all handicapped persons of school age, 34 C.F.R. Section 104.3(k)(2)(i), and it defines an appropriate education to include regular or special education and related aids and services that are designed to meet the individual needs of handicapped persons as adequately as the needs of nonhandicapped persons are met. 34 C.F.R. Section 104.33(b)(1). Related services refer to those services which enable a handicapped student to benefit from the regular or special education which is provided. Thus, where one of the District's handicapped students requires the administration of medication in order to benefit from his or her educational program, the District is obligated to ensure that the medication is administered. The regulation imposes no obligation on the parent to release a recipient from liability in order for the child to receive an appropriate education. Likewise, the regulation contains no provision permitting a recipient to make an appropriate education contingent upon a release of liability from the parent. Accordingly, the District's former medication policy, which conditioned the administration of medication on a waiver of liability, violated the Section 504 regulation, at 34 C.F.R. Section 104.33(a) and (b)(1), insofar as it applied to qualified handicapped persons, including .... (OCR, Ref. 03-90-1047, Region III, 1990)

The school district rescinded its policy and sent notice of this change to all of its principals (January 22, 1990). The desire to protect school personnel is understandable but, nonetheless, is not permissible under the law.

Administration of Medication

OCR considers it the school's responsibility (a) to determine a child's needs for the administration of medication, (b) to administer the medication, and (c) to supervise the administration of the medication, including safeguards, training personnel to administer it, and communicating with the prescribing physician. The Office of Civil Rights has ruled:

> The District, as discussed above, is required to provide [ ], a qualified handicapped student, with any related services, including the administration of medication, he requires to benefit from his regular or special education program. At the beginning of the school year, the District did not determine, in accordance with the placement procedures of 34 C.F.R. Section 104.35(b) and (c), [ ]'s needs for the administration of medication. Subsequently, the District did not supervise the administration of his medication until November 15, 1989. The District, however, did meet with [ ]'s parents on November 15, 1989, and developed procedures for the effective administration of [ ]'s medication. Because the District failed to determine [ ]'s needs for the administration of medication and then administer the medication accordingly until November 15, 1989, the District violated the Section 504 regulation, at 34 C.F.R. Sections 104.33(b)(1) and 104.35(b) and (c). (OCR, Region III, Philadelphia, PA, 1990, Ref. 03-90-1047)

In a separate complaint in California, a school district was found in violation of appropriate management of medication:

> Because [ ]'s handicap seriously interfered with his ability to learn without medication, the District's FAPE[2] obligation clearly required that he receive adequate assistance in taking his medicine. There is substantial evidence that the District took steps to encourage [ ] to take his medication daily. However, by requiring that a ten-year-old child retrieve his own medicine from the nurse's office, and by refusing to provide daily monitoring by an adult, it failed to fulfill its obligation to provide a FAPE. (OCR Region IX, San Francisco, CA, Ref. 09-88-1200, 1988)

A well-designed medication policy for schools is urgently needed, as well as a systematic means for administering medication, monitoring its effects, and communicating with parents and physicians regarding its benefits and possible side effects. The school's involvement in medication is absolutely essential since medical intervention forms the cornerstone of most treatment programs for ADHD and ADD, and medication must, for many students, be taken during the school day.

Other school policies and procedures which have resulted in Section 504 complaints include, among others:

1) Failure to establish standards and procedures for the evaluation and placement of students who, because of their attention disorder, are believed to need special or related services.

---

[2]FAPE - Free and Appropriate Public Education.

2) Failure to provide special education services when students did not qualify for services using P.L. 94-142 criteria for learning disabilities.

3) Inappropriate disciplinary practices including:
    - Spanking (in states which allow it)
    - Inappropriate use of isolation
    - Humiliation

4) Inappropriate suspensions and expulsions of students without determining if the behavior for which a student was being expelled was a manifestation of his handicapping condition.

5) Failure to provide due process to parents of ADHD/ADD children and adolescents.

Summary

A lengthy discussion of educational policies and procedures regarding ADHD/ADD students is beyond the scope of this book. It is, however, relevant to emphasize the importance of safeguards against practices which discriminate against these and other students with individual differences. While policies, or the lack of them, are often the result of uninformed educators and no harm is intended to students, failure, loss of esteem, humiliation and the many other such negative experiences which often occur when problems are unrecognized, can, in fact, do great harm to them. We cannot allow children to be hurt by the negligence of adults.

To fulfill its public responsibility in the best way possible, procedures and policies emanating from informed, thoughtful and caring policymakers are needed at the local, state, and national levels. The majority of those in education truly want to help children. Failure to provide teachers with the necessary tools is, in my opinion, the crime. Only knowledgeable, effective educators can produce competent, contributing students.

Education is helping the child realize his
potentialities.

—Erich Fromm

15

The Teacher's Role in Monitoring Medication

In writing this chapter, it is assumed that the child or adolescent has been carefully evaluated, has been found to have an attention disorder, and a decision to use medication has been made. Generally, the teacher is already quite involved in the evaluation/ treatment process, for she will, in all probability, have completed behavioral checklists and classroom observations and shared those, as well as previously implemented interventions, with the prescribing physician. If those have not been requested, the teacher is urged to send them unsolicited after obtaining written permission from the parents (Figure 15-1), and sending a letter explaining her desire to be a helpful member of her student's treatment team (Figure 15-2).

Teachers play not only an important information-sharing role with the physician, but an important one in identifying the symptoms and encouraging patients to obtain necessary evaluations and appropriate treatment for their child. Videoprograms on ADHD/ADD, books, articles from magazines, and information on local support groups are extremely helpful and should be available from the school library on a check-out basis.

In addition to these roles, educators are also seen by parents as important sources of professional opinion on their child's behavior and on school resources to help with the problems. Referrals for psychological, tutorial and other services are often required from teachers and other school personnel. Parents expect teachers to be knowledgeable, and they rely heavily on their observations and recommendations.

Teachers and school personnel also serve a crucial supportive role in aiding parents acknowledge their child's problems and begin to come to terms with them. Teachers are expected to have recommendations readily available to assist their students at school and to help parents guide their children at home. *Attention Without Tension: The Teacher's Handbook on Attention Disorders* (Copeland & Love, 1990) addresses at length the comprehensive role that educators play, as well as information on home and classroom management strategies.

Medication Monitoring

Having accomplished the preceding objectives, and with the child launched on a multimodal treatment program, the teacher's important role continues. Her assistance in determining the appropriate medication, dose level, time intervals and side effects is generally second to none, except that of the parents. She is the person who sees the child or adolescent the most while he is on the medicine. This is especially true for students who take medicine only twice a day, five days a week. Difficulties at school, whether academic, social, or emotional, have usually been most problematic there. She is, therefore, in the best position to see changes. Many of the benefits of medication, including its positive effect on work rate, attention span, impulsiveness, organization and frustration tolerance, among others, are best judged in the classroom. Likewise, side effects are often most apparent during the time the medication is effective, i.e., during the school day. Thus the teacher becomes, of necessity, the key person monitoring overall medication effects. Without the teacher's input, the physician is without most of the data he needs on which to make ongoing adjustments in the medication regimen.

Most physicians are aware of the teacher's key role and make available to her a *Medication Schedule* (Figure 15.5), as well as a *Side-Effects Checklist* (Figure 15.6), and a behavior checklist (Figure 15.7). The side-effects and behavior checklists may need to be completed on a daily basis initially, followed by weekly reports, and finally only a periodic evaluation every three to four months which is completed prior to the checkup appointment with the student's physician. Any changes in behavior and performance should be shared with both parents and physician and close contact maintained until the child/adolescent improves.

Unlike verbal feedback such as, "He's doing better," or "I don't see a difference," these checklists communicate a wealth of essential information on both the positive effects of the medication and any adverse effects observed in the classroom, thereby assisting the physician in knowing exactly how the medicine is affecting the student. Checklists also save much time and energy trying to make and return phone calls between busy and not easily available professionals—both the teacher and the physician. FAX machines facilitate this process even more. Parents usually complete similar checklists for behavior and other effects observed, which rounds out the physician's understanding of overall medicinal effect. Ideally everyone working with the child will have met or teleconferenced at least once before therapy was begun.

Physicians are urged to contact their patients' teachers (Figure 15.3). If the prescribing physician does not contact the teacher, she is encouraged to contact him and advise him of her willingness to help monitor the medication. Continuing exchange of information until the maximum therapeutic benefit with the fewest side effects has been achieved. Once established, the teacher should complete the behavior checklists, side-effects checklists, and send a report of grades and progress before each periodic checkup. It is helpful for the physician's office to mail these to parents two weeks before their child's checkup.

At this juncture, I must stress that placing on the teacher the entire responsibility for monitoring the effectiveness and potential side effects of medication is neither totally satisfactory nor totally just. Parents are urged to administer medication on weekends, with the approval of the prescribing physician, if not all the time then at least until the appropriate medication, dose and regimen have been determined. Parents are more knowledgeable and more content if they, too, observe the effects of the medication and assist in the monitoring of it. Once the appropriate medication regimen has been determined, they should carefully assess whether to give it for school days only or throughout the week. If the effectiveness of treatment changes, both parents and physician should be notified.

A fully-functioning transdisciplinary team includes, at a minimum, the ADHD/ADD student's teacher, parent and physician. Only with close monitoring by this team can the greatest benefits of medication be achieved. With this treatment approach in place, the stage is set to enhance the student's full development through behavioral, cognitive, social, and educational interventions.

Forms

The following forms are provided to facilitate communication between team members.

<u>**Figure**</u>   <u>**Form**</u>

15.1   *Parent's Written Consent to Communicate with Physician*
15.2   *Teacher's Letter to Physician*
15.3   *Physician's Letter to Teacher/School Personnel*
15.4   *Parent's Written Consent for Physician to Communicate with Teacher/ School Personnel*
15.5   *Medication Schedule*
15.6   *Side-Effects Checklist*
15.7   *Copeland Medication Follow-Up Questionnaire (Teacher/Parent)*

PARENTS' WRITTEN CONSENT TO
COMMUNICATE WITH PHYSICIAN

TO: Dr. _____

_____, my child's teacher, has permission to release academic, behavioral and social/emotional data on my child to you and to discuss his/her difficulties and/or progress with you.

_____
Parent
_____
Address
(___)_____
Phone

_____
Child
_____
School
(___)_____
Phone

Figure 15.1

TEACHER'S LETTER TO PHYSICIAN

Dear Dr._____:

Mr./Mrs. _____ have advised me that they are having _____ evaluated/treated by you. With their permission, I am enclosing copies of behavior checklists, completed by both the parents and me, as well as academic data, and a summary of my intervention efforts with _____. I hope this information is helpful to you.

At _____ School, we believe strongly in a TEAM approach in treating students children who are having difficulties in school. I shall be happy to speak with you or be of any assistance possible in the evaluation and treatment process. As a team, I feel confident we can help _____.

I look forward to hearing from you.

Sincerely,

_____
Teacher
Phone (W)_____

Enclosures: 1)   Copy of Parental Consent
               2)   Student Information

cc: Parents

Figure 15.2

PHYSICIAN'S LETTER TO TEACHER/ SCHOOL PERSONNEL

Re: _____ Student   Parents: _____

Dear _____:

  I am treating your student for _____. He is currently taking _____ as part of the treatment program.
(Elaborate)
  You are a key person in monitoring the effects of all interventions with my patient, and I look forward to our working together for the best interests of _____.
  To assist me in determining appropriate medication, dosage, time intervals needed, benefits and side effects, I have enclosed the following:
  1) *Medication Schedule.*
  2) *Behavior Questionnaire* to be completed on a _____ basis.
  3) A *Side-Effects Checklist* to be completed _____.

  Please complete these and FAX or mail them to me with a copy to my patient's parents.
  I believe very strongly in a team approach to ADHD/ADD and look forward to working with you. Please contact me if you have any questions, comments or suggestions.

     Sincerely,

     _____, M.D.

     Phone _____

     FAX _____

Enclosure: Copy of Parental Consent Forms

cc: Parents

Figure 15.3

PARENT'S WRITTEN CONSENT FOR PHYSICIAN
TO COMMUNICATE WITH TEACHER/SCHOOL PERSONNEL

TO: _____

    Dr. _____, my child's physician, has permission to release medical information and other pertinent data on my child, and to discuss his/her difficulties and/or progress with you and other school personnel.

_____
Parent

_____
Address

_____
Phone

_____
Student

_____
School

_____
Address

_____
Phone

Figure 15.4

(Medication Schedule)

Child's Name _____   **Medication Schedule**   Month _____   Year _____

Instructions re: Medicine

Parents and Teachers:

Please complete Copeland Medication Follow-Up Questionnaire every day, including those days when no medicine is taken.

SUNDAY	MONDAY	TUESDAY	WEDNESDAY	THURSDAY	FRIDAY	SATURDAY

Figure 15.5

ATTENTION DISORDERS (ADHD/ADD)
MEDICATION SIDE EFFECTS

Child/Adolescent's Name_____Date_____Medication_____Tab
Spansule_____ Dose A.M._____ P.M._____Evening_____
Completed by (Name)_____(Position)_____

Side Effects

When medication is used, side effects sometimes occur. If any of the side effects listed below is observed, please indicate which one(s) occurred and the severity of it. If any other side effect occurs, please write it in the space provided.

	Not at All	Just A Little	Pretty Much	Very Much	Don't Know
A. Decreased appetite	___	___	___	___	___
Weight loss	___	___	___	___	___
Insomnia (inability to fall asleep)	___	___	___	___	___
Fitful sleeping	___	___	___	___	___
Difficulty awakening	___	___	___	___	___
Nightmares	___	___	___	___	___
B. Headaches	___	___	___	___	___
Stomachaches	___	___	___	___	___
***Tics* or involuntary motor movements, i.e., eyeblink**	___	___	___	___	___
Dizziness	___	___	___	___	___
Rashes	___	___	___	___	___
Bedwetting	___	___	___	___	___
C. Irritability	___	___	___	___	___
Feeling anxious, "jittery"	___	___	___	___	___
Restlessness	___	___	___	___	___
Tenseness	___	___	___	___	___
Heart racing	___	___	___	___	___
Socially withdrawn	___	___	___	___	___
Sadness	___	___	___	___	___
Other	___	___	___	___	___
_____	___	___	___	___	___

Figure 15.6

COPELAND MEDICATION FOLLOW-UP QUESTIONNAIRE
FOR MONITORING OF MEDICATION
(Parent/Teacher)

Copeland Medication Follow-Up Questionnaire

Teacher/Parent

Weekly Record Form

Copyright © 1991 by Edna D. Copeland, Ph.D.

Child's Name _____

Date _____ month/day to _____ month/day

Completed by _____ Date _____

Please indicate E — excellent; G — good; F — fair; P — poor

Day	Medication Schedule (specify (1) Name of medication; (2) Dose; and (3) Time medication is to be taken)	Attention/ Ability to Focus	Impulse Control	Activity Level (Over/Under)	Compliance/ Cooperation	Organization	Peer/Sibling Relations	Completing and Turning in School Work	Grades
Mon.	a.m.								
	p.m.								
Tues.	a.m.								
	p.m.								
Wed.	a.m.								
	p.m.								
Thurs.	a.m.								
	p.m.								
Fri.	a.m.								
	p.m.								
Sat.	a.m.								
	p.m.								
Sun.	a.m.								
	p.m.								

(Weekly or periodic comments to be written out)

Please put any additional comments on the back of this sheet.

Figure 15.7

16
Medication
Guidelines
for Schools

Schools have not only assumed the role of educating our children, but they have increasingly been thrust into the roles of day-care providers, dietitians, screening agents for immunizations, vaccinations, vision and hearing; and now they must become dispensers of medication as well. While we are, perhaps, burdening the school beyond capacity, there is truly no other social agency which is positioned in America today to become as effective a community resource. As other social institutions have become less central in people's lives, the school assumes ever-increasing importance. I truly believe that schools will become our mental health agencies of the future, especially for children. I encourage this choice, but realize that for schools to be effective education must become a top priority in America. Educators must be given both the essential necessary training and the increased resources if they are to do a credible job. Without such assistance, both parents, teachers and students will be eternally frustrated by a system in which they feel trapped but which is ineffective in meeting their needs.

Regardless of their preparedness for this new role, schools will become increasingly involved in dispensing medication. To be helpful to their students, to avoid unnecessary administrative and legal problems, and to comply with federal regulations will require that carefully crafted procedures and policies be formulated and adopted. The medication guidelines presented on the following pages are merely that—guides. Each school will develop policies consistent with the perceived needs of its students, teachers, local physicians and state and local laws. It is important that school guidelines not conflict with P.L. 94-142 and Section 504 requirements, as discussed previously.

A waiver of liability cannot be obtained for medication, such as Ritalin, which is necessary to treat a "handicapping condition." Schools may wish, on the other hand, to protect themselves with a waiver of liability for over-the-counter medicines which parents may request school personnel to give to their children.

Administration of Medication
Model Guidelines

While schools cannot require parents to sign a waiver of liability, it is very helpful to make certain they understand the school's medication policies and procedures, know whom to contact with questions and concerns, and have a copy of these policies at home. A signed copy in the student's file serves as both a reminder of and proof that the school, in fact, communicated these to each parent.

The following "Notice of Medication Policies and Procedures" outlines suggested ones for each school to consider. It can also serve as the form parents sign to verify that they have read and understand the school's requirements. It is important to emphasize that such policies protect everyone—the student, parents and school personnel.

Notice of Medication Policies and Procedures

I.   ADMINISTRATION OF MEDICATIONS

A.   <u>Forms Required on File</u>
  1.   When prescription medication is to be administered, the physician must complete the appropriate form, Form A (Figure 16.1), and the parent/legal guardian is asked to sign this *Notice of Medication Policies and Procedures.*
  2.   When over-the-counter medicine is to be administered, the parent/legal guardian must complete Form B (Figure 16.2).
  3.   It is requested that parents sign Consent Form C (Figure 15.1) to release information to the physician.
  4.   No medication can be administered until the appropriate forms have been completed and are on file at school.

B.   <u>Administered by</u>: Medication shall be administered only by trained adult school personnel designated solely by the principal. An authorized person will be available on an "on-call basis" at all times.

C.   <u>Medication Storage</u>:   Medication shall be securely stored in a locked cabinet or the school safe and kept in an appropriately labeled container provided by the pharmacist.   The container and label are not the responsibility of the school but of the parent/ legal guardian, pharmacist or physician.   The label shall include:
  - Student's name
  - Name of medication
  - Dosage and times administered
  - Physician's name and phone number

D.   <u>Daily Record</u>:   A daily log will be kept of all medications administered by the school, the amount given and the time dispensed (Figure 16.3).

E. <u>Medication Transport</u>: All medication, except cough drops, must be brought to the school by the parent/legal guardian and must be picked up at the end of the medication period or school year, whichever is earlier.

F. <u>Written Changes in Medication Administration</u>: The school must be notified in writing of any change in medication, dosage or time interval (Form D, Figure 16.4).

G. <u>New Forms Annually</u>: New request forms from the parent/ legal guardian and physician must be completed each year.

H. <u>Communication with Physician</u>: The school will send a Behavior Checklist and a Side-Effects Checklist completed by the teacher to the physician with a copy to the parent at the end of each month unless requested otherwise (Figures 15.6 and 15.7).

II. SCHOOL'S PURPOSE

We, at _____School, desire to help your child in every way possible. We can best serve your child if we work together as a team. Please sign below to signify you understand the medication policies to which we must adhere. Keep one copy for yourself.

If you have any questions, do not hesitate to call your child's teacher, designated person, or principal. We look forward to a successful school year.

III. VERIFICATION

I have read the above and understand _____ School's medication policies and procedures.

_____   _____
Child's Name   Grade/Teacher

_____   _____
Parent/Legal Guardian   Date

COMPONENTS OF RESPONSIBLE
MEDICAL CARE AT SCHOOL

Responsible medical care which benefits students, satisfies legal requirements, and avoids litigation has four major components. They are:

- **Communication**
- **Education**
- **Written Consent**
- **Documentation**

Building positive working relationships always involves attention to the communication which occurs between the parties involved. This aspect of medication administration at school is crucial. When a student requires medication, a designated person, the School Nurse or Counselor, for example, should meet with parents, ascertain their child/adolescent's needs, indicate the school's desire to be of assistance, and give them the name and phone number of the designated person to contact if questions or problems arise. After fully discussing the student's needs, the parents/legal guardian should be advised of the school's medication policies and procedures. They should be encouraged to read the guidelines and to ask any questions about the School's requirements. Once accomplished, parents are asked to sign the appropriate form to signify understanding. They are then encouraged to take a copy home and place it with other important school papers. Communication with parents, educators, and obtaining written confirmation promotes both cooperation and compliance.

Documentation is the final component of a comprehensive medication policy. It is critical that each time medicine is administered the name, dose and time of administration are recorded. Assuming that the medication is administered properly, informed consent and careful documentation are key to avoiding legal liability.

With medication policies and procedures in place and with strict adherence to them, the school can fulfill its medicine-dispensing obligations to students helpfully and efficiently with little concern over potential liability or legal problems. The key is developing a plan and following it.

Examples of Forms Needed For Successful Medication Administration

Figure	Form
16.1	*Physician's Form for Medication and Administration Requirements*
16.2	*Parent's Permission and Waiver of Liability: Over-the-Counter Medication*
15.1	*Parent's Consent Form to Release Information to Physician (p. 282)*
15.4	*Parent's Consent Form to Release Information to Teacher (p. 284)*
16.3	*Daily Log of Medication Administration*
16.4	*Written Notice of Changes in Medication Administration*
15.6	*Side-Effects Checklist (p. 287)*
15.7	*Behavior Checklists (p. 288)*

Summary

Concerns about medication administration are evident throughout the nation. The American Academy of Pediatrics is currently preparing guidelines for both physicians and schools. Educators can be expected to establish policies and procedures at the national, state and local levels which best meet the needs of their students, schools, physicians, other professionals and teachers. The Virginia Task Force Study on "The Effects of the Use of Methylphenidate" (1991) stressed the importance of a collaborative effort between physicians and educators, perceiving this link to be key to assisting ADHD/ADD students perform successfully in school.

With acknowledgment of the medical needs of students during the school day and with the establishment of medication policies and procedures which are carefully devised, which are explicit and easy to follow, which provide for documentation and accountability, and which fulfill the requirements of both IDEA and Section 504 law, schools are positioned to assume another pivotal role in the lives of students, families and the community at large with both proficiency and professionalism.

PHYSICIAN'S FORM FOR MEDICATION
AND ADMINISTRATION

Both state law and all public schools within _____ county require the following information when children need administration of prescription drugs at school. Please complete the following information and forward to the school.

1. Name of student _____ Age _____
                          Last   First   Middle

2. Address _____
             Street   Town/City   Zip

3. School _____ Grade _____

4. School District _____

5. Name of Medication _____ Oral Dosage _____

6. Times at which medication is to be administered _____
   _____

7. Administration of medication to end _____

8. Side Effects (adverse reactions) which should be reported to the physician _____
   _____

9. Special instructions for administration of drug, including sterile conditions, cold storage, etc._____
   _____

_____
Phone

_____ _____
Physician Signature   Emergency Phone

_____ _____
Parent/Guardian's Signature   Parent/Guardian's Phone

NOTE: There must be notification to school employees if any information provided by the physician changes.

           The medication must be delivered to the school by the parent/guardian in the container in which it was dispensed by the prescribing physician or licensed pharmacist.

_____
DATE

Figure 16.1

AUTHORIZATION FOR ADMINISTRATION
OF OVER-THE-COUNTER MEDICATION

With full knowledge of any emergencies, dangers, and risks related to the administration of such medication by the [ ]'s employees, officers, or agents, we, the undersigned, hereby waive all claims which might arise from said administration of medicine to said minor child. We hereby assume full responsibility for the administration of such medication to said minor child and the results thereof. We agree to indemnify and hold harmless _____ school district, _____'s Board of Education, its members, officers, employees, and agents from any and all liability relative to the administration of such medication.

I understand that I must submit a revised statement and sign it if any information/conditions change. It is requested that the form be completed by the parent/legal guardian. It must be completed prior to the administration of any medication.

1. Pupil's name _____ School _____

2. Grade _____ Age _____

3. Address _____

4. Parent/Legal Guardian_____

5. Address _____

6. Phone (H)_____ (W)_____ Emergency_____

Date _____

_____
Parent/Legal Guardian Signature

1. Name of over-the-counter medication(s)_____

_____

2. Dates to administer   From _____ To _____
3. Specific instructions:
   Dosage _____
   Time interval _____
   Time required to dispense_____
   Other_____
4. Possible side effects or negative reactions _____
   Physician's Name_____Phone _____
5. Special instructions (sterile conditions, before meals, etc.):

_____

This form must be completed, signed and dated to be valid. We shall endeavor to assist your child in every way possible.

Figure 16.2

DAILY LOG OF
MEDICATION ADMINISTRATION

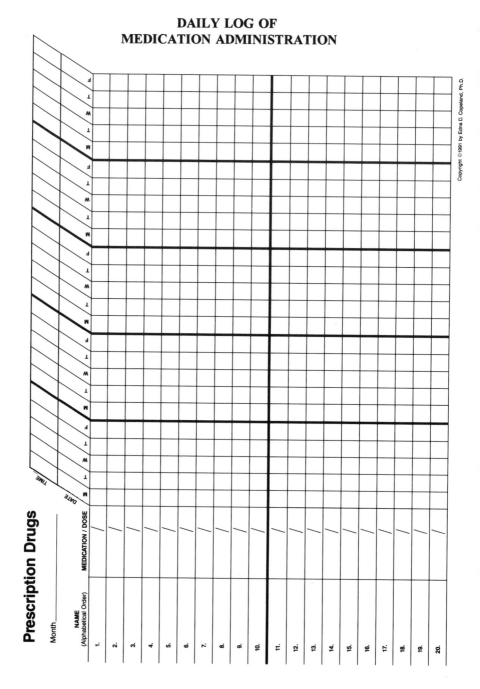

Figure 16.3

MEDICATION CHANGE REQUEST

Name of Child _____ Grade/Teacher_____
  I request the following change in medication (please be very specific):

___ **Medication itself** _____
  _____
  _____

___ **Dose** _____
  _____

___ **Time of administration** _____
  _____

___ **Other** _____
  _____

Change to begin _____
  _____

_____   _____
Signature
Parent/Legal Guardian   **Date**

Figure 16.4

Epilogue

The very real possibility of recognizing and successfully treating the millions of children, adolescents and adults throughout the world who suffer from attention deficit disorders is one which brings a great sense of satisfaction and fruition to those of us who have worked in the field for many years. Just as other medical disorders have succumbed to the discoveries of science, so too will ADHD and ADD. In the future, those with attention disorders will be able to avoid the frustration, failure, anguish, and loss of potential caused by disorders which can be of such little consequence when identified and treated early in a child's life.

For most, medication will contribute greatly to the success of their overall intervention program. Our favorite analogy when explaining attention disorders to children and adolescents is that using medicine for ADHD/ADD is like wearing glasses for visual problems. Medicines for attention disorders must be viewed as neurologic spectacles rather than frightening drugs if we are to make significant advances. In this age of enlightenment, no longer do the blind lead the blind. Neither should those with attention disorders be sentenced to lives imprisoned by ADHD and ADD symptoms. Our hope, instead, is that attention disorders will soon join the legions of other medical disorders which have become manageable problems in living. If this book has contributed in some small way to that process, its mission will have been accomplished.

Appendices

APPENDIX 1

Suggested Readings

A. TEXTS

Accardo, P.J., Blondis, T.A. & Whitman, B.Y. (1991). *Attention Deficit Disorders and Hyperactivity in Children.* New York: Marcel Dekker, Inc.

Barkley, R.A. (1990). *Attention Deficit Hyperactivity Disorder: A Handbook for Diagnosis and Treatment.* New York: The Guilford Press.

Goldstein, S. & Goldstein, M. (1990). *Managing Attention Disorders in Children: A Guide for Practitioners.* New York: John Wiley and Sons, Inc.

Levine, M.D. (1987). *Developmental Variation and Learning Disorders.* Cambridge , Massachusetts: Educators Publishing Service.

B. GENERAL

Copeland, E.D. & Love, V. (1991). *Attention Please: A Comprehensive Guide for Successful Parenting Children with Attention Disorders and Hyperactivity (ADHD/ADD).* Atlanta: Resurgens Press, Inc.

Fowler M.C. (1990). *Maybe You Know My Kid: A Parent's Guide to Identifying, Understanding, and Helping Your Child with Attention-Deficit Hyperactivity Disorder.* Secaucus, New Jersey: Birch Lane Press.

Ingersoll, B. (1988). *Your Hyperactive Child - A Parent's Guide to Coping with Attention Deficit Disorder.* New York: Doubleday.

Silver, L.B. (1984). *The Misunderstood Child: A Guide for Parents of Learning Disabled Children.* New York: McGraw-Hill.

Silver, L.B. (1991). *Attention Deficit Hyperactivity Disorder: A Clinical Guide to Diagnosis and Treatment.* Washington, D.C.: America Psychiatric Press, Inc.

Stewart, M. & Olds, S. (1975). *Raising a Hyperactive Child.* New York: Harper & Row.

Taylor, J.F. (1990). *Helping Your Hyperactive Child.* Rocklin, California: Prima Publishing and Communications.

Weisberg, L.W. & Greenberg, R. (1988). *When Acting Out isn't Acting: Conduct Disorders and ADD.* Washington: PIA Press.

Weiss, G. & Hechtman, L. (1986). *Hyperactive Children Grown Up.* New York: The Guilford Press.

Wender, P.H. (1987). *The Hyperactive Child, Adolescent and adult: ADD Through The Life Span.* New York: Oxford University Press.

C. EDUCATIONAL INTERVENTION

Anderson, W., Chitwood, S. & Hayden, D. (1990). *Negotiating the Special Education Maze: A Guide for Parents and Teachers.* (2nd ed.) Rockville, Maryland: Woodbine House.

Copeland, E.D. (1990). *Attention Disorders: The School's Vital Role.* (Video). Atlanta, GA: Resurgens Press, Inc.

Copeland, E.D. & Walker, R.A. (1994). *Diverse Teaching for Diverse Learners: A Handbook for Teachers and Parents.* Atlanta: Resurgens Press, Inc.

Copeland, E.D. & Love, V. (1990). *Attention Without Tension: The Teacher's Handbook On Attention Disorders (ADHD and ADD).* Atlanta, GA: Resurgens, Inc.

Kavanaugh, J., et al. (Eds.) (1988). *Learning Disabilities: Proceedings of the National Conference on Learning Disabilities.* 1987. Parkton, Maryland: York Press.

Parker, H.C. (1988). *The ADD Hyperactivity Workbook for Parents, Teachers and Kids.* Plantation, Florida: Impact Publications, Inc.

D. BEHAVIOR MANAGEMENT/RESPONSIBILITY

Barkley, R.A. (1987). *Defiant Children: A Clinician's Manual for Parent Training*. New York: Guilford Press.

Becker, W.C. (1971). *Parents Are Teachers*. Champaign, Illinois: Research Press.

E. LANGUAGE/COGNITIVE THERAPY

Healy, J.M. (1987). *Your Child's Growing Mind*. Garden City: Doubleday.

Kendall, P.C., & Braswell, L. (1985). *Cognitive-Behavioral Therapy for Impulsive Children*. New York: Guilford Press.

F. BOOKS FOR CHILDREN AND TEENS

Galvin, M. (1988). *Otto Learns About His Medicine*. New York: Magination Press. (Preschool and Early Elementary)

Levine, M.D. (1990). *Keeping Ahead in School: A Student's Book About Learning Abilities and Learning Disorders*. Cambridge, Massachusetts: Educators Publishing Service, Inc. (Middle and High School)

Moss, D.M. (1989). *Shelley, The Hyperactive Turtle*. Kensington, Maryland: Woodbine House. (Preschool and Early Elementary)

G. ADULT ADD

Barkley, R. (1990). *Attention Deficit Hyperactivity Disorder: A Handbook for Diagnosis and Treatment.* New York: The Guilford Press. Chapter 18.

Hallowell, E. & Ratey, J. (1994). *Driven to Distraction: Recognizing and Coping with Attention Deficit Disorders from Childhood through Adulthood.* New York: Random House.

Hallowell, E. & Ratey, J. (1995). *Answers to Distraction.* New York: Random House.

Kelly, K. & Ramundo, P. (1994). *You Mean I'm Not Lazy, Stupid or Crazy?! A Self-Help Book for Adults with Attention Deficit Disorder.* New York: Simon & Schuster.

Weiss, L. (1992). *Attention Deficit Disorder in Adults: Practical Help for Suffers and Their Spouses.* Dallas, Texas: Taylor Publishing.

Weiss, L. (1994). *The Attention Deficit Disorder in Adults Workbook.* Dallas, Texas: Taylor Publishing.

Wender, P.H. (1987). *The Hyperactive Child, Adolescent and Adult: ADD Through the Life Span.* New York: Oxford University Press. Chapter 7.

APPENDIX 2

Review Articles/Chapters

These review articles are listed in order of comprehensiveness.

Calis, K.A., Grothe, D.R., & Elia, J. (1990). Therapy reviews: Attention-deficit hyperactivity disorder. *Clinical Pharmacy* 9, 632-642.

Zametkin, A.J., & Borcherding, B.G. (1989). The neuropharmacology of attention-deficit hyperactivity disorder. *Annual Review of Medicine*, 40, 447-451.

Brown, R.T., Abramowitz, A.J., Dulcan, M., & Madan-Swain, A. (1989). Attention deficit hyperactivity disorder: Diagnosis, management, prognosis, and current research. *Emory University Journal of Medicine*, 3, 120-131.

Jensen, J.B. & Garfinkel, B.D. (1988). Neuroendocrine aspects of attention deficit hyperactivity disorder. *Endocrinology and Metabolism Clinics of North America*, 17:1, 111-129.

Zametkin, A.J., & Rapoport, J.L. (1987). Neurobiology of attention deficit disorder with hyperactivity: Where have we come in 50 years? *Journal of American Academy of Child and Adolescent Psychiatry*, 26, 676-686.

Donnelly, M., & Rapoport, J.L. (1985). Attention deficit disorders. In J. Wiener (Ed.), *Diagnosis and Psychopharmacology of Childhood and Adolescent Disorders* (pp. 179-197). New York: John Wiley.

APPENDIX 3

Parent Support Group Associations

NATIONAL ASSOCIATIONS

CHADD (Children with Attention Deficit Disorders)   (305) 587-3700
499 N.W. 70th Avenue, Suite 109
Plantation FL 33317

ADDA (Attention Deficit Disorders Association)   (800) 487-2282
19262 Jamboree Boulevard
Irvine, CA 92715

ADDA Group
8091 S. Ireland Way
Aurora, CO 80016

Learning Disabilities Association (LDA)   (412) 341-1515
4156 Library Road
Pittsburgh. PA 15234

Tourette Syndrome Association (TSA)   (718) 224-2999
42-40 Bell Boulevard
Bayside, New York 11361

CANADIAN ASSOCIATIONS

Foundation for Attentional Disorders   (416) 769-7979
57 Pinecrest Road
Toronto, Ontario M6P 3G6

APPENDIX 4

SYMPTOM CHECKLISTS FOR DEVELOPMENTAL DISABILITIES: ADHD/ADD, LD, EMOTIONAL/BEHAVIORAL DISORDERS, ACADEMIC DIFFICULTIES AND MEDICAL PROBLEMS

A. Preschool

B. Elementary

PRESCHOOL CHECKLIST

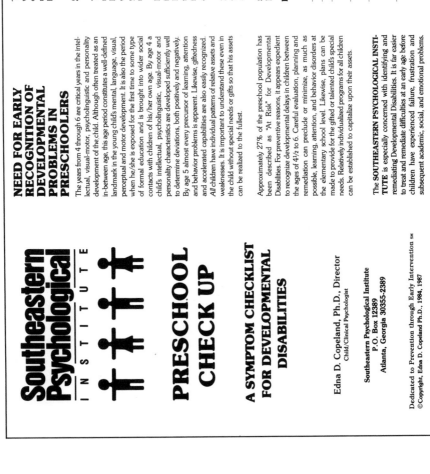

Southeastern Psychological INSTITUTE

PRESCHOOL CHECK UP

A SYMPTOM CHECKLIST FOR DEVELOPMENTAL DISABILITIES

Edna D. Copeland, Ph.D., Director
Child/Clinical Psychologist

Southeastern Psychological Institute
P.O. Box 12389
Atlanta, Georgia 30355-2389

Dedicated to Prevention through Early Intervention ℠
©Copyright, Edna D. Copeland Ph.D., 1984, 1987

NEED FOR EARLY RECOGNITION OF DEVELOPMENTAL PROBLEMS IN PRESCHOOLERS

The years from 4 through 6 are critical years in the intellectual, visual-motor, psycholinguistic and personality development of the child. Although often treated as an in-between age, this age period constitutes a well-defined landmark in the young child's mental, language, visual, perceptual and motor development. It is also the period when he/she is exposed for the first time to some type of formal education and is brought into wider social contacts with children of his/her own age. By age 4 a child's intellectual, psycholinguistic, visual-motor and personality characteristics are developed sufficiently well to determine deviations, both positively and negatively. By age 5 almost every precursor of learning, attention and behavior problems is apparent. Likewise, giftedness and accelerated capabilities are also easily recognized. All children have individual patterns of relative assets and weaknesses. It is important to understand these even in the child without special needs or gifts so that his assets can be realized to the fullest.

Approximately 27% of the preschool population has been described as "At Risk" for Developmental Disabilities. For preventive reasons, it appears expedient to recognize developmental delays in children between the ages of 4½ to 6. Careful evaluation, planning and remediation can preclude or minimize, as much as possible, learning, attention, and behavior disorders at the elementary school level. Likewise, plans can be made to provide for the gifted or talented child's special needs. Relatively individualized programs for all children can be established to capitalize upon their assets.

The **SOUTHEASTERN PSYCHOLOGICAL INSTITUTE** is especially concerned with identifying and remediating Developmental Disabilities. It is far easier to treat and remediate difficulties at an early age before children have experienced failure, frustration and subsequent academic, social, and emotional problems.

The Symptom Checklist for Developmental Disabilities was developed by Dr. Edna D. Copeland after 15 years of clinical practice to help parents and teachers determine whether their children or the children they teach have Developmental Disabilities.

SYMPTOM CHECKLIST

This checklist was developed from the experience of many specialists in the fields which comprise Developmental Disabilities. The questions asked are warning signals of conditions which may interfere with your child's academic, emotional and social adjustment now and in the future.

If you answer "Yes" to as many as 20% of the questions, it may mean that your child has a Developmental Disability. A Developmental Disability does not mean that a child is lacking in intelligence or capability. Rather, it means that a child might have difficulty achieving academically and/or socially at his/her level of ability.

Directions: Place a checkmark (✔) by those questions to which your answer is "Yes". Do not mark questions to which you answer "No".

SYMPTOM CHECKLIST FOR DEVELOPMENTAL DISABILITIES

I. ATTENTION / CONCENTRATION / IMPULSE CONTROL / BEHAVIOR

___ 1. Does your child interrupt frequently?

___ 2. Is your child easily distracted?

___ 3. Is your child up and down frequently during meals?

___ 4. Is your child's work often sloppy although it can be neat if he/she really tries?

___ 5. Does your child move from activity to activity without settling down to any one thing for long?

___ 6. Is there inconsistency in your child's performance, i.e., one day he/she performs a task well; the next day, he/she performs the same task poorly?

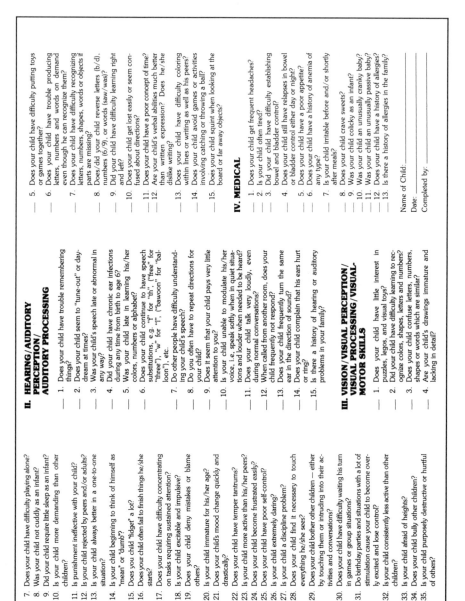

7. Does your child have difficulty playing alone?
8. Was your child not cuddly as an infant?
9. Did your child require little sleep as an infant?
10. Is your child more demanding than other children?
11. Is punishment ineffective with your child?
12. Is your child rejected by peers and/or adults?
13. Is your child always better in a one-to-one situation?
14. Is your child beginning to think of himself as "mean" or "dumb"?
15. Does you child "fidget" a lot?
16. Does your child often fail to finish things he/she starts?
17. Does your child have difficulty concentrating on tasks requiring sustained attention?
18. Is your child excitable and impulsive?
19. Does your child deny mistakes or blame others?
20. Is your child immature for his/her age?
21. Does your child's mood change quickly and drastically?
22. Does your child have temper tantrums?
23. Is your child more active than his/her peers?
24. Does your child become frustrated easily?
25. Does your child have poor self-control?
26. Is your child extremely daring?
27. Is your child a discipline problem?
28. Does your child find it necessary to touch everything he/she sees?
29. Does your child bother other children — either by touching them or intruding into their activities and conversations?
30. Does your child have difficulty waiting his turn in games or group situations?
31. Do birthday parties and situations with a lot of stimulation cause your child to become overly excited and lose control?
32. Is your child consistently less active than other children?
33. Is your child afraid of heights?
34. Does your child bully other children?
35. Is your child purposely destructive or hurtful of others?

II. HEARING/AUDITORY PERCEPTION/ AUDITORY PROCESSING

1. Does your child have trouble remembering things?
2. Does your child seem to "tune-out" or daydream at times?
3. Was your child's speech late or abnormal in any way?
4. Did your child have chronic ear infections during any time from birth to age 6?
5. Was your child late in learning his/her colors, numbers or alphabet?
6. Does your child continue to have speech substitutions, e.g. "f" for "th", ("free" for "three"), "w" for "l", ("bawoon" for "balloon"), etc.
7. Do other people have difficulty understanding your child's speech?
8. Do you often have to repeat directions for your child?
9. Does it seem that your child pays very little attention to you?
10. Is your child unable to modulate his/her voice, i.e. speak softly when in quiet situations and louder when needed to be heard?
11. Does your child talk very loudly, even during normal conversations?
12. When called from another room, does your child frequently not respond?
13. Does your child frequently turn the same ear in the direction of sound?
14. Does your child complain that his ears hurt or ring?
15. Is there a history of hearing or auditory problems in your family?

III. VISION/VISUAL PERCEPTION/ VISUAL PROCESSING/VISUAL-MOTOR SKILLS

1. Does your child have little interest in puzzles, legos, and visual toys?
2. Did your child have difficulty learning to recognize colors, shapes, letters and numbers?
3. Does your child confuse letters, numbers, shapes or words which are similar?
4. Are your child's drawings immature and lacking in detail?

5. Does your child have difficulty putting toys or games together?
6. Does your child have trouble producing letters, numbers and words on demand even though he can recognize them?
7. Does your child have difficulty recognizing letters, numbers, shapes, words or objects if parts are missing?
8. Does/did your child reverse letters (b/d), numbers (6/9), or words (saw/was)?
9. Did your child have difficulty learning right and left?
10. Does your child get lost easily or seem confused about directions?
11. Does your child have a poor concept of time?
12. Are your child's verbal abilities much better than written expression? Does he/she dislike writing?
13. Does your child have difficulty coloring within lines or writing as well as his peers?
14. Does your child avoid games or activities involving catching or throwing a ball?
15. Does your child squint when looking at the board or far away objects?

IV. MEDICAL

1. Does your child get frequent headaches?
2. Is your child often tired?
3. Did your child have difficulty establishing bowel and bladder control?
4. Does your child still have relapses in bowel or bladder control either day or night?
5. Does your child have a poor appetite?
6. Does your child have a history of anemia of any type?
7. Is your child irritable before and/or shortly after meals?
8. Does your child crave sweets?
9. Was your child colicky as an infant?
10. Was your child an unusually cranky baby?
11. Was your child an unusually passive baby?
12. Does your child have a history of allergies?
13. Is there a history of allergies in the family?

Name of Child: _____

Date: _____

Completed by: _____

Southeastern Psychological INSTITUTE

A CHECK UP for ELEMENTARY SCHOOL CHILDREN

A SYMPTOM CHECKLIST FOR DEVELOPMENTAL DISABILITIES

Edna D. Copeland, Ph.D., Director
Child / Clinical Psychologist

Southeastern Psychological Institute
P.O. Box 12389
Atlanta, Georgia 30355-2389

Dedicated to Prevention through Early Intervention

©Copyright, Edna D. Copeland, Ph.D., 1984, 1987

PREVENTION OF LEARNING, BEHAVIOR AND EMOTIONAL DISORDERS THROUGH EARLY IDENTIFICATION, REMEDIATION, TREATMENT AND EDUCATION.

It is becoming increasingly apparent that school failure, behavioral problems, juvenile delinquency, drug and alcohol abuse, and problems have their origins very early in life. Some estimate that as many as 70% of both the learning and emotional problems encountered in adolescents and adults began in unrecognized problems of childhood. Many of these difficulties can be detected by age 6, and younger, as developmental disabilities. These disabilities include learning disorders; communicative disorders; visual-perceptual, visual processing and visual-motor integration deficits; disorders of attention, concentration and perseverance; delayed emotional development; behavioral disorders; and hyperactivity. Subtle physical, visual and hearing problems can also contribute to early school failure and subsequent behavioral and emotional difficulties.

It is the belief of the SOUTHEASTERN PSYCHOLOGICAL INSTITUTE that early identification followed by careful planning, treatment and remediation can eliminate, or significantly minimize, learning, attention, academic, or significantly behavioral problems at the elementary school level when the problems are milder and more amenable to intervention. It can save the child from facing years of school failure which, in turn, can lead to frustration, loss of self-esteem, acting-out, and other emotional difficulties. Early identification and intervention, likewise, spare families the pain and frustration of feeling they are responsible but helpless to change things. In addition, improvement occurs rapidly at younger ages.

Parents are the first to recognize that something is not "exactly right" with their child. However, they frequently do not know whether their concerns are really significant, which things the child will "grow out of", and which warrant professional consultation.

The Symptom Checklist for Developmental Disabilities was developed by Dr. Edna Copeland, after 15 years of clinical practice, to help parents and teachers determine whether their children or the children they teach have developmental difficulties that are either learning, attentional, behavioral, social or emotional in nature.

If you have checked many items and have concerns after completing this questionnaire, you are encouraged to discuss your child's development with his/her teacher and/or pediatrician, or a child psychologist. Addressing even mild developmental delays early is crucial for the child's ultimate welfare. Determining strengths is, likewise, important.

SYMPTOM CHECKLIST

This checklist was developed from the experience of many specialists in the fields which comprise Developmental Disabilities. The questions asked are warning signals of conditions which may interfere with your child's academic, emotional and social adjustment now and in the future.

If you answer "Yes" to as many as 20% of the questions, it may mean that your child has a Developmental Disability. A Developmental Disability does *not* mean that a child is lacking in intelligence or capability. Rather, it means that a child may have difficulty achieving academically and socially at his/her level of ability.

Directions: Place a checkmark (✓) by those questions to which your answer is "Yes". Do not mark questions to which you answer "No".

SYMPTOM CHECKLIST FOR DEVELOPMENTAL DISABILITIES

I. ATTENTION/CONCENTRATION/ IMPULSE CONTROL/BEHAVIOR

— 1. Does your child interrupt frequently?
— 2. Is your child easily distracted?
— 3. Is your child up and down frequently during meals?
— 4. Is your child's work often sloppy although it can be neat if he/she really tries?
— 5. Does your child move from activity to activity without settling down to any one thing for long?
— 6. Is there inconsistency in your child's performance, i.e. one day he/she performs a task well, the next day, he/she performs the same task poorly?

— 7. Does your child have difficulty playing alone?
— 8. Was your child not cuddly as an infant?
— 9. Did your child require little sleep as an infant?
— 10. Is your child more demanding than other children?
— 11. Is punishment ineffective with your child?
— 12. Is your child always better in a one-to-one situation?
— 13. Does your child "fidget" a lot?
— 14. Does your child often fail to finish things he/she starts?
— 15. Does your child have difficulty concentrating on tasks requiring sustained attention?
— 16. Is your child excitable and impulsive?
— 17. Is your child immature for his/her age?
— 18. Does your child's mood change quickly and drastically?
— 19. Is your child more active than his/her peers?
— 20. Does your child become frustrated easily?
— 21. Does your child have poor self-control?
— 22. Is your child extremely daring?
— 23. Is your child a discipline problem?
— 24. Does your child find it necessary to touch everything he/she sees?
— 25. Does your child bother other children — either by touching them or intruding into their activities and conversations?
— 26. Does your child have difficulty waiting his turn in games or group situations?
— 27. Do birthday parties and situations with a lot of stimulation cause your child to become overly excited and lose control?
— 28. Is your child consistently less active than other children?

II. SOCIAL/EMOTIONAL

— 1. Is your child rejected or ignored by peers and/or adults?

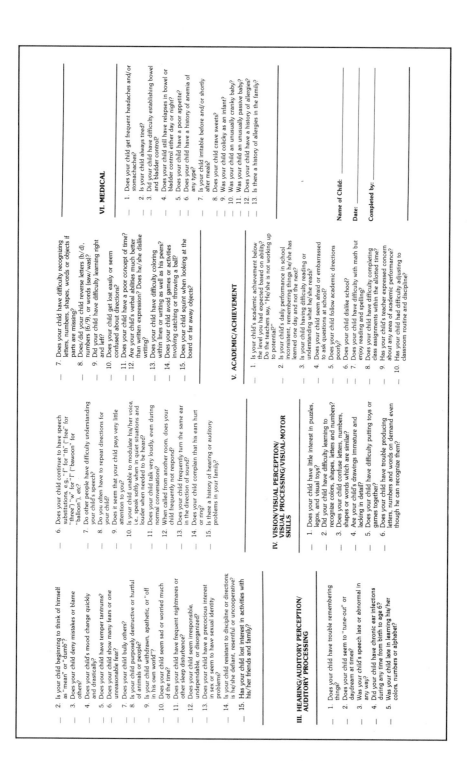

- 2. Is your child beginning to think of himself as "mean" or "dumb"?
- 3. Does your child deny mistakes or blame others?
- 4. Does your child's mood change quickly and drastically?
- 5. Does your child have temper tantrums?
- 6. Does your child show many fears or one unreasonable fear?
- 7. Does your child bully others?
- 8. Is your child purposely destructive or hurtful of animals or people?
- 9. Is your child withdrawn, apathetic, or "off in his own world"?
- 10. Does your child seem sad or worried much of the time?
- 11. Does your child have frequent nightmares or other sleep disturbance?
- 12. Does your child seem irresponsible, undependable, or disorganized?
- 13. Does your child have a precocious interest in sex or seem to have sexual identity problems?
- 14. Is your child resistant to discipline or directions; is he/she defiant, resentful or uncooperative?
- 15. Has your child lost interest in activities with his/her friends and family?

III. HEARING/AUDITORY PERCEPTION/AUDITORY PROCESSING

- 1. Does your child have trouble remembering things?
- 2. Does your child seem to "tune-out" or daydream at times?
- 3. Was your child's speech late or abnormal in any way?
- 4. Did your child have chronic ear infections during any time from birth to age 6?
- 5. Was your child late in learning his/her colors, numbers or alphabet?

- 6. Does your child continue to have speech substitutions, e.g., "f" for "th" ("free" for "three") "w" for "l" ("bawoon" for "balloon"), etc?
- 7. Do other people have difficulty understanding your child's speech?
- 8. Do you often have to repeat directions for your child?
- 9. Does it seem that your child pays very little attention to you?
- 10. Is your child unable to modulate his/her voice, i.e., speak softly when in quiet situations and louder when needed to be heard?
- 11. Does your child talk very loudly, even during normal conversations?
- 12. When called from another room, does your child frequently not respond?
- 13. Does your child frequently turn the same ear in the direction of sound?
- 14. Does your child complain that his ears hurt or ring?
- 15. Is there a history of hearing or auditory problems in your family?

IV. VISION/VISUAL PERCEPTION/VISUAL PROCESSING/VISUAL-MOTOR SKILLS

- 1. Does your child have little interest in puzzles, legos, and visual toys?
- 2. Did your child have difficulty learning to recognize colors, shapes, letters and numbers?
- 3. Does your child confuse letters, numbers, shapes or words which are similar?
- 4. Are your child's drawings immature and lacking in detail?
- 5. Does your child have difficulty putting toys or games together?
- 6. Does your child have trouble producing letters, numbers and words on demand even though he can recognize them?

- 7. Does your child have difficulty recognizing letters, numbers, shapes, words or objects if parts are missing?
- 8. Does/did your child reverse letters (b/d), numbers (6/9), or words (saw/was)?
- 9. Did your child have difficulty learning right and left?
- 10. Does your child get lost easily or seem confused about directions?
- 11. Does your child have a poor concept of time?
- 12. Are your child's verbal abilities much better than written expression? Does he/she dislike writing?
- 13. Does your child have difficulty coloring within lines or writing as well as his peers?
- 14. Does your child avoid games or activities involving catching or throwing a ball?
- 15. Does your child squint when looking at the board or far away objects?

V. ACADEMIC/ACHIEVEMENT

- 1. Is your child's academic achievement below the level you had expected based on ability? Do the teachers say, "He/she is not working up to potential?"
- 2. Is your child's daily performance in school inconsistent, remembering things he/she has learned one day and not the next?
- 3. Is your child having difficulty reading or understanding what he/she reads?
- 4. Does your child seem afraid or embarrassed to ask questions at school?
- 5. Does your child follow academic directions poorly?
- 6. Does your child dislike school?
- 7. Does your child have difficulty with math but enjoy reading and spelling?
- 8. Does your child have difficulty completing class assignments within the allotted time?
- 9. Has your child's teacher expressed concern about any area of academic performance?
- 10. Has your child had difficulty adjusting to classroom routine and discipline?

VI. MEDICAL

- 1. Does your child get frequent headaches and/or stomachaches?
- 2. Is your child always tired?
- 3. Did your child have difficulty establishing bowel and bladder control?
- 4. Does your child still have relapses in bowel or bladder control either day or night?
- 5. Does your child have a poor appetite?
- 6. Does your child have a history of anemia of any type?
- 7. Is your child irritable before and/or shortly after meals?
- 8. Does your child crave sweets?
- 9. Was your child colicky as an infant?
- 10. Was your child an unusually cranky baby?
- 11. Was your child an unusually passive baby?
- 12. Does your child have a history of allergies?
- 13. Is there a history of allergies in the family?

Name of Child: _____

Date: _____

Completed by: _____

APPENDIX 5

Sources of Tests Discussed in Chapter 4

A. Continuous Performance Test (CPT)

There are many varieties of this instrument which have been developed as versions of the original continuous Performance Test by Roswald and Associates.

T.O.V.A.©
Test of Variables of Attention
Universal Attentions Disorders
4281 Katella Avenue, #215
Los Alamitos, CA 90720

Gardner Steadiness Test
Lafayette Instrument Company
P.O. Box 1279
LaFayette, IN 47902

Gordon Diagnostic System (GDS)
(Vigilance Task and Delay Task)
Gordon Diagnostic System
P.O. Box 746
DeWitt, NY 13214

B. Matching Familiar Figures Test (MFFT)

Jerome Kagan, Ph.D.
William James Hall
Harvard University
33 Kirkland Street
Cambridge, MA 02138

C. Pediatric Early Elementary Examination, (Peeramid) and Pediatric Examination of Educational Readiness at Middle School. *Structured Interviews*, especailly for pediatricians, by Melvin Levin, M.D.

Educators Publishing Service, Inc.
75 Moulton Street
Cambridge, MA 02138-1104

APPENDIX 6

Selected Bibliography
Coping with the Grief
of ADHD/ADD and LD

Fowler, Mary Cahill (1990). *Maybe You Know My Kid: A Parent's Guide to Identifying, Understanding, and Helping Your Child with Attention-Deficit Hyperactivity Disorder.* Secaucus, New Jersey: Birch Lane Press.

Simons, Robin (1987). *After the Tears: Parents Talk about Raising a Child with a Disability.* New York: Harcourt Brace Jovanich.

APPENDIX 7

TSA and Suggested Readings in Tourette Syndrome:

Tourette Syndrome Association (TSA)
42-40 Bell Boulevard
Bayside, New York 11361
(718) 224-2999

Suggested Reading

Brunn, R.D., Cohen, D.J., & Lechman, J.F. (1990). *Guide to the Diagnosis and Treatment of Tourette Syndrome*. Bayside, NY: TS Association.

Buehrens, A. (1991). *Hi, I'm Adam*. Duarte, CA: Hope Press.

Chase, T. A., Friedhoff, A.J. & Cohen, D.J. (1991). "Tourette Syndrome: Genetics, Neurobiology and Treatment" in *Advances in Neurology*, Vol. 58. NY: Science Publishing.

Comings, D.E. (1990). *Tourette Syndrome and Human Behavior*. Duarte, CA: Hope Press.

Haerle, T. (Ed.) (1992). *Children with Tourette Syndrome: A Parent's Guide*. Rockville, MD: Woodbine Press.

Hughes, S. (1990). Ryan: *A Mother's Story of Her Hyperactive/Tourette Syndrome Child*. Duarte, CA: Hope Press.

Seligman, A.W. & Hilkevich, J.S. (1992). *Don't Think About Monkeys—Extraordinary Stories by People with Tourette Syndrome*. Duarte, CA: Hope Press

APPENDIX 8

U.S. DEPARTMENT OF EDUCATION
OFFICE FOR CIVIL RIGHTS
REGIONAL CIVIL RIGHTS OFFICES

Region I

Connecticut, Main, Massachusetts, New Hampshire, Rode Island, Vermont

Office for Civil Rights, Region I
U.S. Department of Education
John W. McCormack POCH
Room 222, 01-0061
Boston, Massachusetts 02109-4557
(617) 223-9662; TDD (617) 223-9695

Region II

New Jersey, New York, Puerto Rico, Virgin Islands

Office for Civil Rights, Region II
U.S. Department of Education
26 Federal Plaza, 33rd Floor
Room 33-130-1010
New York, New York 10278-0082
(212) 264-4633; TDD (212) 264-9464

Region III

Delaware, District of Columbia, Maryland, Pennsylvania, Virginia, West Virginia

Office for Civil Rights, Region III
U.S. Department of Education
3535 Market Street
Room 6300, 03-2010
Philadelphia, Pennsylvania 19104-3326
(215) 596-6772; TDD (215) 596-6794

Region IV

Alabama, Florida, Georgia, North Carolina, South Carolina

Office for Civil Rights, Region IV
U.S. Department of Education
P.O. Box 2048, 04-3010
Atlanta, Georgia 30301-2048
(404) 331-2954; TDD (404) 331-7816

Region V

Ilinois, Indiana, Minnesota, Michigan, Ohio, Wisconsin

Office for Civil Rights, Region V
U.S. Department of Education
401 South State Street
Room 700C, 05-4010
Chicago, Illinois 60605-1202
(312) 886-3456; TDD (312) 353-2541

Region VI

Arkansas, Louisiana, New Mexico, Oklahoma, Texas, Mississippi

Office for Civil Rights, Region VI
U.S. Department of Education
1200 Main Tower Building
Suite 2260, 06-5010
Dallas, Texas 75202-9998
(214) 767-3959; TDD (214) 767-3639

Region VII

Iowa, Kansas, Missouri, Nebraska, Kentucky

Office for Civil Rights, Region VII
U.S. Department of Education
10220 N. Executive Hill Blvd.
8th Floor 07-6010
Kansas City, Missouri 6413-1367
(816) 891-8026; TDD (816) 374-6461

Region VIII

Colorado, Montana, North Dakota, South Dakota, Utah, Wyoming

Office for Civil Rights, Region VIII
U.S. Department of Education
Federal Building
1244 Speer Blvd., Suite 310, 08-7010
Denver, Colorado 80204-3582
(303) 844-5695; TDD (303) 844-2417

Region IX

Arizona, California, Hawaii, Nevada, Guam, Trust Territory of the Pacific Islands, American Samoa

Office for Civil Rights, Region IX
U.S. Department of Education
Old Federal Building 09-8010
50 United Nations Plaza, Room 239
San Francisco, California 94102-4102
(415) 556-7000; TDD 556-6806

Region X

Alaska, Idaho, Oregon, Washington

Office for Civil Rights, Region X
U.S. Department of Education
925 Second Avenue
Room 3310, 10-9010
Seattle, Washington 98174-1099
(206) 220-7880; TDD (206) 220-7907

Glossary

ANOREXIA - loss of appetite.

ARACHNOID - the middle of the three membranes covering the brain and spinal cord with a cobweb-like texture.

ATTENTION - All the processes related to one's ability to discriminate adequately and to selectively respond to the various stimuli received by the brain at any given moment.

AXON - A nerve fiber which extends from the cell body of a neuron and carries the nerve impulse to a receptor neuron.

BASAL GANGLIA - several large masses of gray matter embedded deep in the white matter of the cerebrum. They regulate voluntary movements at a subconscious level.

BIPOLAR DISORDER - a disorder characterized by manic and depressive episodes.

BRAIN DOMINANCE - the preference for using one half of the brain over the other.

CEREBELLUM - the largest part of the hind brain which coordinates muscle movements.

CEREBRAL CORTEX - the intricately folded outer layer of the cerebrum responsible for perception, memory, thought, intellect and voluntary activity.

CEREBRAL HEMISPHERE - one of two paired halves of the cerebrum.

CEREBROSPINAL FLUID - the fluid surrounding the brain and spinal cord.

CHOLINE - a basic compound important for the synthesis of lecithin and other phospholipids, and acetylcholine.

CORPUS CALLOSUM - the bundle of tissue separating the two halves of the brain.

DENDRITE - one of the shorter branching processes of the cell body of a neuron important in synapses with other neurons.

DSM-IV™ - Diagnostic and Statistical Manual of Mental Disorders - Fourth Edition.

DURA MATER - the thick, outermost membrane of the three membranes surrounding the brain and spinal cord; it is next to the skull.

DYSLEXIA - a developmental disorder affecting a person's ability to learn to read and write.

DYSPHONIA - difficulty in speaking due to a disorder of the larynx, vocal cords, tongue, or mouth.

ECLAMPSIA - the occurrence of one or more convulsions, not caused by epilepsy or cerebral hemorrhage, in a woman with pregnancy-induced hypertension. It can result in coma, and it is dangerous to mother and baby.

ENDOGENOUS - arising within, or derived from, the body.

ENURESIS - the involuntary passing of urine, especially bed-wetting at night.

ETIOLOGY -the cause of a specific disease.

FRONTAL LOBE - the frontal part of each cerebral hemisphere. Responsible for the control of voluntary movement.

FRONTAL SYSTEM - includes frontal lobes, thalamus, hypothalamus, the limbic system and the basal ganglia. Responsible for controlling emotions, judgment, creativity, and will.

GRAY MATTER - the darker colored tissue of the central nervous system, composed mainly of the cell bodies of neurons. It covers the entire surface of the brain.

HYPERTHYROIDISM - overactivity of the thyroid gland.

HYPOGLYCEMIA - deficiency of glucose in the blood stream.

HYPOMANIA - a mild degree of mania. Elated mood leads to faulty judgment; behavior lacks the usual social restraints; speech is rapid; person is intense and/or irritable.

HYPOTHALAMUS - the region of the forebrain linked to the thalamus and the pituitary gland. It controls body temperature, thirst, hunger, eating, water balance, hormonal regulation and autonomic nervous activity.

HYPOTHYROIDISM - subnormal activity of the thyroid gland.

LIMBIC SYSTEM - set of structures and networks in the brain involved in the expression of mood and instinct. It governs the self-preservation instinct, and links thoughts and emotions.

MEDULLA OBLONGATA - the "reptile" brain responsible for regulation of the heart and blood vessels, respiration, salivation and swallowing.

MOTOR AREA - region of the cerebral cortex that is responsible for initiating nerve impulses that bring about voluntary activity.

NARCOLEPSY - an extreme tendency to fall asleep involving hallucinations/cataplexy.

NEUROLEPTIC DRUGS - drugs used principally to regulate symptoms of psychosis.

NEURON - nerve cell.

NEUROTRANSMITTER - a chemical substance released from nerve endings to transmit impulses across synapses to other nerves. Common ones include: dopamine, acetylcholine, serotonin.

NOREPINEPHRINE (noradrenalin) - a hormone; also a neurotransmitter.

NUCLEUS - the part of the cell that contains DNA.

OCCIPITAL LOBE - the lobe that receives and sends out visual information.

OTITIS MEDIA - inflammation of the middle ear.

PARIETAL LOBE - the "somatosensory" area. It receives information on bodily sensations and modulates spatial orientation.

PIA MATER - innermost of the three membranes surrounding the brain and spinal cord. It contours each fissure and sulcus of the surface of the brain.

PLANUM TEMPORALE - structure beneath the cerebral hemispheres related to language comprehension and production.

PREMOTOR CORTEX - the area where complex movements are organized.

PSYCHOTROPIC - describes drugs that affect mood, including antidepressants, sedatives, stimulants, and tranquilizers.

RECEPTOR - structure on the post-synaptic cell that is specific for one type of neurotransmitter.

RETICULAR ACTIVATING SYSTEM - a system of nerve pathways in the brain concerned with states of alertness and attention. The system integrates information from all of the senses and the brain and then determines the activities of the brain and the body.

RETICULAR FORMATION - a network of nerve pathways throughout the brain stem, connecting motor and sensory nerves to the cerebellum and the cerebrum.

SEROTONIN - a neurotransmitter, related to sleep.

SULCUS - an infolding of the brain.

SYNAPSE - the minute gap across which nerve impulses pass from one neuron to the next. An impulse is transmitted by the release of a neurotransmitter into the gap.

TEMPORAL LOBE - the region of the cortex concerned with sound and spoken language.

THALAMUS - one of two masses that lie deep in the cerebral hemispheres in each side of the forebrain. The thalami relay sensory messages to the cortex.

TOXEMIA - blood poisoning caused by toxins formed by a bacterial infection.

WHITE MATTER - nerve tissue of the central nervous system. In the brain, the white matter is beneath the gray matter.

References

Abikoff, H., & Gittelman, R. (1985). The normalizing effects of methylphenidate on classroom behavior of ADHD children. *Journal of Abnormal Child Psychology, 13*, 33-44.

Aldrich, M. (1990). Narcolepsy. *New England Journal of Medicine, 323*, 389-394.

Aman, M., & Kern, R. (1989). Review of fenfluramine in the treatment of developmental disabilities. *Journal of the American Academy of Child and Adolescent Psychiatry, 28*, 549-565.

American Academy of Pediatrics (AAP). (1985). Committee on drugs report: Behavioral and cognitive effects of anticonvulsant therapy. *Pediatrics, 76*, 644-647.

American Psychiatric Association. (1987). *Diagnostic and statistical manual of mental disorders* (3rd ed., rev.). Washington, DC: APA.

American Psychiatric Association. (1994). *Diagnostic and statistical manual of mental disorders (fourth edition)*. Washington, DC: APA.

Andreasen, N. (1984). *The broken brain: The biological revolution in psychiatry*. New York: Harper & Row.

Atlanta Constitution. (1987). Task force to study needs of hyperactive pupils. *The Atlanta Constitution*, 13 April, 15(A).

Atlanta Constitution. (1987). Parent sues over use of Ritalin to treat pupils. *The Atlanta Constitution*, 10 November, 33(A).

Atlanta Constitution. (1987). State may curb Ritalin use if consumption doesn't drop. *The Atlanta Constitution*, 8 June, 1(E).

Atlanta Journal and Constitution. (1987). Ritalin: Miracle or nightmare? Hyperactivity drug made one boy exemplary student, another school terror. *The Atlanta Journal and Constitution*, 29 November, 12(D).

August, G., & Garfinkel, B. (1989). Behavioral and cognitive subtypes of ADHD. *Journal of the American Academy of Child and Adolescent Psychiatry, 28*, 739-748.

Baker, L., & Cantwell, D. (1987). A prospective psychiatric follow-up of children with speech/language disorders. *Journal of the American Academy of Child Psychiatry, 26*, 546-553.

Ballinger, C., Varley, C., & Nolan, P. (1984). Effects of methylphenidate on reading in children with attention deficit disorder. *American Journal of Psychiatry, 141*, 1590-1593.

Barkley, R. (1977a). The effects of methylphenidate on various measures of activity level and attention in hyperkinetic children. *Journal of Abnormal Child Psychology, 5*, 351-369.

Barkley, R. (1977b). A review of stimulant drug research with hyperactive children. *Journal of Child Psychology and Psychiatry, 18*, 137-165.

Barkley, R. (1981). *Hyperactive children: A handbook for diagnosis and treatment*. New York: Guilford Press.

Barkley, R. (1988). The effects of methylphenidate on the interactions of preschool ADHD children with their mothers. *Journal of the American Academy of Child and Adolescent Psychiatry, 27*, 336-341.

Barkley, R., & Cunningham, C. (1979a). The effects of methylphenidate on the mother-child interactions of hyperactive children. *Archives of General Psychiatry, 36,* 201-208.

Barkley, R., & Cunningham, C. (1979b). Stimulant drugs and activity level in hyperactive children. *American Journal of Orthopsychiatry, 49,* 491-499.

Barkley, R., Karlsson, J., Strzelecki, E. & Murphy, J. (1984). Effects of age and Ritalin dosage on the mother-child interactions of hyperactive children. *Journal of Consulting and Clinical Psychology, 52,* 750-758.

Barkley, R., McMurray, M., Edelbrock, C., & Robbins, K. (1989). The response of aggressive and nonaggressive ADHD children to two doses of methylphenidate. *Journal of the American Academy of Child and Adolescent Psychiatry, 28,* 873-881.

Biederman, J., Baldessarini, R., Wright, V., Knee, D., & Harmatz, J. (1989a). A double-blind placebo controlled study of desipramine in the treatment of ADD: I. Efficacy. *Journal of the American Academy of Child and Adolescent Psychiatry, 28,* 777-784.

Biederman, J., Baldessarini, R., Wright, V., Knee, D., Harmatz, J., & Goldblatt, A. (1989b). A double-blind placebo controlled study of desipramine in the treatment of ADD: II. Serum drug levels and cardiovascular findings. *Journal of the American Academy of Child and Adolescent Psychiatry, 28,* 903-911.

Bowden, C., Deutsch, C., & Swanson, J. (1988). Plasma dopamine B-hydroxylase and platelet monoamine oxidase in attention deficit disorder and conduct disorder. *Journal of American Academy of Child and Adolescent Psychiatry, 27,* 171-174.

Bower, B. (1988). Hyperactivity: The family factor. *Science News,* 18 June, 399.

Bower, B. (1990). The ticcing link: Many mental disorders and a few crucial genes may tie into Tourette's syndrome. *Science News, 138* (21 July), 42-44.

Bradley, C. (1937).   The behavior of children receiving Benzedrine. *American Journal of Psychiatry, 94*, 577-585.

Bronheim, S. (1990). *An educator's guide to Tourette's Syndrome.* Booklet. Bayside, NY: Tourette Syndrome Association.

Brown, R., Abramowitz, A., Dulcan, M., & Madan-Swain, A. (1989). Attention deficit hyperactivity disorder: Diagnosis, management, prognosis and current research. *Emory University Journal of Medicine, 3*, 120-131.

Brown, T., & Sexson, S. (1989). Cardiovascular responses in attention deficit hyperactivity disordered adolescents. *Journal of Adolescent Health Care, 3*, 120-131.

Brunn, R., Cohen, D., & Leckman, J. (1990). *Guide to the diagnosis and treatment of Tourette Syndrome.* Bayside, NY: TSA Association.

Calis, K., Grothe, D., & Elia, J. (1990). Therapy reviews: Attention-deficit hyperactivity disorder. *Clinical Pharmacy, 9*, 632-642.

Callahan, M. (1988). Busy days, sleepless nights. *Parents Magazine, 63* (August), 177ff.

Cantwell, D. (1972). Psychiatric illness in the families of hyperactive children. *Archives of General Psychiatry, 27*, 414-427.

Cantwell, D. (1985). Hyperactive children have grown up. *Archives of General Psychiatry, 42*, 1026-1028.

Carey, P. (1983). *Determination of a range of concern for mobile source emissions of formaldehyde based only on its toxicological properties.* Ann Arbor, MI: U.S. Environmental Protection Agency. Technical report EPA-AA-TSS 83-5, July, 1983.

Carroll, J., Jefferson, J., & Greist, J. (1987). Psychiatric uses of lithium for children and adolescents. *Hospital Community Psychiatry, 38*, 927-928.

Casat, C., Pleasants, D., & Van Wyck Fleet, J. (1987). A double-blind trial of bupropion in children with attention deficit disorder. *Psychopharmacology Bulletin, 23*, 120-122.

Citizens Commission on Human Rights (Sponsored by Church of Scientology) (1987). *How psychiatry is making drug addicts out of America's school children* (CCHR Information Letter #1). Los Angeles: Author.

Cohen, D., et al., (Eds.). (1987). *Tourette's syndrome and tic disorders.* New York: John Wiley.

Coleman, W., & Levine, M. (1988). Attention deficits in adolescence: Description, evaluation, and management. *Pediatrics in Review, 9,* 287-298.

Collier, C., Soldin, S., Swanson, J., MacLeod, S., Weinberg, F., & Rochefort, J. (1985). Pemoline pharmacokinetics and long-term therapy in children with attention deficit disorder and hyperactivity. *Clinical Pharmacokinetics, 10,* 269-278.

Collins, B., Whalen, C., & Henker, B. (1980). Ecological and pharmacological influences on behaviors in the classroom. The hyperkinetic syndrome. In S. Salzinger, J. Antrobus, & J. Glick (Eds.), *The ecosystem of the "sick" child.* New York: Academic Press.

Comings, D. (1990). *Tourette syndrome and human behavior.* Duarte, CA: Hope Press.

Conners, C. (1979). The acute effects of caffeine on evoked response, vigilance, and activity level in hyperkinetic children. *Journal of Abnormal Child Psychology, 7,* 145-151.

Conners, C. (1980). *Food additives and hyperactive children.* New York: Plenum Press.

Conners, C. (1990). *Food and behavior.* Presented at second annual CH.A.D.D. conference, Washington, DC, 9 November. Audiotape. Plantation, FL: Ch.A.D.D.

Conners, C., & Taylor, E. (1980). Pemoline, methylphenidate and placebo in children with minimal brain dysfunction. *Archives of General Psychiatry, 37,* 922-932.

Copeland, E. (1989). *Attention disorders: The school's vital role.* Videoprogram. Atlanta, GA: Resurgens Press, Inc.

Copeland, E., & Love, V. (1991). *Attention, please! A comprehensive guide for successfully parenting children with attention disorders and hyperactivity (ADHD/ADD).* Atlanta, GA: Resurgens Press, Inc.

Copeland, E., & Love, V. (1990). *Attention without tension: The teacher's handbook on attention disorders (ADHD and ADD).* Atlanta, GA: Resurgens, Inc.

Copeland, E. & Walker R. *(1994). Diverse Teaching for Diverse Learners: A Handbook for Teachers and Parents.* Atlanta, GA: Resurgens Press, Inc.

Copps, Stephen C. (1992). *The Attending Physcian - Attention Deficit Disorders: A Guide for Pediatricians and Family Physicians.* Atlanta, GA: Resurgens Press, Inc.

Cowen, E., Pederson, A., Babigan, H., Izzo, L., & Trost, M. (1973). Long-term follow-up of early detected vulnerable children. *Journal of Consulting and Clinical Psychology, 41,* 438-446.

Cowley, G., Springen, K., Gordon, J., & Koehl, C. (1991). A Prozac backlash. *Newsweek,* 1 April, 64-67.

Cowley, G., Springen, K., Leonard, E., Robins, K., & Gordon, J. (1990). The promise of Prozac. *Newsweek,* 26 March, 37-41.

Crook, W. (1985). *Tracking down hidden food allergy.* Jackson, TN: Professional Books.

Cunningham, C., Siegel, L., & Offord, D. (1985). A developmental dose-response analysis of the effects of methylphenidate on the peer interactions of attention deficit disordered boys. *Journal of Child Psychology and Psychiatry, 26,* 955-971.

David, O., Clark, J., & Voeller, K. (1972). Lead and hyperactivity. *Lancet,* 28 October, 900-903.

Demilio, L. (1989). Psychiatric syndromes in adolescent substance abusers. *American Journal of Psychiatry, 146,* 1212-1214.

DeNelsky, G., & Denenberg, V. (1967). Infantile stimulation and adult exploratory behavior: Effects of handling upon tactual variation seeking. *Journal of Comparative and Physiological Psychology, 63,* 309-312.

Denson, R., Nanson, J., & McWatters, M. (1975). Hyperkinesis and maternal smoking. *Canadia n Psychiatric Association Journal, 20*, 183-187.

Dickey, C. (1991). Why can't we understand the Arabs. *Newsweek*, 7 January, 26-27.

Donnelly, M., & Rapoport, J. (1985). Attention deficit disorders. In J. Wiener (Ed.), *Diagnosis and psychopharmacology of childhood and adolescent disorders* (pp. 179-197). New York: John Wiley.

Donnelly, M., Zametkin, A., & Rapoport, J., Ismond, D, Weingartner, H., Lane, E., Oliver, J., Linnoila, M., & Potter, M. (1986). Treatment of childhood hyperactivity with desipramine: plasma drug concentration, cardiovascular effects, plasma and urinary catecholamine levels, and clinical response. *Clinical Pharmacology Therapy, 39*, 72-81.

Douglas, V., Barr, R., O'Neil, M., & Britton, B. (1986). Short-term effects of methylphenidate on the cognitive, learning, and academic performance of children with attention deficit disorder in the laboratory and classroom. *Journal of Child Psychology and Psychiatry, 27*, 191-211.

Dulcan, M. (1990). Using psychostimulants to treat behavioral disorders of children and adolescents. *Journal of Child and Adolescent Psychopharmacology, 1*, 7-20.

Dykman, R., McGrew, J., Harris, T., Peters, J., & Ackerman, P. (1976). Two blinded studies of the effects of stimulant drugs on children: Pemoline, methylphenidate and placebo. In R.T. Anderson and C.G. Halcomb (Eds.), *Learning disability/minimal brain dysfunction syndrome.* (pp. 217-235). Springfield, Il: Thomas.

Education for All Handicapped Children Act. U.S. Code. 1982. Title 20, secs. 1232, 1401, 1405, 1406, 1411-1420, 1453.

Elia, J. (1989). In "Helping children with attention disorders" by Dixie Farley, *FDA Consumer*, 23 (1), 11-15.

Egger, J., Carter, C., Graham, P., Gumley, D., & Soothill, J. (1985). Controlled trial of oligoantigenic treatment in the hyperkinetic syndrome. *Lancet*, 9 March, 540-545.

Famularo, R., & Fenton, T. (1987). The effects of methylphenidate on school grades in children with attention deficit disorder without hyperactivity: A preliminary report. *Journal of Clinical Psychiatry, 48*, 112-114.

Federal Register, Vol. 45, No. 92, May 9, 1980. "Rules and Regulations," 30936-30955, GPO 892-250.

Feingold, B. (1975). *Why your child is hyperactive*. New York: Random House.

Ferry, P., Banner, W., & Wolf, R. (1986). *Seizure disorders in children*. Philadelphia: J.B. Lippincott Co.

Friedman, J., Carr, R., Elders, J., Ringdahal, I., & Roache, A. (1981). Effect on growth in pemoline treated children with attention deficit disorder. *Medical Journal Dis. Child, 135*, 329-332.

Garfinkel, B., Webster, C., & Sloman, L. (1981). Responses to methylphenidate and varied doses of caffeine in children with attention deficit disorders. *Canadian Journal of Psychiatry, 26*, 395-401.

Georgia Department of Education. (1987). *Report to Dr. Werner Rogers by Attention Deficit Disorder Study Group* (appointed by the Department of Education), 10 August. Atlanta, GA: author.

Gittelman-Klein, R. (1974). Pilot clinical trial of imipramine in hyperkinetic children. In C.K. Conners (Ed.), *Clinical use of stimulant drugs in children*. Amsterdam Excerpta Medica, 193.

Gittelman-Klein, R., & Feingold, I. (1983). Children with reading disorders. II. Effects of methylphenidate in combination with reading remediation. *Journal of Child Psychology and Psychiatry, 24*, 193-212.

Gold, B. (1990). School was a nightmare for Tracey. *Redbook* (March), 46-49.

Golden, G. (1988). The relationship between stimulant medication and tics. *Pediatric Annals, 17*, 405-408.

Goldstein, S., & Goldstein, M. (1990). *Managing attention disorders in children*. New York: John Wiley & Sons.

Gray, D., & Kavanaugh, J. (1985). *Biobehavioral measures of dyslexia*. Parkton, MD: York Press.

Gross-Glenn, K., Duara, R., Yoshii, R., et al. (1986). PET-scan studies during reading in dyslexic and non-dyslexic adults. *Neuroscience, 146,* 33-35.

Hagerman, R., & Falkenstein, A. (1987). An association between recurrent otitis media in infancy and later hyperactivity. *Clinical Pediatrics, 5,* 253-257.

Hart, S., & McKenzie, A. (1989). Inspirational obstruction blown away. *Biomedicine,* 7 October, 233.

Harter, M., Diering, S. & Wood, F. (1988). Separate brain potential characteristics in children with reading disability and attention deficit disorder: Relevance-independent effects. *Brain and Cognition, 7,* 54-86.

Hartsough, C., & Lambert, N. (1985). Medical factors in hyperactive and normal children: Prenatal, developmental, and health history findings. *American Journal of Orthopsychiatry, 55,* 190-210.

Healy, J. (1987). *Your child's growing mind*. Garden City, NJ: Doubleday.

Hebb, D. (1947). The effects of early experience on problem solving at maturity. *American Psychologist, 2,* 306-307.

Hechtman, L., Weiss, G., & Perlman, T. (1984). Young adult outcome of hyperactive children who received long-term stimulant treatment. *Journal of American Academy of Child Psychiatry, 23,* 261-269.

Henker, B., Astor-Dubin, L., & Varni, J. (1986). Psychostimulant medication and perceived intensity in hyperactive children. *Journal of Abnormal Child Psychology, 14,* 105-114.

Hoge, S., & Biederman, J. (1986). A case of Tourette's syndrome with symptoms of attention deficit disorder treated with desipramine. *Journal of Clinical Psychiatry, 47,* 478-479.

Holborow, P., & Berry, P. (1986). Hyperactivity and learning difficulties. *Journal of Learning Disabilities, 19,* 426-431.

Holdsworth, L., & Whitmore, K. (1974). A study of children with epilepsy attending ordinary schools: I. Their seizure patterns, progress, and behavior in school. *Developmental Medicine and Child Neurology, 16*, 746-758.

Horachek, H. (1991). Wellbutrin - a new drug for treating ADD. *A.D.D. Ventures*, February, 11.

Huessy, H., & Wright, A. (1970). The use of imipramine in children's behavior disorders. *ACTA Paedopsychiatrica, 37*, 194-199.

Hunt, R. (1987). Treatment effects of oral and transdermal clonidine in relation to methylphenidate: An open pilot study in ADD-H. *Psychopharmacology Bulletin, 23*, 111-114.

Hunt, R., Capper, L., & O'Connell, P. (1990). Clonidine in child and adolescent psychiatry. *Journal of Child and Adolescent Psychopharmacology, 1*, 87-102.

Hynd, G., & Semrud-Clikeman, M. (1989). Dyslexia and brain morphology. *Psychological Bulletin, 106*, 447-482.

Hynd, G., Semrud-Clikeman, M., Lorys, A., Novey, E., & Eliopulos, D. (1990). Brain morphology in developmental dyslexia and attention deficit disorder/hyperactivity. *Archives of Neurology, 47*, 919-926.

Interagency Committee on Learning Disabilities. (1987). *Learning disabilities: A report to the U.S. Congress* (pp. 194-217). Washington, DC: GPO.

Jensen, J., & Garfinkel, B. (1988). Neuroendocrine aspects of attention deficit hyperactivity disorder. *Endocrinology and Metabolism Clinics of North America, 17:1*, 111-129.

Johnston, C., Pelham, W., Hoza, J., & Sturges, J. (1988). Psychostimulant rebound in attention deficit disordered boys. *Journal of American Academy of Child and Adolescent Psychiatry, 27*, 806-810.

Kalachnik, J., Sprague, R., Sleator, E., Cohen, M., & Ullmann, R. (1982). Effect of methylphenidate hydrochloride on stature of hyperactive children. *Developmental Medicine Child Neurology, 24*, 586-595.

Kaplan, B., McNicol, J., Conte, R., & Moghadam, H. (1989). Dietary replacement in preschool-aged hyperactive boys. *Pediatrics, 83*, 7-17.

Kealy, E.R. (1990). Questions still remain on attention deficit disorders. (Commentary). *Education Week*, 28 November, 23.

Kelly, P., Cohen, M., Walker, W., Caskey, O., & Atkinson, A. (1989). Self-esteem in children medically managed for attention deficit disorder. *Pediatrics, 83*, 211-217.

Kinsbourne, M., & Caplan, P. (1979). *Children's learning and attention problems*. Boston: Little, Brown & Co.

Klee, S., Garfinkel, B., & Beauchesen, H. (1986). Attention deficits in adults. *Psychiatric Annals, 16*, 52-56.

Klein, R., & Mannuzza, S. (1988). Hyperactive boys almost grown up. *Archives of General Psychiatry, 45*, 1131-1134.

Klóve, H. (1984). Discussion in L.J. Bloomingdale (Ed.), *Attention deficit disorder: Diagnostic, cognitive and therapeutic understanding* (pp. 60-67). New York: Spectrum Publications, Inc.

Kohn, A. (1989). Suffer the restless children. *The Atlantic Monthly, 264* (November), 90-100.

Kohn, A. (1989). Suffer the restless children. *Education Week*, 22 November.

Kramer, P.D. (1993). *Listening to Prozac*. New York: Viking Press.

Leber, P. (1988). Letter to Ciba-Geigy Corporation, 12 May. Rockville, MD: U.S. Department of Health and Human Services, FDA.

Levine, M., & Melmed, R. (1982). The unhappy wanderers: Children with attention deficits. *Pediatric Clinics of North America, 29*, 105-120.

Licamele, W., & Goldberg, R. (1989). The concurrent use of lithium and methylphenidate in a child. *Journal of the American Academy of Child and Adolescent Psychiatry, 28*, 785-787.

Locke, J. (1762). *On the conduct of the understanding*. Section XXX.

Long, M. (1987). What is this thing called sleep? *National Geographic, 172* (December), 787-821.

Lou, H., Henriksen, L., Bruhn, P., Borner, H., & Nielsen, J. (1989). Striatal dysfunction in attention deficit and hyperkinetic disorder. *Archives of Neurology, 46*, 48-52.

Love, A., & Thompson, M. (1988). Language disorders and attention deficit disorders in young children referred for psychiatric services: Analysis of prevalence and a conceptual synthesis. *American Journal of Orthopsychiatry, 58*, 52-64.

Maloney, S. (1982). Indian Brook to reopen Wednesday. *Plymouth (MA) Old Colony Memorial*, 7 October, 1.

Marshall, P. (1989). Attention deficit disorder and allergy: A neurochemical model of the relation between the illnesses. *Psychological Bulletin, 106*, 434-436.

Masland, R., & Masland, M. (1988). *Prevention of reading failure.* Parkton, MD: York Press.

Mattes, J. (1980). The role of frontal lobe dysfunction in childhood hyperkinesis. *Comprehensive Psychiatry, 21*, 358-369.

McClellan, J., Rubert, M., Reichler, R., & Sylvester, C. (1990). Attention deficit disorders in children at risk for anxiety and depression. *Journal of the American Academy of Child and Adolescent Psychiatry, 29*, 534-339.

McIntyke, H. (1982). *The primary care of seizure disorders.* Woburn, MA: Butterworth Publishers.

McNutt, B., Ballard, J., & Boileau, R. (1976). The effects of long-term stimulant medication on growth and body composition of hyperactive children. *Psychopharmacology Bulletin, 12*, 13-14.

Mesulam, M. (1986). Frontal cortex and behavior. *Annals of Neurology, 19*, 320-325.

Miller, J. (1990). E.D. moves to halt aid to Georgia district, state agency. *Education Week*, 5 September, 34, 39.

Morrison, J., & Stewart, M. (1971). A family study of hyperactive child syndrome. *Biological Psychiatry, 3*, 189-195.

Needleman, H., Gunnoe, C., Leviton, A., Reed, R., Peresie, H., Maber, C., & Barrett, P. (1979). Deficits in psychologic and classroom performance of children with elevated dentine lead levels. *New England Journal of Medicine, 300*, 689-695.

Nelson, K., & Ellenberg, J. (1979). Apgar scores and long-term neurological handicap. *Annals of Neurology, 6,* 1982 (abstract).

Newsweek Staffwriter, (1988). Good news for hyperactive children. *Newsweek,* 15 February, 60.

New York Times. (1987). Sharp increase in sales of Ritalin. New York Times, 5 May, 3(3).

OCR Complaint 09-88-1072. (1989). Region IX, San Francisco, CA: Office of Civil Rights, U.S. Department of Education.

OCR Complaint 09-88-1200. (1989). Region IX, San Francisco, CA: Office of Civil Rights, U.S. Department of Education.

OCR Complaint 03-90-1047. (1990). Region III, Philadelphia, PA: Office of Civil Rights, U.S. Department of Education.

Okimoto, J., & Stegall, P. (1987). *Boomerang kids.* New York: Pocket Books.

Parker, H. (1988). *The ADD hyperactivity workbook for parents, teachers and kids.* Plantation, FL: Impact Publications, Inc.

Pelham, W. (1987). What do we know about the use and effects of CNS stimulants in ADD? In J. Loney (Ed.), *The young hyperactive child: Answers to questions about diagnosis, prognosis and treatment.* New York: Haworth Press.

Pelham, W., & Bender, M. (1982). Peer relationships and hyperactive children: Description and treatment. In K. Gadow & I. Bailer (Eds.), *Advances in learning and behavioral disabilities (Vol. 1).* Greenwich, CT: JAI Press.

Pelham, W., Bender, M., Caddel, J., Booth, S., & Moorer, S. (1985). Methylphenidate and children with attention deficit disorder: Dose effects on classroom, academic and social behavior. *Archives of General Psychiatry, 42,* 948-952.

Pelham, W., Sturges, J., Hoza, J., Schmidt, C., Bijlsma, J., Milich, R., & Moorer, S. (1987). Sustained release and standard methylphenidate effects on cognitive and social behavior in children with attention deficit disorder. *Pediatrics, 4,* 1987, 491-501.

Physicians' Desk Reference. (1994). Oradell, NJ: Medical Economics Company, Inc.

Pleak, R., Birmaher, B., Gavrilescu, A., Abichandini, A., & Williams, D. (1988). Mania and neuropsychiatric excitation following carbamazepine. *Journal of the American Academy of Child and Adolescent Psychiatry, 27,* 500-503.

Pliszka, S. (1987). Tricyclic antidepressants in the treatment of children with attention deficit disorder. *Journal of the American Academy of Child and Adolescent Psychiatry, 26,* 127-132.

Pond, E., & Gilbert, C. (1987). A support group offers help for parents of hyperactive children. *Children Today* (November/December), 23-26.

Popper, C. (1989). Diagnosing bipolar vs. ADHD. *Journal of the American Academy of Child and Adolescent Psychiatry.* Reprinted in *Challenge, A Newsletter of the Attention Deficit Disorder Association, 4,* September/October, 1990, 1-2.

Porrino, L., Rapoport, J., Behar, D., Sceery, W., Ismond, D., & Bunney, W., Jr. (1983). A naturalistic assessment of the motor activity of hyperactive boys: I. Comparison with normal controls. *Archives of General Psychiatry, 40,* 681-687.

Price, R., Leckman, J., Pauls, D., et al. (1986). Gilles de la Tourette's syndrome: Tics and central nervous system stimulants in twins and non-twins. *Neurology, 36,* 232-237.

Quinn, P., & Rapoport, J. (1975) One-year follow-up of hyperactive boys treated with imipramine or methylphenidate. *American Journal of Psychiatry, 132,* 241.

Rapoport, M., DuPaul, G., Stoner, G., & Jones, T. (1986). Comparing classroom and clinic measures of attention deficit disorder: Differential, idiosyncratic and dose-response effects of methylphenidate. *Journal of Consulting and Clinical Psychology, 54,* 334-341.

Rapp, D. (1979). *Allergies and the hyperactive child.* New York: Simon & Schuster.

Raskin, L., Shaywitz, S., Shaywitz, B., et al. (1984). Neurochemical correlates of attention deficit disorder. *Pediatric Clinics of North America*, 54, 714-718.

Rehabilitation Act of 1973, Section 504. *U.S. Code*. 1982. Title 29, sec. 794.

Reichard, C., & Elder, T. (1977). The effects of caffeine on reaction time in hyperkinetic and normal children. *American Journal of Psychiatry*, 26, 133-143.

Restak, R. (1984). *The brain*. New York: Bantam Books.

Riddle, M., Hardin, M., Cho, S., Woolston, J., & Leckman, J. (1988). Desipramine treatment of boys with attention deficit hyperactivity disorder and tics: Preliminary clinical experience. *Journal of the American Academy of Child and Adolescent Psychiatry, 27*, 811-814.

Riddle, M., Nelson, J., Kleinman, C., Rasmusson, A., Leckman, J., King, R., & Cohen, D. (1991). Case study: Sudden death in children receiving Norpramin: a review of three reported cases and commentary. *Journal of the American Academy of Child and Adolescent Psychiatry, 30*, 104-108.

Riddle, K., & Rapoport, J. (1976). A 2-year follow-up of 72 hyperactive boys. *Journal of Nervous and Mental Disorders, 162*, 126-134.

Rosemond, J. (1989). Is your child hyperactive? What parents need to know. *Better Homes & Gardens* (April), 38.

Rosensweig, M. (1966). Environmental complexity, cerebral change and behavior. *American Psychologist, 21*, 321-332.

Ross, D., & Ross, S. (1982). *Hyperactivity: Current issues, research, and theory*, 2d ed. New York: John Wiley & Sons.

Safer, D., & Allen, R. (1973). Factors influencing the suppressant effects of two stimulant drugs on the growth of hyperactive children. *Pediatrics, 51*, 660-667.

Safer, D., Allen, R., & Barr, E. (1972). Depression of growth in hyperactive children on stimulant drugs. *New England Journal of Medicine, 287*, 217-220.

Safer, D., & Krager, J. (1988). A survey of medication treatment for hyperactive/inattentive students. *Journal of the American Medical Association, 260*, 2256-2258.

Salanto, M., & Wender, E. (1989). Does methylphenidate constrict cognitive functioning? *Journal of the American Academy of Child and Adolescent Psychiatry, 28*, 897-902.

Salholz, E. (1987). Behavior pills: Disciplining unruly kids with a potent drug. *Newsweek, 109* (April 20), 76.

Schachar, R., Taylor, E., Wieselberg, M., Thorley, G., & Rutter, M. (1987). Changes in family function and relationships in children who respond to methylphenidate. *Journal of the American Academy of Child and Adolescent Psychiatry, 26*, 728-732.

Schechter, M., & Timmons, G. (1985). Objectively measured hyperactivity: II. Caffeine and amphetamine effects. *Journal of Clinical Pharmacology, 25*, 276-280.

Schnackenberg, R. (1973). Caffeine as a substitute for schedule II stimulants in hyperactive children. *American Journal of Psychiatry, 130*, 796-798.

Schrag, P., & Divoky, D. (1970). *The myth of the hyperactive child.* New York: Pantheon Books.

Schwartz, S. (1964). Effect of neonatal cortical lesions and early environmental factors on adult rat behavior. *Journal of Comparative and Physiological Psychology, 57*, 72-77.

Seabrook, C. (1990). CDC: Lead levels still poisoning kids. *The Atlanta Constitution*, 17 July, 1(A).

Segal, J., & Segal, Z. (1988). The "hyper" child. *Parents* (December), 215.

Shaywitz, B., Shaywitz, S., Anderson, G., Jatlow, P., Gillespie, S., Sullivan, B., Riddle, M., Leckman, J., & Cohen, D. (1988, September). D-Amphetamine effects on central noradrenergic mechanisms in children with attention deficit hyperactivity disorder. *Presentation made at the seventeenth national meeting of the Child Neurology Society, Halifax, Canada.*

Shaywitz, S. (1986). Prevalence of attentional deficits and an epidemiologic sample of school children (unpublished raw data). In J. Kavanaugh & T. Truss (Eds.), *Learning Disabilities: Proceedings of the National Conference, 1988*, (pp. 369-546). Parkton, MD: York Press.

Shaywitz, S., & Shaywitz, B. (1988). Attention deficit disorder: Current perspectives. In J. Kavanaugh and T. Truss, Jr. (Eds.), *Learning disabilities: Proceedings of the national conference* (1987) (pp. 369-523). Parkton, MD: York Press.

Shimberg, E. (1979). *Coping with Tourette syndrome: A parent's viewpoint.* Pamphlet. Bayside, NY: Tourette Syndrome Association, Inc.

Silver, L. (1991). *Attention deficit hyperactivity disorder: If it's for real, why all the confusion?* Address to LDA National Conference, February 27. Chicago, IL.

Silverstein, F., Parrish, M., & Johnston, M. (1982). Adverse behavioral reactions in children treated with carbamazepine (Tegretol). *Journal of Pediatrics, 101*, 785.

Skeels, H., & Dye, H. (1939). A study of the effects of differential stimulation on mentally retarded children. *AAMD Proceedings, 63*, 114-136.

Smith, L. (1976). *Improving your child's behavior chemistry.* New York: Prentice-Hall.

Spedalle, S. (1989). Hyper, not just active? Drug-free therapies gaining popularity. *Essence* (May), 114ff.

Speltz, M., Varley, C., Peterson, K., & Beilke, R. (1988). Effects of dextroamphetamine and contingency management on a preschooler with attention deficit hyperactivity disorder and oppositional defiant disorder. *Journal of American Academy of Child and Adolescent Psychiatry, 27*, 175-178.

Spitz, R. (1945). Hospitalism: An inquiry into the genesis of psychiatric conditions in early childhood. *Psychoanalytic Study of the Child, 1*, 53-74.

Sprague, R., & Sleator, E. (1977). Methylphenidate in hyperkinetic children: Differences in dose effects on learning and social behavior. *Science, 198,* 1274-1276.

Stevenson, R., Pelham, W., & Skinner, R. (1984). State-dependent and main effects of methylphenidate and pemoline on paired-associate learning and spelling in hyperactive children. *Journal of Consulting and Clinical Psychology, 52,* 104-113.

Sterling, D. (1990). Families struggle with kids' hyperactive behavior. *USA Today,* 6 February, 4(D).

Stern, L. (1988). Your child's health: Is your child really hyperactive? *Woman's Day,* 4 October, 26.

Still, G. (1902). The Coulstonian Lectures on some abnormal physical conditions in children. *Lancet, 1,* 1008-1012.

Stoff, D., Friedman, E., Pollock, L., et al. (1989). Elevated platelet MAO is related to impulsivity in disruptive behavior disorders. *Journal of American Academy of Child and Adolescent Psychiatry, 28,* 754-760.

Storm, G. (1983). Alternative therapies. In M. Levine, W. Carey, A. Crocher & R. Gross (Eds.), *Developmental-behavioral pediatrics.* Philadelphia: W.B. Saunders Company.

Swanson, J. (1988). Discussion in J. Kavanaugh and T. Truss, Jr. (Eds.), *Learning disabilities: Proceedings of the national conference* (1987) (pp. 542-546). Parkton, MD: York Press.

Swanson, J., & Kinsbourne, M. (1980). Food dyes impair performance of hyperactive children on a laboratory learning test. *Science, 207,* 1485-1487.

Swanson, J., Learner, M., & Cantwell, D. (1986). Blood levels and tolerance to stimulants in ADHD children. *Clinical Neuropharmacology (Supp.), 9.*

Swanson, J., Sandman, C., Deutsch, C., et al. (1983). Methylphenidate hydrochloride given before breakfast. I. Behavioral, cognitive, and electrophysiologic effects. *Pediatrics, 72,* 49-55.

Teicher, M. (1990). Emergence of intense suicidal preoccupation during fluoxetine treatment. *American Journal of Psychiatry, 147,* 207-210.

Thomas, S. (1990). Give attention deficit disorders their due. (Letter to editor). *Education Week*, 24 October, 26.

Toufexis, A. (1989). Worries about overactive kids. *Time*, 16 January, 65.

Tourette Syndrome Association Medical Committee. (1989). *Questions and answers on Tourette Syndrome*. Pamphlet. Bayside, NY: Tourette Syndrome Association.

Trimble, M., & Thompson, P. (1982). Anticonvulsant drugs, cognitive function, and behavior. *Epilepsia*, 23 (5), October, 531-544.

U.S. Office of Child Development. (1971). *Report of the 1971 conference on the use of stimulant drugs in the treatment of behaviorally disturbed young school children*. Washington, DC: GPO.

Vatz, P., & Weinberg, L. (1988). The hyperactive myth and drugs in the classroom. *USA Today*, September, 89-90.

Virginia Departments of Education, Health Professions, Mental Health, Mental Retardation and Substance Abuse Services. (1991). *The effects of the use of methylphenidate. Report of the task force on the use of methylphenidate in the treatment of attention deficit hyperactivity disorder diagnosed children*. House Document No. 28. Richmond, VA: General Assembly of Virginia.

Walker, S. (1974). Drugging the American child: We're too cavalier about hyperactivity. *Psychology Today* (December), 43-49.

Weiss, G. (1990). Hyperactivity in childhood. *New England Journal of Medicine, 323*, 1413-1415.

Weiss, G., & Hechtman, L. (1986). *Hyperactive children grown up*. New York: The Guilford Press.

Weiss, G., Kurger, E., Danielson, U., & Elman, M. (1975). Effect of long-term treatment of hyperactive children with methylphenidate. *CMA Journal, 112*, 159-163.

Weisskopf, M. (1990). Hypersensitivity to chemicals called rising health problem. *The Washington Post*, 10 February.

Wender, P. (1987). *The hyperactive child, adolescent and adult: ADD through the life span*. New York: Oxford University Press.

Wender, P., Wood, D., Reimherr, F., & Ward, M. (1983). An open trial of pargyline in the treatment of attention deficit disorder, residual type. *Psychiatric Research, 9*, 329-336.

Werner, E. (1989). Children of the garden island. *Scientific American* (April), 106-111.

Werry, J., Aman, M., & Lampen, E. (1975). Haloperidol and methylphenidate in hyperactive children. *ACTA Paedopsychiatrica, 42*, 441-449.

Werry, J., Aman, M., & Diamond, E. (1980). Imipramine and methylphenidate in hyperactive children. *Journal of Child Psychology and Psychiatry, 21*, 27-35.

Whalen, C., Henker, B., Castro, J., & Granger, D. (1987). Peer perceptions of hyperactivity and medication effects. *Child Development, 58*, 816-828.

Whalen, C., Henker, B., & Dotemoto, S. (1981). Teacher response to the methylphenidate (Ritalin) versus placebo status of hyperactive boys in the classroom. *Child Development, 52*, 1005-1014.

Whalen, C., Henker, B., Dotemoto, S., Vaux, A., & McAuliffe, S. (1981). Hyperactivity and methylphenidate: Peer interaction styles. In K. Gadow & J. Loney (Eds.), *Psychological aspects of drug treatment for hyperactivity* (pp. 381-415). Boulder, CO: Westview Press.

Whalen, C., Henker, B., & Finck, D. (1981). Medication effects in the classroom: Three naturalistic indicators. *Journal of Abnormal Child Psychology, 9*, 419-433.

Whalen, C., Henker, B., & Hinshaw, S. (1985). Cognitive-behavioral therapies for hyperactive children: Premises, problems and prospects. *Journal of Abnormal Child Psychology, 13*, 391-410.

Whalen, C., Henker, B., Swanson, J., Granger, D., Kliewer, W., & Spencer, J. (1987). Natural social behaviors in hyperactive children: Dose effects of methylphenidate. *Journal of Consulting and Clinical Psychology, 55*, 187-193.

Whitehouse, D., Shah, U., & Palmer, F. (1980). Comparison of sustained release and standard methylphenidate in the treatment of minimal brain dysfunction. *Journal of Clinical Psychiatry, 41*, 282-285.

Wiener, J. (1985). *Diagnosis and psychopharmacology of childhood and adolescent disorders.* New York: Wiley Interscience.

Willerman, L. (1973). Activity level and hyperactivity in twins. *Child Development, 44*, 288-293.

Wisner, J. (1985). *Diagnosis and psychopharmacology of childhood and adolescent disorders.* New York: Wiley Interscience.

Wolkenberg, F. (1987). Out of a darkness. *New York Times Magazine,* 11 October, 62.

Zametkin, A. (1990). *Neurobiology of ADD.* Presented at second annual CH.A.D.D. conference, Washington, DC, 9 November. Audiotape. Plantation, FL: CH.A.D.D.

Zametkin, A., & Borcherding, B. (1989). The neuropharmacology of attention-deficit hyperactivity disorder. *Annual Review of Medicine, 40*, 447-451.

Zametkin, A., Nordahl, T., Gross, M., King, A., Semple, W., Rumsey, J., Hamburger, S., & Cohen, R. (1990). Cerebral glucose metabolism in adults with hyperactivity of childhood onset. *New England Journal of Medicine, 323*, 1361-1366.

Zametkin, A., & Rapoport, J. (1987). Neurobiology of attention deficit disorder with hyperactivity: Where have we come in 50 years? *Journal of American Academy of Child and Adolescent Psychiatry, 26*, 676-686.

Zametkin, A., Rapoport, J., Murphy, D., et al. (1985). Treatment of hyperactive children with monoamine oxidaseinhibitors, I: Clinical efficacy. *Archives of General Psychiatry, 42*, 962-966.

Zamula, E. (1988). Taming Tourette's tics and twitches. *FDA Consumer, 22* (7), 27-30.

Subject Index

A

Academic achievement, 130
  in content areas, 122-127
  and medication, 123, 127, 132
  negative effect of ADHD/ADD on, 122-127
  progress reports, 183, 205
Academic performance, 114
  and ADHD/ADD, 38, 40
  and medication, 97, 99, 103, 109-110, 132
  and Ritalin and Dexedrine, 78-79
  screening, 77
Academic problems, 72, 109-110
Achenbach Child Behavior Checklists, 146
Activity-level problems, 6, 7, 8, 9, 10, 12, 101-103, 165, 271
  component of attention disorders, 7, 9
  and Dexedrine, 78
  and diagnosis, 102

  and medication, 97, 101-103
  and norepinephrine deficiency, 210
  and Ritalin, 78, 142
ADD
  co-occurrence of depression and anxiety with, 221
  misdiagnosed, 221
Addiction, 196
  and Cylert, 163
  and Desoxyn, 196
  and Dexedrine, 163
  and Prozac, 227
  and Ritalin, 163
Adolescent, 5, 96, 97, 98, 99, 100, 103, 123, 132, 134, 135, 142, 149
  drugs for, should be investigated rigorously, 224-225
  and psychological aspects of medication, 154-155
  and sports, 128
  study of, and interventions, 84
  suggested readings for, 154, Appendix 1

Adults with ADHD/ADD, 5, 12-14, 96
  and benefits of medication, 99
  hyperactive, 24-25, 108-109, 162
  and success, 108-109, 156
Aggression
  and Clonidine, 238
  and major tranquilizers, 249, 250, 256, 259
  and Prozac, 208, 229
Aggressiveness
  and anticonvulsants, 56
  and Catapres, 97
  and Tegretol, 278
Agitation
  and Ritalin, 168
  and Dexedrine, 193
Alcohol, 53, 73, 100
  abuse, 188
  and danger of Tofranil, 214
Allergies, 56, 59, 60-62, 86, 87, 90, 91, 124, 143, 151, 152, 177
  and effect on dosage, 172-173
  and need to try many medications, 179
  and sensitivity to medication, 173-174
  to dyes, 167-168
  to Ritalin, 168
Amphetamine, 189, 190, 193, 206
Anger, 11, 13, 28, 66, 73, 254
  angry outbursts, 256, 257
    and Tegretol, 254
    length of, 256-257
    thought disorganization during, 257
Anorexia
  and Prozac, 228
  and stimulants, 176
Antibiotics, 87, 130
Anticonvulsant or anticonvulsant medications, 56-57, 87, 97
  and Cylert, 200
  effect of, on attention system, 56
  and Ritalin, 170
  and seizure disorders, 278
Antidepressants
  and effect on norepinephrine, 162, 166, 289
  mechanism of, 166
  second-line treatment, 208
Antihypertensive, 170, 237
Anxiety, 212, 221, 231
  about drugs, 87-89

  and Dexedrine, 193
  and Prozac, 228, 230
  and Ritalin, 168
Aplastic anemia, 203
Appetite
  decreased (anorexia), 315
    and Cylert, 203
    and Dexedrine, 177-178
    and Ritalin, 174, 177-178
    and stimulants, 176
  and Prozac, 228
  suppression, and antidepressants, 208
Arithmetic, 122
  disorder, 274
  problems with, 275
  subtest, 118, 119, 121, 124, 125
Arousal, over- and under -, 9, 32
  component of attention disorders, 7, 9
  effect of medication on hypothalamus, 28
  highly aroused and Clonidine, 237, 242
  overarousal and environmental toxins, 57-60
  underaroused ADD, 31, 37
Ataxia and Tegretol, 278
Attention, -al, 17, 25, 29
  auditory, 42, 126
  definition of, 40
  efficiency, 61, 69, 74
    measuring, 76-77
  improved with medication, 78, 96, 97, 98-99, 213
  and limbic system, 28-29
  poor, 12, 31, 56, 66, 71, 76, 78, 97, 98, 106, 120, 127, 165
  role of RAS in, 30-32
  span, short, 10, 12, 62, 120
  sustained, effect of MAOI on, 233
  sustained measuring, 76-77
  system, 32, 40, 56, 96
  tasks and Ritalin, 142
Axon, 32, 35
Auditory
  attention task, 42
  CPT, 42
  discrimination, 44
  instruction, 132
  memory, 126
    measuring, 116-117
    problems with short-term,

associated with ADHD/ADD,
26-27
processing problems, 11, 13, 114-115
system and temporal lobes, 26-27
Autonomic nervous system, 198
narcolepsy and, 288
Automatisms, 278

B

Barkley's Home Situations Questionnaire,
146
Basal ganglia, 19, 25, 27, 28, 29, 53, 273
BEAMS, 49
Bedwetting, 271, 315
and antidepressants, 207, 211
and Tofranil, 271
Beery-Buktenica Test of Visual-Motor
Integration, 126
Biphetamine, 190
Bipolar disorder, 55, 193, 241
and ADHD, co-existing treatment,
259-260
distinguishing between,
and attention deficit disorder,
255-259
family history of, and Tofranil, 212
Block design subtest, 118, 119, 121, 124,
125
Blood pressure, 169-170, 183, 191, 204,
205, 218, 235, 243, 244
Blood tests
and Cylert, 203
differential platelets count, 183, 205,
218
elevated serum liver enzyme test, 200
liver function, 203
platelet counts, 235
SGOT, 203
SGPT, 203
SMAC, 183, 218
Brain
assymetry, 42
comparison studies of LD and ADD,
42-43
damage to, 18, 20, 23, 25, 28, 49, 50,
52, 53, 54, 57, 58
and development of habits, 34-35
dysfunction of, 18, 23, 25, 26, 28, 31-
32, 135
exterior of, 18, 19, 20
injury to, 20, 25-26, 39, 49, 50, 52-54

and medication, 86-87, 162, 164-166
Brain Dominance, 20-21
in dyslexics, 42
and role in schools, 21, 62-63
Brown v. Board of Education of Topeka,
295
Bruxism, 281
Bulemia, 228

C

Caffeine
as treatment, 260-261
compared to stimulants, 261
Carbamazepine, see Tegretol.
Cardiac
conduction defect, 213, 224
dysrrhythmia, 244
Cardiac arrhythmias, 285
and tricyclics, 213
Cardiac toxicity and Norpramin, 222-224
Cardiovascular effect of Clonidine, 243
Cataplexy, 5, 289
Catapres, 97, 239, 275
availability of, 239, 240
history of use, 237
Catapres TTS, 240
availability of, 240
dosage, adjusting, 240
duration of, 242
form of, 239
Catecholamines, 209
Causes of ADHD/ADD
abnormalities of neurotransmitters,
26, 29, 30, 37-38, 41, 96, 97, 148,
162, 166
abnormalities of neurotransmission,
37, 41, 165
allergies, 50, 60-62, 90
biologic variables, 67
complex partial seizures, 56-57
cultural factors, 50, 63-67
damage to brain, 6, 18, 20, 23, 25-26,
50, 52-54
diet, 50, 60-62
differences in brain structures, 18, 20-
38, 49, 53
dysfunction in brain, 18, 23, 24, 25,
26, 28, 31, 135, 162
educational factors, 46
educational practices, 50, 62-63, 88
emotional factors, 63-67, 73

environmental toxins, 50, 57-60, 73, 90
exact, still unknown, 67-68
food intolerances, 50, 60-62, 90
genetic inheritance, 46, 50-51
heredity, 50-51
inappropriate expectations, 73
many potential, 67
neurochemical, 30, 39, 40, 44, 49, 68, 95
neurophysiological, 17-40, 48, 86, 134-135
no single, 49, 67-68
nutrition, 50, 60-62
organic factors, 6, 50, 52-54
physiological, 49-60, 85, 88, 188
psychosocial variables, 67
social factors, 50, 63-67
stress, 50, 66-67
Characteristics of ADHD/ ADD
activity level problems, 6, 7, 9, 10, 12, 78, 101-103, 165, 271
acts before thinking, 10, 12
angry outbursts, 11, 13, 66
argumentative, 10, 13
arousal problems, 7, 9
assignments incomplete, 11,
attention, poor, 6, 12, 31, 56, 66, 71, 73, 76, 78, 97, 98, 106, 120, 127, 165
attention-getting behavior, 9, 11, 103, 106, 128
auditory memory problems, 11, 13, 26-27, 114-115
auditory processing problems, 11, 13
class clown, 11
cognitive problems, 9, 11
concentration, poor, 31, 66, 98, 99, 106, 118, 120, 127, 165, 271, 274
daydreaming, 10, 12
disorganization, 10, 12, 13, 66, 133, 135
disregards socially-accepted standards of behavior, 10, 13
distractibility, 6, 9, 10, 12, 71, 75, 76, 98, 99, 118, 120, 122, 274
emotional difficulties, 9, 11, 13
excitability, 10, 12
family interaction problems, 9, 11, 13, 72, 97, 129-130, 135-137
fidgeting, 274

handwriting, 11, 13, 133
hyperactivity, 6, 10, 12, 79, 97, 98, 100, 101-102
immaturity, 9
of behavior, 11, 13, 38
of judgment, 13, 38, 100
impulsive, -ity, 6-8, 9, 10, 12, 23, 31, 56, 57, 76, 77, 78, 79, 97, 100-101, 106, 120, 122, 127, 128, 134, 136, 165
inattention, 6-8, 9, 10, 12, 56, 57, 66, 78, 79, 99, 271, 284
learning problems, 11, 13
lethargy, 10, 12, 227
low frustration tolerance, 10, 11, 12, 13, 31, 66, 100-101, 128
low self-esteem, 11, 13
noncompliance, 9, 10, 13, 71, 101, 103-104, 106, 136
overactivity, 7, 9, 10, 12, 76, 97, 101-102, 104, 111, 127, 128
poor peer relations, 9, 11, 13, 75, 76, 97, 128-129
underactivity, 7, 9, 10, 12, 97, 102-103, 111, 127, 227
visual-motor problems, 9, 11, 75-76, 120, 275
work-rate problems, 13, 133
CH.A.D.D., 162, 187, 298
Chlorpromazine
Side effects, 145-147, 183, 205, 218, 307, 308, 309, 315, 320
Symptom, 145-147
Use of, 145-147
Chemicals, 57, 59, 60, 86
Chores, 135
Chromosome tests, 73
Church of Scientology, 47
Circadian rhythm, 282
Civil rights, 296-303
to nondiscrimination on basis of handicap, 296
Choline,
and Alzheimer's Disease, 37
Class clown, 11, 142-143
Classroom modifications, 90, 92, 93, 108, 134
management strategies, 306
Clomipramine, 275, 276
Clonazepam, 56
Clonidine
advantages of, 244-245, 246-247

and aggression, 238, 241, 242
availability of, 239-240
benefit
    maximum time to, 242
    compared to stimulants, 242-245
and blood pressure, 170, 243, 246
combined with stimulants, 245
compared to stimulants, 242-245
and conduct disorder, 238
description, 239-240
and distractibility, 245
dosage, 242-243
effect, duration of, compared to
    stimulants, 245
and explosivenesss, 238
for attention disorders, 237
and hyperarousal, 242, 244-245
hypertensive, 239, 241, 243
and inattentiveness, 245
indications for, 237-238, 244-245
mechanism of action, 240-241
and oppositional behavior, 238
and overfocused disorder, 238-239,
    242
and panic anxiety, 241
and post-traumatic stress disorder,
    241
second-line agent, 141
sedative effect, 242, 246
side effects, 243, 244, 246
and social phobia, 241
and Tourette syndrome, 237, 238,
    242, 245-246, 271, 275
useful in disorders with "high
    arousal," 241-242, 244
Clorgyline, 233
Cocaine, 53, 171
Coding subtest, 118-119, 121
Cognitive, 9, 11, 308
    abilities and tricyclic antidepressants,
        213
    ADD, 40
    behavior modification, 129, 135
    cognition, 9, 29, 99
    control over impulses, 100
    emphasis in parenting programs, 135,
        136
    functioning, effect of medication on,
        109-110
    looseness, 255
        abilities, 258
        processing, 257

processing, effect of medication on,
    132
specific cognitive training, 100
stimulation, 239
strategies, 101, 134
style continuum, 238
tasks and Ritalin, 142
therapy, 129, 275
and Tourette Syndrome, 270, 275
College, 151
    students with ADHD/ADD identified,
        123
Complex partial seizures, 56-57
    causing ADHD/ADD, 56
    and Tegretol, 254
    See also, Seizures, Seizure Disorders
Compliance, 65, 71
    and medication, 104, 136
    of preschoolers improved with
        recommended medication, 89, 91,
        150-151, 152, 156
    with stimulants, 101
Comprehension subtest, 118-119, 121, 124-
    125
Computation, 120
Computerized brain scan, 49
Concentration, 165, 271
    and attention system, 40
    deficiency of norepinephrine, 210
    improved by medication, 97, 99, 115-
        122, 127
    poor, 31, 98, 106, 274
    problems, 118
        and effect on measures, 118-122
    and reading, 43
    role of RAS in, 30-32
    and stress, 66
Conduct disorder, 231, 238, 255
    and differences in MAO, 232
    and potential benefit of MAOI's, 232
Conference, interpretive, 77-79
Conners Abbreviated Teacher
    Questionnaire, 106, 107
Conners Parent Questionnaire, 146
Conners Parent Rating Scale, 104
Conners Rating Scale, 261
Conners Teacher Questionnaire, 146
Conners Teacher Rating Scale, 104
Consequences, 35, 64, 65
    consistent, 134
    logical, 134
    natural, 134

negative vs. positive, 134-135
predictable, 134
Constitutional Slow Growth Syndrome, 182
Cooperation, 83, 97, 126
lack of, 13
Cooperativeness, 97, 103, 106
and medication, 136
teaching, 136
Continous performance tasks, 76
See also, CPT, 42
Continuous Performance Test, Appendix 5
Coordination, 76
motor, improved by Ritalin and Dexedrine, 78
Copeland Medication Follow-up Questionnaires for (Teachers/Parents), 182-183, 204-205, 218, 309, 320, 322
and behavior checklist, 305, 307-308, 320-322
Copeland Symptom Checklist for Adult Attention Deficit Disorders, 12-14
Copeland Symptom Checklist for Attention Deficit Disorders (for Children and Adolescents), 10-11, 14, 146
Coping patterns, 72
strategies, 135
Counseling, 127, 146, 151-156, 275
for children, 146, 151, 154-156
for parents, 127, 146, 151, 152-153
CPT, 42, 76, Appendix 5
Crack, 53
Cultural factors, influence of, 50, 63-67
Curriculum, a, 62
Cylert
and abuse potential, 196, 197, 201
administration of
and build-up effect, 201
compared to Dexedrine and Ritalin, 201-202
discontinuing, 199, 203
frequency of, 201-202
time of, 201
and weekends, 201-202
alternate stimulant, 141
and antihistamines, 193
and aplastic anemia, 203
availability of, 198
and benefit of, 198
and buildup in plasma, 143, 149, 197,
199, 202
classification of, 197
close monitoring necessary, 204
compared to other stimulants, 197-198, 203, 204
compared to Ritalin and Dexedrine, 197, 199, 201, 204
contraindications, 199-203
disadvantages of, 204
dyes in, 198
effectiveness
duration of, 199
maximum therapeutic, time to, 199
efficacy of, 161
and elevated liver enzymes, 203
follow-up schedule, 204
for children under six, 199
forms of, 198
frequency of use, 197
history of, 140, 197
long-term effects, 140, 200
mechanism of action, 197, 198
medication follow-up visit checklist, 204, 205
and narcolepsy, 288-289
need for monitoring, 200, 201
rebound, 202
safety of, 161, 200
side effects, 202-204
and Tourette syndrome, 200
when to consider, 141, 196, 197-198, 200, 201

D

Daily log of medication administration, Fig. 16.3, 319-321, 326
Danger, 259
insensitive to, 11, 13
Daycare, 65 , 317
Daydreaming, 10, 12, 97, 113, 142
Decongestants and Tofranil, 214, 215
Delivery
aspects of, as cause of ADD, 52
Dendrites, 32, 33, 35-36
Denial, 256
Department of Education
compliance guidelines for schools, 297
and jurisdiction over schools, 297-298
Dependence, drug, 201

Depression, 51, 103
  and antidepressants, 180, 207, 210-212
  and clonidine, 244
  may mimic ADHD/ADD, 55, 168
  and medication, 180
  narcolepsy misdiagnosed as, 5
  and Norpramin, 221
  in parents with ADD, 51
  and Prozac, 226, 227
  and Ritalin, 168, 180
Densensitization, 87
Desipramine hydrochloride, see Norpramin.
Desoxyn
  abuse potential, 196
  available sizes of, 196
Destructiveness, 256, 259
Detroit Test of Learning Aptitude-Revised, 116, 117, 126
Development, developmental
  delayed physical, 11
  disabilities, 54,
  disorder, 72
  goals, 135-137
  handicap, 78
  history, 8, 72
  immaturity and shorter attention span, 62
  intellectual, 76
  issues, importance of, 69-70
  learning patterns, 72
  neurological, see Neurological development
  pediatrician, 69-79
  problems, and diagnosis, 78
  questionnaires, 72
  quotient, 33
  tasks, discussed, 74-77
Deviation quotient, 124
Dexedrine
  abuse of, 189, 190, 195-196
  abuse potential, 196
  administration of, 194-195
    compared to Cylert, 199
    compared to Ritalin, 194-195
    frequency of, 195
    schedule issues in, 195
    time of, 194
      relationship to meals, 194
    and adolescents in psychiatric facilities, 195
  and antihistamines, 193

approved for children three to five, 169, 190, 192
  and aspirin sensitivity, 192
  availability of, 189
  available sizes of, 190, 192
  benefits of, 78-79, 190
  and build-up in bloodstream, 143, 149, 163, 194
  and caffeine, compared, 261
  checklist for medication follow-up, 183
  classification, 190
  close monitoring necessary, 196
  compared to Ritalin, 140-141, 189, 191, 193, 194-195
  contraindications, 193, 195, 204
  and cost factor, 196
  dyes in, 192
  effect on norepinephrine, 38, 191
  efficacy of, 161, 192
  Elixir, 192, 194, 195
  frequency of use, 197
  generic form of, 190
  history of, 140, 189
  and impulsive, risk-takers, 195
  indications for, 192-193
  lack of response to, 141
  mechanism of, 140, 191
  and motor tics, 193
  and narcolepsy, 179, 193, 288
  and obesity, 192
  poor response to, and Pondimin, 206
  procedure for trial of, 140-141
  rebound, 195
  regulation of, 190
  side effects, 140, 195
    appetite suppression, 177-178, 195
    compared to Ritalin's, 195, 201
    and depression, 180
    difficulty falling asleep, 178
    "glassy-eyed" effect, 180
    growth suppression, 180-182, 195
    headaches, 179, 194
    and lethargy, 180
    sleep disturbance, 178-179
    stomachaches, 179, 194
  therapeutic blood levels not available for, 163
  and tolerance, 163
  and Tourette syndrome, 271
  warnings same as Ritalin, 168-171, 193

Dexedrine Spansule
186, 192-195
Dextroamphetamine sulfate, see Dexedrine.
Diabetes, 87
Diagnosis of ADHD/ADD, 68, 72-77, 88
American Academy of Pediatrics recommendations, 8
assessment, 74-77, 78, 115-127
DSM-IV criteria, 7-8
evaluation process for, 72-77
developmental pediatrician's role in, 69-79
initial interview with parents, 72-73
inaccurate, 102, 180
interpretive conference regarding, 77-79
interview with child, 74-77
neurodevelopmental exam, 74-77
school history, 72-73
symptom checklists, 10-14
use of developmental tasks, 74-77
Diet, 50, 90
and effect on behavior, 61-62
effectiveness in treating ADHD/ADD, 61-62
Differential platelets count, 183, 205
Digit span subtest, 118, 119, 121, 125
Dilantin, 57
Directions
following, 75, 76
and medication, 114-115, 126
oral, 126
Disability, 75, 78, 297
Discipline, 11, 51, 63, 64, 65, 67, 83
Disciplinary practices, inappropriate, 303
Disinhibition, 23, 100
Disobedience, 10
Disorganization, 10, 12, 13, 18, 135
and brain dominance, 21
and deficient RAS, 31
and stress, 66
improved by medication, 99, 101, 133
Distractibility, 9, 10, 12, 71, 75, 76, 274
component of attention disorders, 6
and deficient reticular activating system, 31
and dysfunction in prefrontal area, 25
and effect on measures of intelligence, 118-122
improved with medication, 98-99, 115, 219, 245

internally, 115, 120
quotient, 119, 120, 123, 124, 125,s e e Freedom from Distractibility Quotient
Divorce, 65
Dizziness, 315
Documentation
component of responsible medical care at school, 321-323
for insurance, 77
of developmental problems, 78
required by prescribing physician, 91-92
DOE, see Department of Education
Dopamine, 29, 36, 37
deficiencies in, 166
and Dexedrine, 191
effect of clonidine on, 241
dopaminergic, 197
implicated in ADHD/ADD, 29, 37, 162, 166
and MAO-B drugs, 233
MAOIs and necessity of avoiding foods containing, 234
and Parkinson's Disease, 29, 37
and Pondimin, 206
and schizophrenia, 29
and stimulant medications, 161
Tourette Syndrome and excess of, 273
and tricyclic antidepressants, 207
and Wellbutrin, 261
Dopamine beta-hydroxylase, 232
Downers, 188
Downey, in re, 296
Down's Syndrome, 32
Driving automobile, 98, 100
Drug holidays, 149, 194
Drugs and drug abuse, 91, 100, 187-189
and alcohol, 188
and amphetamines, 190-191
and Cylert, 197, 201
and Desoxyn, 196
and Dexedrine, 193, 195, 196
effect of, 53
more common in untreated ADHD/ADD, 188
and Prozac, 226
and Ritalin, 144, 164
and stimulants, 89, 187-189
DSM-III, III-R and IV, 6-9,41
Due process, 303
Dugan vs. State of New Hampshire, 294

Dyes
    in Cylert, 198
    in Dexedrine, 192
    in Ritalin, 167-168
    testing for sensitivity to, 167-168
    in tofranil, 211
Dyslexia, 41, 44, 109, 274
    decreased glucose metabolism study, 42
    effect of medication on, 43
    studies of brain structures in, 42-43
Dysphoria, 258

E

Ear infections, 55-56, 61, 177, 285
Eating disorders
    and antidepressants, 207
    and Prozac, 228
    and Wellbutrin, 262
ECG, see Electrocardiograms, 254
Eclampsia, 52
Education, -al
    about medication, 152-156
    classroom modifications, 90
    compulsory, 294
    concern for overidentification of ADHD/ADD, 8
    creating attentional difficulties, 62-63
    definition of ADHD/ADD, 294
    Department of,
        guidelines, 297
        See also, Department of Education
    free and appropriate public, 300, 302
    free and public, established, 295
    history, 8
    is component of responsible medical care at school, 321-322
    issues, 62-63, 75
    needs of students with attention disorders, 293-294
    on overfocused disorder, 238
    requirement modifications, 275
    rights of handicapped to,
        alternative services appropriate to individual needs, 295-296
    services, 78
    special services, 53, 294, 300, 301
    system, 53
Education of the Handicapped Act, 40-41, 295-297, 298, 303

Education Week, 48
Educator, see Teacher/Educator
    See also, School
EEG, 42, 73, 235, 254, 277
EHA, see Education of the Handicapped Act
Electrocardiograms
    and tricyclics, 213, 218
Electrolyte measurements, 235
Emotion,-al
    -ally disturbed children, 189
    acceptance, 85-86
    control and medication, 28
    disorder, 97
    as factor in intervention, 78
    factors, 63-67
    and frontal system, 25
    growth, 79
    and hypothalamus, 28
    improved, 126
    lability, 255, 259
    and limbic system, 28-29
    problems, 5, 9, 11, 13, 41, 49
        and Tourette syndrome, 270-271
    and temporal lobes, 26
    and thalamus, 28
Encephalitis, 6, 52
Endocrinologist, 182
Energy level, high, 255, 257
Enuresis, see Bedwetting.
Environment, -al, 45, 46, 49, 54
    allergies, 90
    home, 65-66
    toxins cause ADHD/ADD symptoms, 50, 57-60. See also, Toxins
Environmental manipulation, 239
Enzymes, 200, 203-204
Epilepsy, 49, 56
    petit mal, 276-277. See also, Seizures, absence
    psychomotor, 278
    temporal lobe, 278. See also, Seizures, complex partial
    and Tourette syndrome, 270
Epinephrine and Tofranil, 214
Equal protection, 295
ERP, 42
Evaluation
    intellectual, 119, 122
    medical, 8, 54-55
    psychological, 92, 113
    process, 72-77

school standards and procedures for, 303

Examination
neurodevelopmental, 74-77
neurologic, 8
See also, Evaluation

Excitability, 10, 12

Exercise
physical, 63

Explosive
ADHD/ADD children, 97

Explosiveness
and clonidine, 238

Extracurricular activities, 127, 131

Eye/hand coordination, 75, 76

F

Failure
sense of in parents with ADHD/ ADD, 51

Family
benefits of medications for, 130, 131
effect of Attention Deficit Disorder on, system, 71-72, 129-130
fragmentation of, 65-66, 73
interaction problems, 9, 11, 13, 72, 97, 129-130, 135-137
and interpretive conference with physician, 77-79

FDA, 47, 186, 212, 246, 261

Fenfluramine hydrochloride. See also, Pondimin

Fetal Alcohol Syndrome (FAS), 53

Fetal distress as causative factor in ADD, 52

FFD, See also, Freedom from Distractibility Quotient

Fine-motor function
assessing, 75
control, 106, 112
importance of, skills, 75
and medication, 111-114
task, 184-185

Fluoxetine hydrochloride, 275, See also, Prozac

Focusing, 97, 116, 245

Follow-up, 89, 182, 204
benefits of, 79, 144-145, 146-147
Copeland Questionnaire, 182, 183, 204, 205, 309, 320, 322
medication use requires, 78, 151

Visit Checklist for Physicians and Parents, 183, 205, 218
Cylert, 205
Ritalin/Dexedrine, 183

Food additives, 60

Food intolerances, 50, 90
and Attention Deficit Disorder, 61-62, 127

Formaldehyde, 59-60

Frustration, 10, 11, 12, 101, 113, 258
and family, 13
low tolerance of,
and deficient RAS, 31
and impulsivity, 100
and peer relations, 128-129
and stress, 66

G

Generic, 39, 40, 186, 187
and Cylert, 197
and Dexedrine, 190
and Imipramine, 209
medications, 164, 186-187, 197, 228
and Prozac, 228
and Ritalin, 164, 186

Genetics, 45, 46, 50-51.

Geometric design subtest, 124

Gilles de la Tourette Syndrome, see Tourette Syndrome

Glaucoma, 222
and Dexedrine, 193
and Ritalin, 168

Glucose, 48
in dyslexics, 42
metabolism rate in hyperactives, 24-25, 42, 162

Goldstein Behavioral Observation Checklist, 146

Gordon Diagnostic System, 76

Growth
Constitutional Slow Growth Syndrome, 182
and Cylert, 203
and stimulants, 177, 180-182, 195

H

Habit, 34-35, 37-38

Haldol, 97, 275
dosage, 252
side effects, 252

and Tourette syndrome, 252-253
Hallucinations, 287
Haloperidol, see Haldol.
Handicap, -ing, 78-79, 300-301
    and appropriate alternative edu-
        cation, 295, 296
    and attention disorders, 293
    and civil rights, 296, 302
    and Educating the Handicapped Act,
        295-297
Handwriting, 75, 106, 184
    alternatives to, 133-134
    examples of, 111-113
    and medication, 111, 114, 115, 133-
        134
    problems with, 11, 13, 127
    skills improved by Ritalin and
        Dexedrine, 78
Headaches, 174, 215, 258, 315
    and Dexedrine, 193-194
    and MAOIs, 235
    migraine, and antidepressants, 207
    and Prozac, 230
    and Ritalin, 172, 174
    and stimulants, 176-177, 179
Hearing, 21, 72, 317
    Ear infections, 55-56, 61
    See also, Auditory system
Heart disease, 213, 285
    and major tranquilizers, 250-251
Heart rate, 183, 235
    and Cylert, 204, 205
    and Norpramin, 218
    problems and tricyclics, 213
    and Ritalin, 170
    and Tofranil, 218
Height, 183, 205, 218
    and Cylert, 203
    and stimulants, 180-182
Hepatic
    disorder, 199
        and Tofranil, 214
    dysfunction, 203
    failure, 204
Hepatitis, 203
Heroin, 53
HLA antigens
    in narcolepsy, 287
Holidays
    and special events, 148-149
        drug, 79, 149,

Home
    environment, 65
    managing ADHD/ADD symptoms at,
        135-137
Homework, 142
Hormonal functions, 28
Huntington's chorea, 29
Hyperactive, hyperactivity, 10, 12, 18, 20,
    23, 46, 190, 254, 296
    and anticonvulsants, 56-57
    child can exhibit normal level of
        activity, 102
    Congressional investigation, 46-47
    difficult situations for, 102
    and ear infections, 55-56
    and effect of medication, 97, 98, 100,
        146, 219
    and effect of stimulants, 101, 189
    and encephalitis, 52
    and glucose metabolism rate study,
        23-25, 48, 162
    in fathers and uncles, 51
    and impulsivity in adulthood, studied,
        100
    and major tranquilizers, 248, 250
    involvement of frontal lobes in, 23-24
    key element from childhood for
        success in adults with, 108-109
    and medication, researched, 100-101
    most troublesome setting for, 102
    overactivity in DSM-IV™ criteria, 7-8
    and premature infants, 53
    questioned, 47-48
    and Ritalin and growth, 181
    studied in twins, 51
    and sleep apnea, 285-286
    and substance abuse, 188
    as symptom, 6, 79
    as target symptom, 142
    and Tourette syndrome, 270, 271, 273
Hyperarousal, 244-245
    and major tranquilizers, 251
Hyperkinetic Reaction of Childhood, 6
Hypertension, 255, 285
    and Cylert, 204
    and Dexedrine, 193
    rebound, 244
    and Ritalin, 169-170
Hyperthyroidism, 55
    and Dexedrine, 193
Hypoglycemia, 55

Hypomania
    and Prozac, 208, 229-230
Hypotension and Clonidine, 243-244
Hypothalamus, 19, 20, 25, 29
    and ADHD/ADD, 28
    effect of medication on function of, 28
    role of, 28
Hypothyroidism, 55, 87
    thyroid test, 73

I

IDEA, see Individuals with Disabilities
    Education Act
Imipramine hydrochloride, see Tofranil
Immaturity, 9
    of behavior, 11, 13, 38, 100
    developmental, 63
Immunizations, 317
Impulsive, impulsivity, 6, 9, 23, 29, 34, 35,
    76, 91, 106, 134, 136, 165, 254, 255,
    256, 258, 259
    deficient RAS and, 30-31
    and differences in MAO activity, 232
    disorder and substance abuse, 188
    and effect on intelligence measures,
        118, 120, 122
    and environmental toxins, 57-60
    and epilepsy, 56
    improved by medication, 97, 100-101,
        127, 219
    impulse control and medication, 112,
        113, 213
        and reading, 43
    in adulthood, 100
    in DSM-IV™, 7-8, 12-13
    and norepinephrine deficiency, 210
    and peer relations, 128-129
    and potential benefit of MAOIs, 232,
        233
    as symptom, 7, 8, 10, 12, 73, 78, 79
Inattention, 5, 9, 10, 12, 57, 142, 255
    attention difficulties as symptoms, 73,
        78, 79
    in DSM-IV™ criteria, 7-8
    and dysfunction in prefrontal area, 25
    improved by medication, 97, 98, 99,
        189, 245
    and lead, 57
    and sleep, 284
    and stress, 66
    and Tourette, 271

Individuals with Disabilities Education Act
    (IDEA), 297
    See also, Education of the
        Handicapped Act
Information subtest, 118, 119, 121, 124,
    125
Inhibition, 23, 25, 37
Insomnia, 281, 315
    and Cylert, 202
    and Prozac, 230
    remedies for, 285
    and Ritalin, 175
    and stimulants, 176
Insulin, 87
Intelligence
    assessments, by school, 74
    group administered tests, do not
        reflect true ability of ADHD/
        ADD student, 122
    measures of, by physician, 77
    tests, 118-127
    See also, Measurements/Tests
Intelligence quotient (I.Q.), 33, 74
    areas affected by ADHD/ADD in
        measures of, 118-122, 123, 124-
        125
Irritability, 11, 13, 254, 257, 315
    and anticonvulsants, 56
    and antidepressants, 208
    and sleep apnea, 285
    and stimulants, 176-177

J

Jaundice, 203
Judgment
    common sense, 120
    and frontal system, 25, 273
    immaturity of in ADHD/ADD, 13, 38,
        100
    poor, consequences of, 100

K

L

Lability, 208
Labor
    aspects of, as cause of ADD, 52
Language, 11, 21, 26, 56, 74, 75-76
    abilities, measuring, 120, 126
    consultant, 71

development and medication, 41-42
disorders, 40, 44, 56, 258
   and co-occurrence of ADHD/
     ADD in preschoolers, 41-42,
     192
   and study of brain structures, 42-
     43
evaluations by school, 74
problems, effect of, 75-76
   processing, 26, 75-76, 114-115
processing and medication, 115, 132
Large muscle skills, 76
Law, 77, 100, 294-296
Lead, 50, 57-59, 73
Learn, effect of medication on ability to,
   109-110, 132
Learning, disabilities, 5, 47, 90, 258
   children with ADHD/ADD and/or,
     109-110
   compared to attention disorders, 40-
     44
   and co-occurrence of attention
     disorders, 40-41, 43-44, 109-110,
     192
   and discrepancy requirements, 123,
     294
   and eligibility for special education,
     40-41
   and lead, 58
   medication does not substantially
     improve true, 43, 110, 133
   premature infants at risk for, 53
   require specific remediation, 110
   and Tourette syndrome, 271, 273,
     274, 275
Learning, kinesthetic, 128, 132
   modalities, 110
   problems, 10, 11, 13, 49, 69, 188
   strengths and weaknesses, 90
   strengths enhanced, 123
   style, 73
Legal Issues,
   administration of medication, 300-
     302, 318
   civil rights of handicapped, 296-298
   disciplinary practices, 303
   DOE vs. OCR jurisdiction over
     schools, 297-298
   evaluation and placement procedures,
     303
   historical perspective on, 294-296
   jurisdiction, 297, 298

neurological disorders included under
   "other health impaired" of EHA
   (P.L. 94-142), 298
and parent groups, 297, 298
and requirement of waiver of liability,
   299-301, 318
rights of ADHD/ADD students, 296
Section 504, P.L. 93-112,
   Rehabilitation Act of 1973, and
   civil right to learn, 293, 296, 297
applies to students with ADD's,
   293
and specific inclusion of attention
   deficit disorders in Section 504,
   297, 298
Lethargy, 10, 12, 13, 28, 57, 180
Liability, school, 299-301, 319, 321
   avoiding, 321, 322
   waiver of, 299-301
Limbic system, 19, 25, 28, 29, 31, 96, 273
Limit-setting, 257
   Difficult for parents with ADD, 51
Listening, 102
   and medication, 115
   problems, 75
Lithium, 163
   alone not effective for ADHD, 259-260
   and bipolar disorder and Tegretol,
     254
   for bipolar disorders, 259
   with stimulants for co-existing bipolar
     disorder and ADHD, 259-260
Litigation, 293, 294, 296
Liver, 197, 200
   dysfunction and Cylert, 203
   enzyme studies, 204
   function testing, 203, 205, 216, 218,
     235
Lobes, temporal, 23, 25, 26-27, 278

M

Mania, 254
Manic-depressive illness, see Bipolar
   disorder
Magnetic resonance imaging (MRI), 42, 49
Major depressive disorder, 227-228
   and Prozac, 227-228
   and residual ADHD/ADD, 230
MAOIs, see Monoamine Oxidase
   Inhibitors
   advantage over stimulants, 208

and desipramine, 222
duration of effect, 208
effect on sustained attention, 233
enzymes and serotonin, dopamine,
    and norephinephrine, 232
follow-up procedures for, 235
indications, 235
list of foods to avoid, 234
mechanism of, 166, 232, 233
and narcolepsy, 289
Nardil and Parnate most frequently
    used, 234
and norepinephrine, 166, 232
and Prozac, 228
and Ritalin, 171
second-line agent, 141
side effects, 235
and serotonin, 207, 233
and sleep, 208
and tricyclics contraindicated, 213
uses of, 207-208
See also, Nardil, Parnate
Matching Familiar Figures Test, 77
Math disorders, 44
    affected by ADHD/ADD, 122-127
    computation, 109
    SAT, 123
Mazes subtest, 118, 119, 124, 125
Media, 47, 88, 294
Medical history, 9, 72
    evaluation, 54
Medication, see Treatment/Interventions
    psychotropic, see Tranquilizers, major
Medulla, 20, 26, 32
Mellaril, 97
Memory, 11, 109
    auditory short-term, 26-27, 115-118,
        120, 126
    and medication, 115-122, 126
    in narcolepsy, 287
    and oral directions, 127
    and Ritalin, 142
    short-term,
        and effect on measures, 118-122
        and medication, 97
    visual, 27
    visual attention span, 126
Mercury, 50
Metabolic rate and dosage of medication,
    153, 172-173, 199, 214
Metabolism
    of glucose, 24-25, 42, 48, 162

Methamphetamine   hydrochloride,   see
    Desoxyn.
Methylphenidate hydrocholride, See also,
    Ritalin
Methylxanine, caffeine, see Caffeine
Minimal brain dysfunction (MBD), 6
Monoamine oxidase inhibitors, see MAOIs
Mood
    changes, 257
    disorders, 255-256, 257
        and co-existing ADHD, 255-256,
            257
        treatment of, 259-260
    effect of antidepressants, 208
    swings, 11, 13
        and Tofranil, 175, 212
Mothers, 11
    and medicine and improved relations
        with, 129-130
    very young, as causative factor in
        ADD, 52
Motor
    abilities, 74
    control, 122
    coordination improved by Ritalin and
        Dexedrine, 78
    persistence, measuring, 77
    restlessness, 10, 12, 23, 73, 97, 255,
        281
    skills and Tourette syndrome, 270, 271
    speed, 75
MRI scan, 42, 49
Multi-modal, see Treatment intervention
Multiple Sleep Latency Test, 287

N

Narcolepsy, 55, 96, 168, 179, 279, 281
    and abnormal REM sleep, 288
    chronic underarousal of, 287
    diagnosis of, 287-288
    genetically based, 287, 288
    and mean sleep latency, 287-288
    misdiagnosis of, 287
        produces symptoms of under-
            aroused ADD, 287
    and Multiple Sleep Latency Test, 287
    neurochemical, cause of, 288
    treatments for, 193, 288-289
Nardil
    availability of, 234
    contraindications, 234

dosage, 234
effectiveness, time to follow-up for, 235
side effects, 235
warnings about food and drugs containing tyramine and dopamine, 234
National Tourette Syndrome Association, 272, 276, Appendix 7
Neurochemical, 30, 40, 68, 95
effect of Dexedrine, 140
effect of Ritalin, 140
imbalance and attention, 39
Neurochemistry
different from norm in attention disorders, 49
different from norm in narcolepsy, 287, 288
Neurological development, 63
delayed in ADHD/ADD, 38
key in school placement and academic performance, 38, 62, 133
and medication, 133
shorter attention spans in neurologically immature, 62
Neurological disorders, 269-279
Neurologist, 71, 145, 169, 200, 278
and multiple medical disorders, 278
Neuron, 32-33, 34, 35, 36, 37, 40, 41
cortical, 40, 43
excitatory, 35, 37
inhibitory, 37
messenger, 165
receptor, 36, 165
transmitter, 165
Neuronal connections and need for experience and stimulation to increase number of, 33
functioning as whole, 39
Neuronal patterns, 34
Neuron
receptor, 233
transmitter, 233
Neurophysiology, 86, 162
and poor response to punishment, 134-135
Neurotransmission, 38
Neurotransmitters, 132, 136
activity altered in narcolepsy, 288
ADHD/ADD caused by disorder of, 37-38, 96, 148
and antidepressants, 166

and Dexedrine, 191
disorders caused by problems with, 29, 37
function of, 36-38, 43
increased availability of, and improved attention span, 99
and MAOIs, 166
medication can alter abnormalities in, 38, 44, 96, 97
and need to define precise effect of each medication, 162
and organization, 133
process in overfocused, 238
and Ritalin, 191
specificity of, 37, 67-68
and stimulants, 162, 164, 166
Tourette syndrome caused by disorder of, 273
See also, Choline, Dopamine, Serotonin, Norepinephrine
Night terrors, 281, 282
Nightmares, 258, 281, 315
Night-owl syndrome, 282
Noncompliance, 9-10, 13, 65, 71, 101, 103, 104, 106, 136
Norepinephrine
action of, 165
and attentional symptoms, 161
and behavioral symptoms, 161
and Clonidine, 241
deficiencies in, 165-166
and Dexedrine, 191
increases availability of, 38
implicated in ADHD/ADD, 37, 162, 165 166, 210
and MAO-B drugs, 232, 233
Norpramin prevents re-uptake of, 38
and Pondimin, 206
and Prozac, 227
Ritalin increases availability of, 38, 165
and stimulant medications, 161, 164-166, 210, 288
and Tofranil, 214, 219
and tricyclic antidepressants, 207
and Wellbutrin, 261
Norpramin
adolescents and danger of overdose, 220
advantages of, 210
approved by FDA for use in depression, 219

availability of, 220
benefit:risk ratio, 222
benefits of, 222
and cardiac toxicity, 222
careful monitoring essential, 220, 225-226
compared to imipramine, 219
compared to Tofranil, 208
contraindications, 222
deaths associated with, 219
discontinuation, 220
dosage, 220
effect on norepinephrine, 38, 210
effectiveness of, 219
for depression and anxiety co-occurring with ADD, 221
indications, 221
long-term effectiveness of, 225
mechanism of, 210
and medication follow-up visit checklist, 218
not approved for children under twelve, 222
researched for use in ADHD/ ADD, 221
side effects, 222, 225
therapeutic blood levels, 220
and tics, 219, 225, 275
and Tourette syndrome, 225
warnings
    deaths investigated, 222-224
    recommendation of investigation, 224
Notice of medication policies and procedures, 318-320
Nucleus, 32, 35
Nurse, school, 321
Nutrition, 50, 60-62

O

Obesity, 193
Object assembly subtest, 118, 119, 121, 125
Obsessive-compulsive disorders
    and antidepressants, 207
    and Clomipramine, 276
    and Prozac, 228
    and serotonin, 37
    and Tourette syndrome, 228, 273, 274
    traits, 274
Occipital lobes, 22, 27

Office of Civil Rights, 293, 296, 298, 299, 301, 302, Appendix 8
    complaints registered, 296
    established, 296
    findings on Section 504 complaints, 299, 300, 301, 302, 303
    and jurisdiction over schools, 297, 298
Ondine's Curse, 281
Oppositional defiant disorder, 255
Orap, see Pemacide
Organic factors as cause of ADD/ADHD, 48, 50, 52-54
    not believed to contribute substantially, 54
Organization, organizational, 21, 65, 66, 67, 83, 89, 90, 91, 121
    assistance and supervision, 133, 275
    and brain dominance, 21
    can be learned, 101, 13
    lack of, and medication, 115, 133
    more difficult for parents with ADD, 51
    problems in Tourette syndrome, 275
    skills, acquiring, 135
    temporary/sequential, 76
Orton-Gillingham Society, 109
Otis-Lennon Test of Mental Ability, 122
Otitis media, 55-56
Overactivity, 7, 9, 10, 12, 76, 97, 132
    in academic setting, 102
    and behavior problems, 104-108, 130
    and clonidine, 237, 238
    in DSM-III-R, DSM-IV™ criteria, 7-8
    improved with medication, 97, 101-102, 127-128
    and peer relations, 128-129, 130
    and poor response to punishment, 135
    in sports, 127-128
Overaroused, see Arousal, aroused
Overfocused behavior, 37
    ADD, 97
    and clonidine, 242
Overfocused disorder, 111, 238, 239
    adverse effect on stimulants on, 237, 238
    characteristics of, 238, 239
    and clonidine, 238, 239, 242
    importance of differentiating from ADD, 238, 239
    intervention for, 239
    and work rate problem, 238, 239
Overinhibited, 238

Overstimulated, -ion 11, 13, 107, 257

P

Paddling, 303
Pain, insensitivity to, 11, 13, 26
Paranoia, 256
PARC v. Commonwealth of Pennsylvania, 295
Parents, 4, 48, 53, 99, 100, 101, 106, 173, 174, 175, 176, 177, 271
  and anger, 85
  and benefit of support groups, 150, 152
  concerns about child's
    medication, 173, 180-181
    social relationships, 128
  considering treatments, 84-85, 88, 89-90, 139-140, 150
  counseling for, 146, 151, 152-153, 172
  difficulties of, 51
  divorced, 73
  education about ADHD/ADD for, 89, 150
  effect of ADHD/ADD child on, 71-72, 129-130
  emotions of, before diagnosis, 11, 72
  expectations, 136-137
  fears, 73
  and finding physician for ADHD/ADD, 70-72
  and grief, 85
  groups and legal action, 297
  and home behavior management, 135-137
  and marital problems, 73, 130
  and medication, 139-140, 145-148, 150, 153-155
  and need for
    emotional support, 89
    follow-up, 144-145, 147-151
  and need to obtain knowledge of treatment choices, 52, 85, 91, 150, 152-153
  negative behavior of, 130
  non-compliance with recommended medications, 150-151, 152-156
  poor parenting, 5
  psychological needs of, 151
  and reaction to ADHD/ADD diagnosis for child, 85-86
  relationship with physician, 69-70, 72
  and reluctance to use medications, 86-89, 93
  and school's administration of medication, 318, 320, 321
  separated, 73
  and self-diagnosis, 171
  and self-medication, 171
  single, 65
  and sports, 128
  studies of, 51
  support groups for, 52
  supporting parents, 79
  and teacher, 305-306
  and team role, 152-153
  and Tourette syndrome, 270, 273
  training programs for, 134-135, 136
  and waiver of liability, 299-300, 301
  with ADHD/ADD, 50-52
Parietal lobe, 22, 25-26
Parkinson's Disease, 29, 37
Parnate, 233-235
Pediatrician, 86, 102, 145, 182, 278
  and appointment time, 71, 74
  as collaborative partner, 79
  developmental, 69-79
  evaluation process used by, 72-77
  how to find, 70-71
  and interpretive conference, 77-79
  for multiple medical problems, 278
  needs for, 70-72
  role of, 71, 78-79
Peeramid, 74
Peer relations
  and ADHD/ADD, 128
  and medications, 97, 128-129
  poor, 9, 11, 13, 72, 75, 76, 128
  -ships, 79, 131
Pemacide (Orap), 252-253
Pemoline, see Cylert
Perceptual
  abilities, 74
  difficulties, 274
  organization deviation quotient, 124
  skills and Tourette syndrome, 270
Performance scores, 118, 119, 121, 123, 124, 125
Pertofrane, see Norpramin
Pesticides, 50, 59
PET, 49
Pharmacodynamics
  definition, 163
  and therapeutic windows, 163

Pharmacokinetics
  definition, 163
Pharmacotherapy, 132
  See also, Intervention, medical
Phenelzine sulfate, see Nardil
Phenobarbitol, 56-57
Phenylethylamine, 233
Phenytoin, 56
Photosensitization and Tofranil, 214
Physician, 4, 48, 68, 69, 87, 91, 92, 162, 164, 169, 170, 171, 181, 270
  and American Academy of Pediatrics guidelines for, 322
  checklist for medication follow-up visit, 182, 183, 204, 205, 218
  and check-up, 145, 307
  choosing appropriate, 69-72
  choosing target symptoms for medication, 139-140
  and counseling, 152-156
  and importance of collaborative effort with educators, 322-323
  and issue of medication for non-school times, 148-149
  making decision to use medication, 141-143
  for multiple medical disorders,
  need for careful monitoring of medication by, 144-145, 146, 147, 151, 181-182
  and need for follow-up visits, 144-147, 151, 182
  and philosophy of medication, 147-148
  and procedure for deciding which medication is best, 140-141
  and reassessment of medication, 147
  responsible for prescribing and monitoring medication, 71, 144-145, 182
  role of prescribing, in team, 145
Physician's Desk Reference (PDR), 164, 190, 203, 212, 278
Physiology, 46, 48
  ADHD/ADD as problems in, 49-50, 63
  of children different from adults, 244
Pia mater, 19, 20
Picture completion subtest, 118, 119, 121, 124, 125
Picture arrangement subtest, 118, 119, 121, 125
Pierce v. Society of Sisters, 295

Pituitary problems, 55
P.L. 93-112, See also, Rehabilitation Act of 1973
P.L. 94-142, See also, Education of the Handicapped Act
Planning, 75, 273
  ability, 10, 12
  and fine-motor function, 75
  must be taught, 101
Planum temporale, 42-43
Plasma
  concentration, 220
  levels, 184, 199, 215
Plessey v. Ferguson, 295
Pneumonia, 86
Polypharmacy, 169
Ponderax, see Pondimin
Pondimin, 206
Poor reality testing, 256
Positive reinforcement
  to assist learning process, 35
  substituted for punishment, 104, 134-135
  and successful parenting programs, 134-135, 136
Post-maturity, 52
Post traumatic stress disorder, 241
Predictability, 65, 66, 67, 98
Prefrontal areas, 22, 25
Prefrontal cortex, 96
  decreased glucose metabolism rate in, 24-25
Pregnancy, 73
  conditions of, as cause of ADD, 52
  pre- and post-natal complications of, 53
Prematurity, 53, 73
Premotor cortex, 22, 23-25, 96
Preschoolers, 41, 101, 192
Prescriptions, 197, 325
Pressure to succeed, 67
Primary sensory cortex, 26
Processing,
  auditory, 114-115
  information, 76
  visual, 76
Prozac, 97
  and addiction, 227
  advantages of, 228
  administration,
    frequency of, 228
  and aggression, 229

and anxiety, 228
benefits of, for ADHD/ADD, 227
and bulemia,
cautions for patients and families, 231
compared to other antidepressants, 229
contraindications, 228
drug interactions, 230
dyes in, 226
efficacy of, 227-228
history of, 208, 226
and hypermania, 229-230
indications, 227-228
mechanism of, 227
and obsessive-compulsive disorder, 228
and Tourette syndrome, 228
and potential for abuse, 226-227
residual ADHD/ADD and depression, 230
risk of, 229-230, 231
and serotonin, 207
side effects, 227, 230
and sleep, 208
use in depression, 226, 227-228, 229-230
Psychiatric
disorder, 97, 278
illness
narcolepsy misdiagnosed as, 287
and Tourette, 270
Psychiatrist, 71, 145, 182, 260, 278
Psychoeducational evaluation, 113, 115
Psychological
aspects of giving and taking medication, 154-155
consultant, 71
counseling, 276
evaluation, 113, 115
expert, 75
patterns, 72
services, 78, 302
testing, 92
Psychopharmacology, -ists, 162
Psychosocial, 8, 46
Psychostimulant, see stimulant
Psychotherapy
usefulness of, 78
Psychotic symptoms, 256
Punishment, 10, 104, 134-135

Q

Questionnaires, see Checklists and Measures/Tests

R

Reaction time
improved by Ritalin and Dexedrine, 78
Reading, 56, 75, 76, 109, 118, 275
affected by ADD's, 122-127
comprehension, and medication, 132
disabled and medication, 115
disorders and ADD's in preschoolers, 192
and study of brain structures, 42-43
oral, and medication, 132
skills and medication, 43
Reasoning
abstract verbal, 120
common sense, 120
Rebound, 176, 184-185, 194, 195, 202
Receptor, 36, 39, 40, 68
Rehabilitation Act of 1973, 293, 296-297
See also, See P.L. 93-112; Section 504
Reinforcement, 104
ADHD patients respond positively to, 135
positive, 104, 136
Remediation, 44
of gaps and delays, 123, 133
for LD, 110
Renal disorders and Tofranil, 214
Renal function test, 235
Respiratory stimulation, 191
Responsibility, 63, 65, 67, 83, 151
ADD not excuse for lack of, 155
and medication, 135
program, 121, 127, 135
underdeveloped sense of, 13
Restlessness, 10, 23, 73, 142, 315
as symptom, 78
improved with medication, 97
See also, Motor restlessness
Reticular activating system, 19, 28
effect of anticonvulsants on, 56
effect of stimulants on, 31-32
and limbic system, 29
part of reticular formation, 31-32

results of deficiency in, 31
role as monitor of stimuli, 31-32
"gatekeeper," 30
Ritalin, 84, 96, 121, 127, 140, 142, 163, 164
    abuse of, 144, 170-172, 187-189
    and activity level, 142
    administration of
        and benefit period, 172-173, 184
        duration of effectiveness, 166,
            172-173, 184
        frequency of, 175
            relationship to meals, 172-
            173
        schedule issues in, 175
    adverse reactions of, 141, 172, 176-
        182
    and attentional tasks, 142
    availability of, 166-167
    and behavioral tasks, 142
    benefits of, 78-79
    and blood pressure, 170
    and build-up in bloodstream, 143,
        149, 163
    and caffeine, compared, 261
    checklist for medication follow-up
        visit, 183
    children under six, 169
    and cognitive tasks, 142
    combined with other medications, 169
    combining with Ritalin-SR, 185-186
    compared to Cylert, 199
    compared to Dexedrine, 140-141, 190,
        191, 194, 195
    contraindications, 168
    and depression, 168, 180
    dosage
        adjusting, 143-144, 166, 173
        for allergic children, 173-174, 179
        and body weight, 174
        efficacy of, 161, 164, 169
    and drug interactions, 170, 193
    dyes in, 167-168
    and family relations, 129-130
    and growth, 169
    and handwriting, 112, 184
    history of, 140
    and hypertension, 169-170, 204
    and increased heart rate, 170
    investigation of, 47
    lack of response to, 141, 190, 193
    legal classification of, 164
    and long-term use, 169

    and memory task, 142
    and motor tics, 168, 176
    and narcolepsy, 168, 179, 288
    not physiologically addictive, 163, 187
    prescriptions and refills for, 164
    primary use of, 168
    rebound, 177, 184, 195
    safety of, 161, 164, 169, 187
    and seizures, 169
    side effects of appetite suppression,
        176-178
    compared to Dexedrine, 194-195
        growth suppression, 180-182
    headaches, 174, 179, 172
    increase in heart rate, 170
    sleep problems, 174, 175, 178-179
    stomachaches, 174, 172, 179
    and task force study, 144, 170-171,
        187
    taste of, 175
    and thought disturbance, 168
    and tolerance, 163
    and Tourette syndrome, 168, 176, 271
Ritalin-SR, 107
    advantages of, 184-185
    available size of, 184
    combining with Ritalin, 185-186
    compared to Dexedrine Spansule, 194-
        195
    compared to Ritalin, 184
    disadvantages of, 184
    dosage, 173, 175-176
    and dyes, 167
    form of, 166-167
    frequency of administration, 173, 175
    length of effectiveness, 173, 184
    time of administration, 173
    time to effectiveness, 173
    variations in metabolism of, 184
Routine, 73, 91
    difficulty for parents with ADD, 51
    for taking medication, 150-151
Running, excessive, 10

S

Sadistic impulses, 256
Sadness, 315
Salicylates, 61
SAT, see Scholastic Aptitude Test
Schizophrenia, 29
Scholastic Aptitude Test, 123

School
    attendance compulsory, 294
    and attention disorders, 8, 46, 62-63,
       66, 83, 92-93, 132-135, 293-322
    and activity-level problems, 102
    achievement, poor, 9, 11, 73, 75, 122-
       127
    behavior, 79, 135
    components of responsible medical
       care at, 321, 322
    counselor, 145, 321
    curriculum too advanced, 62
    classroom modification, 90, 92, 108
    delayed entrance into, 133
    dropout rates and lead, 58
    educational practices, 50, 62-63
    environment, effect of, 108
    failure, 109
    field trips, 79
    holidays, 79
    and impulsivity, 100
    integration, 295
    lack of provisions for students with
       attention disorders, 293-294
    liability of, 322
    medication guidelines for, 317-327
    nurse, 74, 302, 321
    and overfocused disorder, 238, 239
    performance, 79
       and medication, 97, 99, 110-115
       related to language competence,
       75
    placement, 8, 38, 63, 66, 90, 132, 133
    poor judgment, 100
    principal, 74, 301
    private, and government's right to
       regulate, 295
    public law required establishment of,
       294
       free and, 295
    related problems and limitations of
       medicine, 132-135
    retention, 133
    segregation, 295
    and self-esteem, 131
    "separate but equal" 295
    special education, 294
    and traditional classes given up, 65-66
Section 504, 41, 293, 297-302, 318, 323
    complaints, 298-303
    history of, 297
    ignorance of, 298

    other causes for complaints about
       schools, 302, 303
    violations, 300-302
Sedative, 56
Seizures, seizure disorders, 55, 87, 276-279
    absence,

       and stimulants, 278
       and EEG, 277
       effect of, 277
       misperceived, 277
       and "spacey"-ness, 277
    ADHD/ADD secondary to, 55, 56-57
    and antidepressants, 229
    attention deficit symptoms exacer-
       bated by anticonvulsants for, 56
    and carbamazepine, 278
    complex partial, 56-57, 97, 276, 277,
       278
    and Cylert, 200
    grand mal, 57,
       implications of, 279
    medical treatment of, with co-existing
       attention disorders, 277-278
    mistaken for attention disorders, 276,
       277
    and Prozac, 229
    and Ritalin, 169
    and stimulants, 278
    and Tegretol, 56-57, 97, 278-279
    and Wellbutrin, 261
Self-advocacy, 79
Self-control, 71, 98
    loss of, 28, 108
    and testing, 77
Self-discipline, 65, 83, 128
    lacking in ADHD/ADD children, 99
    and medication, 135
    and need for teaching, 135
Self-esteem, 75, 76, 106, 107
    low, 11, 13
    and medication, 130-131
    and weight, 178
    and Tourette syndrome, 274
Senses, and
    occipital lobes, 27
    parietal lobes, 26
    temporal lobes, 26-27
    thalamus, 28
Sensivity, 173
    decreased, 26
    to drugs, 143, 153

to dyes in Ritalin, 167-168
hypersensitivity to Ritalin, 168
Sensory cortex, 22, 26
Sensory screening, 8
Sentences subtest, 124
Septohippocampal system, 135
Sequencing, 75
Serotonin
    and action of Prozac on, 227
    antidepressants increase availability
        of, 275
    antidepressants inhibit reuptake of,
        289
    effect of clonidine on, system may
        inhibit aggressive behaviors or
        thoughts, 241
    and involvement in pathophysiology
        of ADHD
    and MAO-A drugs, 233
    and narcolepsy, 288-289
    and obsessive-compulsive disorder, 37
    and overfocused behavior, 37
    and Pondimin, 206
    and Prozac, 207
    Prozac blocks reuptake of, 227
    results of deficiency in, 273
    and Tourette Syndrome, 37, 273, 275
    and Wellbutrin, 261
Sexual hyperawareness, 259
Siblings, 11
    ADHD child affects, 71-72, 129-130
    considerations for, 130
Side effects of medication
    checklists, 145-147, 205, Fig. 15.6,
        308, 309, 315, 320, 322, and
        Appendix 4
    and effect on compliance, 151, 152
    as factor in benefit:risk ratio, 139-
        140, 152
    and need for education about, 152
    and need for monitoring, 144-145,
        146, 151, 182
    See also, individual medication
        names.
Similarities subtest, 118, 119, 121, 124, 125
Skill-development program, 104, 135-136
Skull, 18, 19
Sleep
    and antidepressants, 208
    and attention centers, 179, O
    apnea, 281, 284, 285, 286, 287
    biological clock, 282

adjusting, 282
    difficulty, 281
    deprivation, 282, 283, 284, 285
    disorders, 281-289
        See also, Narcolepsy.
    latency, 258
    machine, 178, 283, 284
    myoclonus, 281
    nightmares in, 315
    and night-owl syndrome, 282
    overnight, pattern, 258
    paralysis, 289
    reduced need for, 10, 12, 281
    restless, 10, 283
    REM, 287, 288
    and Tofranil, 212
    too much sleep and ADD, 179, 283
Sleepwalking, 274, 281, 281
SMAC, 183, 216
Social, socially
    acceptable interactions, 104, 258-259
    activities, 76
        and impulsivity, 100
        and poor judgment, 100
    behavior and medication, 128-129, 134
    consequences significant, 78
    cues and expectations, sensitivity to,
        improved by medication, 97
    decisions and delayed neurological
        development, 38, 133
    distress, 51
    expectations, conforming to, 104
    function interference and intervention,
        78
    influence of, factors, 50, 63-67
    interventions, 104, 108, 129, 130, 134,
        308
    intuitive understanding lacking, 128-
        129
    relationships and ADHD/ ADD, 128
        and Tofranil, 213
    resources, 54
    skills, as predictor of long-term
        adjustment, 130
        lacking, 128-129, 134
        training, 104, 108, 129, 130, 134
Sore throats, 285
Spatial skills, 21
Special education, 40-41, 53, 294, 300, 301,
    302, 303,
    personnel, 145, 303
    and 504 complaints, 303

Speech, 21, 126, 127
  consultant, 71
Spelling, 109, 122
Sports, 97, 101
  and effects of medication, 127-128
Step-families, 65
Stimulants, stimulant medication, 40, 55,
  86, 89, 121, 135
  See also, Cylert, Dexedrine, Ritalin
Stimulation, 44
  cognitive, 239
  early, critical to later ability, 33-34
  emotional, 239
  excessive, 34
Stimulus, 35, 76, 165
Stomach
  aches, 172, 174, 179, 258, 315
    and Cylert, 203
    and Dexedrine, 193-194
    and Ritalin, 179
  pain and stimulants, 177
Stress, 5, 50, 86, 91, 130
  associated with ADHD is chronic, 72
  influence of, 66-67
  intolerance, 259
Structure, 67, 89, 91, 121
  benefits of, 64-65
  must be taught, 101, 133
Study skills, 75
Subcortical brain structures, 19, 27-29
  See also, Thalamus, Hypothalamus,
    Limbic system, and Basal ganglia
Substance abuse
  and ADD's, 187-189
Successive approximation, 150
  to determine dosage, 163
Sudden infant death syndrome, 281
Sugar, 60
Sulci (sulcus, sing.), 23
Support groups, 52, 86
  and Appendix, 3
  and benefits of, 150, 152
Suspension, 303
Sweating, excessive, 235
Sympathomimetic amines and Tofranil,
  214
Synapse, 35, 36, 38, 41, 162, 165, 166
Synaptic cleft, 35, 38, 161, 209

T

Talking
  excessive, 10, 12
  out of turn, 10
Tardive dyskinesia, 245
  and major tranquilizers, 251
Teacher, 305-316
  and formulation of policies, 322-323
  and importance of collaborative effort
    with physicians, 322-323
  and lack of
    knowledge about Section 504,
      298-299
    training in attention disorders,
      294
  role in monitoring medication, 145,
    146-147, 305-316
  and Tourette syndrome, 273
Teaching
  methods, 62, 132, 294
  strategies for LD, 110
Team
  approach, 71, 145
  manager, 145, 146, 182
  members of, 308
  and parents, 152-153
  and teacher, 305
Teenager, see Adolescent.
Teeth grinding, see Bruxism
Tegretol, 56-57, 97
  careful differential diagnosis needed,
    254-255
  and aggressiveness, 279
  results with attention deficit disorders,
    254
    and absence seizures, 254
    and complex partial seizures, 254,
      255
  and seizures, 278-279
  side effects of, 279
  and stimulants, 254
  uses of, 254
Television, 66, 102
Temperament, 50, 73
Temper Tantrums, 257
  causes, 257
  severe problem with, 259
Temporal lobes, 25-27
Temporal/Sequential organization, 76
Testing, Tests, see Measures/Tests
Thalamus, 19, 20, 25

role of, 27-28
Theophylline, 57
Therapeutic windows, 163
Therapist, 145, 152
Thioridazine, see Mellaril
Thorazine, 97
Thought
    disorders and Dexedrine, 193
    disturbance and Ritalin, 168
    processes disorganized, 257
Thyroid, 222
Thyroid tests, 73, 183
    hypothyroidism, 55, 87
Thyroxin, 87
Tics, 97, 269-270, 315
    and Clonidine, 275, 237, 238
    complex, 272
    and Cylert, 200
    and desipramine, 225
    and Haldol, 275
    motor, 272
    and Norpramin, 219, 275
    Ritalin and motor, 168
    simple, 272
    and stimulants, 177, 269-270, 275
    and Tofranil, 270, 275
    in Tourette Syndrome, 269, 270, 271,
        272, 273
    vocal, 272
Time
    reaction, 78
    sense of, 30
    sequences, 76
Time-out, 135, 142
Tofranil
    Ampules, 209, 211
    Availability of, 211
    Bedwetting, 207, 211
    Benefits of, 212, 214
    Classification of, 209
    Compared to Norpramine, 207
    Contraindications, 213-214, 215
    Dosage, 211-214
    Effect on norepinephrine, 38, 210
        study of, 208-209
    Effectiveness, long term, 213, 216
    Manufacturers, 209
    Mechanism of, 209-211
    Pamoate, 209
    Response to, compared to stimulants,
        213
        and learning, 213

    and motor performance, 213
    and social relationships, 214
    Risks greater than for stimulants, 216-
        217
    Second-line agents, 212
    Side effects, 215-217
    Utilization, 207, 209, 211
Tofranil-PM, 211
Tolerance, 153
Tomography
    emission-computed, 53
    positron emission (PET), 49
Touch cueing, 108
Tourette syndrome, 254
    attention disorders secondary to, 55
    characteristics of, 270, 272-273
    and Clonidine, 237, 238, 242, 245-246,
        271, 275-276
    and Cylert, 200
    desipramine and, 225
    and Dexedrine, 271
    and dopamine, 273
    and fluoxetine, 275
    and Haldol, 252
    and hyperactivity, 274
    incidence of, 272
    and misdiagnosis of, 270
    and neurotransmitter abnormalities,
        273
    and Norpramin, 275
    onset of, 271
    and Ritalin, 168, 177, 271
    and serotonin, 37, 273
    severity of, 273
    and sexual acting-out, 274
    and sleep disorders, 274
    and stimulants, 200, 237, 269-271, 275
    symptoms, 270-273
    and tics, 269-273
    and Tofranil, 216, 271, 275
    treatment of co-existing attention
        disorders, 271, 274, 275, 276
        of learning disabilities, 270, 274,
            275
        of hyperactivity, 271, 274
    treatments for, 245-246, 275-276
Toxemia, 52, 73
Toxins, 50, 86
    as cause of ADD/ADHD symptoms,
        57-60
    See also, Lead; Formaldehyde;
        Pesticides; Mercury

Tranquilizers, 97, 188
major, 249-254
Haldol (haloperidol), 250. See also, Haldol
history of, 250
and hyperactivity, 249, 250, 251
hyperarousal, 251
Mellaril (thioridazine), 250
primary use, 249
side effects, 251
Stellazine (trifluoperazine), 250
Thorazine (chlorpromazine, 250
used for severe behavioral problems in children, 250
use in ADHD, 249, 250, 253-254
See also, Thorazine; Mellaril; Haldol
Transcyclopromine sulfate, see Parnate Tablets
Tricyclic antidepressants, 43, 96, 207-216
advantages over stimulants, 208
as second-line agent, 141, 212, 211
and attention, 213
and behavioral scales, 213
build-up, 214, 215
and cardiac toxicity, 222-224
and clinical assessment, 213
close monitoring of, critical, 217
and cognitive abilities, 213
and comprehensive cardiac assess--ment, 224
contraindications, 213-215
and dopamine, 207
and duration of effect, 208
and drug abuse, 208
and holiday use, 215
and impulse control, 213
investigation of, 223-224
long-term effectiveness not known, 216
low doses of, 211
mechanism of, 210
more research recommended, 224-225
and narcolepsy, 279
and norepinephrine, 207
pulse checked during treatment of, 224
rebound, 215
and Ritalin, 171
scientific evidence for use in ADHD/ADD, 212
and sleep, 208

Trifluoperazine, see Stellazine
Tutoring, 110, 133, 302
Tyramine
MAOIs and necessity of avoiding foods containing, 234

U

Underachievement
of parents with ADD/ADHD, 51
pattern of, 123
relative to ability, 11, 13
Underactive, -ity, 7, 9, 10, 12, 142, 238
ADD, 97, 102, 111, 127
and rebound fatigue, 176
improved by medication, 97, 102-103, 127-128
in academic setting, 102
need to identify and treat, 102-103
and sleep problems, 179, 284
in sports, 127-128, 285
and written work, 111
Underaroused, 7, 9, see Arousal, aroused
ADD, 37, 277, 283, 285, 287
Urinary retention, 216, 222

V

Verbal scores/tests, 118-119, 121, 124
comprehension deviation quotient, 124
I.Q. score, 119, 121, 123, 124, 125
method, 133, 134
reasoning, abstract, 120
SAT, 123
Verbal performance, 113
Vesicles, 36, 165
Vigilance
improved by Ritalin and Dexedrine, 78
improved with medication, 97
Virginia
Task Force Study, 51, 144, 171-172, 187, 323
Vision/visual, 21, 27, 72, 317
attention span, 126
blurred, 215-216, 287
detail, 120
double, 287
hallucinations, 287
learner, 132
memory
problems, 27

long-term, 120, 127
short-term, 127
method, 133-134
motor,
integration, 126
problems, 9, 11, 44, 75-76, 275
tasks, 120
problems of, compared to ADHD/ADD, 49, 87, 97, 130, 151, 155
processing, 76, 127
retrieval, 127
Vocabulary subtest, 118, 119, 121, 124, 125
Vocalization
in hyperactive boys and stimulant medication, 101
Volition, 293
and frontal system, 25

W

Wechsler Intelligence Scale for Children-Revised (WISC-R), 118-121
scores affected by ADHD/ADD, 118-122
medication, 121-122
Wechsler Preschool and Primary Scale of Intelligence Revised (WPPSI-R), 124-125
scores affected by ADHD/ ADD, 124-125
Weight, 183, 205, 218, 258
and Cylert, 203
and Ritalin, 174
Weight loss, 177, 315
and Cylert, 203
and Dexedrine, 177-178, 189
and MAOIs, 235
minimizing, 177
and Prozac, 228, 230
and Ritalin, 177-178
and stimulants, 176-177, 180-182
Wellbutrin, 261-262
Wholistic learning, 21
nature of ADHD/ADD child, 136
Wolf v. State of Utah, 295
Woodcock Reading Mastery, 127
Word-processor, 114, 133
attack, 126, 127
identification, 126, 127
Work
assignments, not completed, 13

completion, 110-111, 115
ethic, 63-65, 135
rate, 113
excessively slow, 13, 118, 120, 238, 239
problems, 11
and medication, 133-134
rushes through work, 11, 13
written
modification of, requirements, 111, 114
reducing, 134
WRAT-R
scores affected by ADHD/ ADD, 122-123, 126